HIGH-PERFORMANCE SPORTS CONDITIONING

Bill Foran, Editor

Contents

HIGH-PERFORMANCE SPORTS CONDITIONING

Bill Foran, Editor

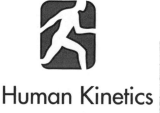

Human Kinetics

Library of Congress Cataloging-in-Publication Data

High-performance sports conditioning / [edited by] Bill Foran.
    p. cm.
  Includes index and bibliographical references.
  ISBN 0-7360-0163-8
   1. Physical education and training. 2. Physical fitness. 3. Exercise. 4. Physical
fitness--Study and teaching. I. Foran, Bill.

GV711.5 .H59 2001
613.7'11'--dc 21

99-088063

ISBN-10: 0-7360-0163-8
ISBN-13: 978-0-7360-0163-2
Copyright © 2001 by Human Kinetics, Inc.

Developmental Editors: Kent Reel and Julie Rhoda; **Assistant Editors:** Kim Thoren and Carla Zych; **Copyeditor:** Bob Replinger; **Proofreaders:** Erin Cler and Julie A. Marx; **Indexer:** Nan N. Badgett; **Permission Manager:** Cheri Banks; **Graphic Designer:** Fred Starbird; **Graphic Artists:** Kim Maxey and Tara Welsch; **Art Manager:** Craig Newsom; **Illustrator:** Mic Greenberg; **Photo Editor:** Clark Brooks; **Cover Designer:** Jack W. Davis; **Photographer (cover):** Tom Roberts; **Photographer (interior):** Please see page vi for credits; **Printer:** Versa Press

Human Kinetics books are available at special discounts for bulk purchase. Special editions or book excerpts can also be created to specification. For details, contact the Special Sales Manager at Human Kinetics.

Printed in the United States of America   20 19 18 17 16

The paper in this book is certified under a sustainable forestry program.

Human Kinetics
Web site: www.HumanKinetics.com

United States: Human Kinetics, P.O. Box 5076, Champaign, IL 61825-5076
800-747-4457
email: humank@hkusa.com

Canada: Human Kinetics, 475 Devonshire Road Unit 100, Windsor, ON N8Y 2L5
800-465-7301 (in Canada only)
email: info@hkcanada.com

Europe: Human Kinetics, 107 Bradford Road, Stanningley, Leeds LS28 6 AT, United Kingdom
+44 (0) 113 255 5665
email: hk@hkeurope.com

Australia: Human Kinetics, 57A Price Avenue, Lower Mitcham, South Australia 5062
08 8372 0999
e-mail: info@hkaustralia.com

New Zealand: Human Kinetics, P.O. Box 80, Torrens Park, South Australia 5062
0800 222 062
e-mail: info@hknewzealand.com

Photo Credits

The Functional Training Advantage

Sports training has progressed rapidly over the last 40 years. Innovative scientists such as Tudor Bompa have advanced new principles of training to help make conditioning more systematic and productive. Practitioners such as Boyd Epley have demonstrated the value of training experts working full time with sports teams; Epley literally put more power into Nebraska Cornhusker football, leading other teams and programs to follow suit. And organizations such as the National Strength and Conditioning Association (NSCA) and the American College of Sports Medicine (ACSM) have gained credibility and members as the field has become more professional and more accepted.

Because of these achievements off the field and convincing evidence on the field, the value of expert sports exercise prescription is no longer questioned. The only unknown is, how much better can it get? Some believe that athletes' bodies will soon hit a "ceiling," a point at which physiological and anatomical limits can be extended no further. Others wink and whisper that as long as ergogenic aids are so accessible athletes will continue to define new limits of performance.

High-Performance Sports Conditioning takes a different tack. In this book we've assembled an expert panel of scientists and practitioners to present the present and future of sports conditioning: functional training. Traditional training resulted in athletes with adequate aerobic and anaerobic capacity, sufficient musculature—lean or bulky depending on whether the amount of weight or the number of reps was emphasized, and fair to poor flexibility. In other words, athletes could pass a general physical exam and achieve acceptable scores on fitness tests. All very fine, but what did such training contribute to athletes' ability to play their sport? Unfortunately, the gains were less than satisfactory.

The functional training advantage is this: After establishing a solid fitness base, athletes do conditioning activities that are designed for the specific purpose of *enhancing their individual performance in their sport*. The intensity, duration, and frequency of aerobic and anaerobic work are tailored to the endurance and power demanded in the activity. Resistance training zeroes in on the movement patterns, loads, and length of activity required of the athletes' musculature during practice and competition. Stretching exercises are specific to the joints, connective tissue, and musculature most active in the sport and serve to develop dynamic, multidirectional range of motion instead of static, single-plane flexibility. Moreover, this new type of training also enhances those sports performance factors that used to be thought of as part of an athlete's "natural talent" and as being resistant to much conditioning-induced development. Not only are speed, agility, coordination, balance, and other key factors being improved markedly through effective functional training programs, but the drills and activities used to develop such attributes involve movement patterns and skills specific to the sport and perhaps even to a designated position.

As you read *High-Performance Sports Conditioning*, the physical benefits of functional training will become as apparent to you as they are to those who implement such conditioning programs. But another very real and important benefit of functional training is that it keeps athletes sharper mentally and more motivated through each practice. Training activities are no longer seen as punishment and as being separate from actually playing the sport; now, each conditioning exercise and drill is seen as contributing directly to performance.

The first part of *High-Performance Sports Conditioning* establishes the key components of athlete conditioning, explains how to test for baseline fitness levels, and covers each major performance factor in depth. The second part of the book takes the next step toward effective design and application of a functional training program, developing drills and workouts that promote both skills and conditioning, and putting all of the pieces together with consideration for the peak performance periods targeted throughout the annual training calendar. A closing chapter addresses the very real challenge of how to help an athlete who is returning from injury regain or exceed his or her preinjury performance level.

Functional training bridges the gap between the training room and playing field. It is the result of many years of work by outstanding scientists and practitioners, many of whom have contributed to this book. And it's much more than a fad; it's a proven approach to conditioning that produces the best possible sports performance. You can use this book in many ways, as a reference, course text, or training manual. The important thing is to use it often and get the functional training advantage.

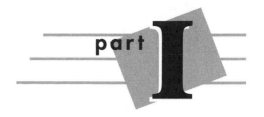

part I

Developing the Sports Performance Foundation

What aspects of sports conditioning are most important to assess and train in to produce the highest athletic performance? You'll find out in the ten chapters in part I.

Dr. William Kraemer and Ana Gómez start with chapter 1, "Establishing a Solid Fitness Base," an overview of how we've come to know what we know about solid conditioning, training principles, and the physiology of performance. The chapter discusses the nine basic sports performance factors: power, strength, speed, agility, coordination, quickness, flexibility, local muscular endurance, and cardiovascular aerobic capacity. Gray Cook's chapter 2, "Baseline Sports-Fitness Testing," tells you how to perform a functional movement screen on athletes to assess their overall mobility and stability and functional performance.

Nikos Apolostopoulos covers "Performance Flexibility" in chapter 3 by introducing an innovative technique he developed called micro-Stretching®. This type of stretching is not a quick warm-up stretching routine, but rather a training session in itself covering 14 total-body stretches. Steven Scott Plisk explains the basics of movement mechanics, a muscle's rate of force development, and power in chapter 4, "Muscular Strength and Stamina." He then provides training methods for improving athletes' maximum strength, strength endurance, and speed strength. In chapter 5, "Explosive Power," Donald A. Chu presents 15 plyometric exercises that offer a sure way to develop explosive power.

The quickest athlete will dominate in any one-on-one situation. In chapter 6, "Lightning Quickness," Peter Twist covers four types of factors that affect an athlete's quickness: biomechanical, anatomical and physiological, neuromuscular, and bioenergetic. He then provides 18 drills that improve athletes' quickness. E. Paul Roetert's chapter 7, "3-D Balance and Core Stability," explains why athletes can improve their performance by enhancing their muscular balance, dynamic balance, and core stability. The 28 single-joint, multijoint, dynamic, and stabilizing exercises provided in the chapter relate specifically to stabilizing the body during athletic performance.

In chapter 8, "Agility and Coordination," Mark Verstegen and Brandon Marcello cover the foundations needed to improve these two building blocks of movement. They offer six agility drills and sport-specific drills for 12 sports. George Dintiman's "Acceleration and Speed" (chapter 9) focuses first on recognizing the factors that can limit acceleration and speed, then on how to test and evaluate an athlete's strengths and weaknesses, and finally on some speed improvement training programs, including four form-training drills and 13 speed-enhancing exercises. In chapter 10, "Aerobic Capacity for Endurance," Jack Daniels covers seven principles of aerobic training and explains how to measure athletes' current aerobic capacity.

chapter

1

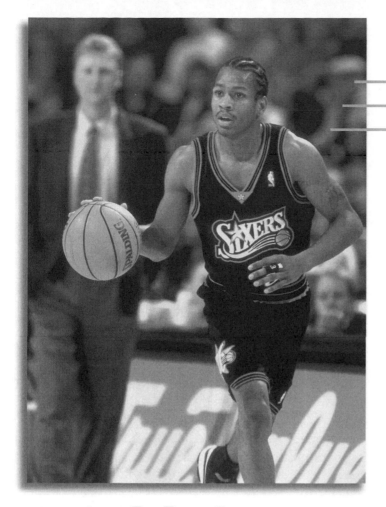

Establishing a
Solid Fitness Base

William J. Kraemer and Ana L. Gómez

Significant advances have been made in the process of physical conditioning for sport over the past 50 years. In the 1950s and 1960s it was common for athletes in team sports such as football and basketball to "play themselves" into shape. Even athletes in individual sports did not commonly embrace the concept of year-round conditioning in the 1940s, 1950s, and even into the 1960s. For example, several 10K runners in the 1948 Olympic Games had trained for only six months before the event.

Gradually, competitors and coaches began to attribute the success of certain individuals and teams to their intense physical conditioning: perhaps it was true that conditioning could provide an edge in competition. Yet the scientific underpinnings for many conditioning methods were in their infancy. The common

3

methods of communication about training techniques involved copying the champion performer and word of mouth in the gym. In addition, muscle magazines in the area of "physical culture" provided information to athletes on training techniques.

As competitive demands started to rise (e.g., the first sub four-minute mile was run, the first 500-pound clean and jerk was lifted, the first sub 2:10.00 marathon was achieved) at all levels in athletics, interest in physical conditioning as the focal component of a sports training program became more important. The major sports of football and basketball were becoming big business in the 1970s on both the major college and professional levels. Any organization that hoped to succeed needed athletes who could perform at high levels and, in the professional ranks, athletes who could stay healthy and have long careers.

By the late 1970s the concept of a strength and conditioning coach had become formalized with the founding of the National Strength Coaches Association in 1978. Renamed the National Strength and Conditioning Association (NSCA) a few years later, one of its specific missions was to encourage the exchange of ideas among strength and conditioning coaches. At first, this desire by coaches for new knowledge and research in strength and conditioning for athletes was limited because most of the scientific studies in the 1960s and 1970s focused on cardiovascular and aerobic conditioning methods. Only a few scientists had studied the effects of strength training on performance. By the late 1980s the study of anaerobic metabolism, strength training, and other athletic attributes such as agility became popular and, more important, accepted as a valid line of investigation in the scientific world. The "art" of coaching strength and conditioning had now become more of a profession. The knowledge base for so-called clinical judgments in the development of training programs could be based on scientific facts and athletic testing. Among strength and conditioning professionals, debate could be based on facts rather than the philosophies and anecdotal observations that had been the basis for almost all training theory up to the early 1980s.

Another focal point and original mission of the NSCA in 1978 was to bridge the gap between the coach and the laboratory scientist. The coach was becoming a professional, capable of prescribing exercise in a manner similar to the way a physician treats disease in his or her patients. The prescription process includes reviewing the athlete's history, conducting preliminary testing, determining goals, and ultimately matching a specific training program to initial needs. Using the knowledge base established by scientific studies, the coach evaluates the efficacy of potential programs to meet specific goals in developing the conditioning program for the athlete (Fleck and Kraemer 1997). The success of the program is then evaluated with further assessments, and program elements are changed to meet the dynamic needs and goals of the athlete over time (Kraemer and Fry 1995). Thus, a strength and conditioning program becomes a dynamic process that requires attention to the ever-changing knowledge base, continual evaluation of progress toward specific training goals, and management of each athlete's total conditioning program.

With the advent of professional certification (the CSCS offered by the NSCA) in strength and conditioning, this composite job has achieved unique status in the field of coaching. The strength and conditioning specialist has become an important element of the athletic support staff, taking a place alongside the athletic trainer, sport nutritionist, sport physical therapist, and team physician.

The 1980s and 1990s brought continued expansion of study in the field and an explosion of technology that could be applied to strength and conditioning. Almost all collegiate athletes and elite athletes in the professional ranks now participate in year-round conditioning programs. Coaches are hungry for new training ideas and new equipment to use as conditioning tools in the weight room, gym, and on the field.

By the 1990s, many products had become available to aid athletic performance and prevent injury across several professions in the field now commonly called sports medicine. Over 150 equipment companies now sell various machines for strengthening and conditioning athletes. The invention of new products has escalated in the field of sports medicine. Medications, surgical techniques, and therapies are available to treat and prevent injuries. The clothing, shoes, equipment, and competition venues (tracks, swimming pools, etc.) used by athletes in training and competition have also improved each year to help boost athletic performance. Olympic gold medalist Rafer Johnson commented that he would have loved to have worn a pair of shoes like those that athletes run in today when he competed in the decathlon in Rome in 1960. He feels he could have boosted his performance with this simple addition of new technology. Sport nutrition also became more broadly recognized in the 1990s as an important dimension of the athlete's training program. Thus, many elements that support the development of athletes have improved, helping athletes raise the bar on performance. Nevertheless, central to this whole phenomenon has been the quality and type of exercise stimuli used to prepare the athlete's body for elite competition.

A COMPREHENSIVE SPORTS-FITNESS BASE

Developing a sports-fitness base is important for both the performance and the health of the athlete (Hoffman, Sheldahl, and Kraemer 1998). A comprehensive program, which addresses each aspect of the athlete's physical and mental capabilities, is imperative for total success. Total conditioning was another concept promoted by the NSCA in its infancy. A comprehensive approach to the athlete was influenced by the perceived approach taken by the former Soviet Union and Eastern Bloc countries in developing their athletes (Mateyev 1972; Medvedyev 1988). In this approach to athlete development, sport coaches, physicians, and sport scientists teamed up to get the most out of an athlete—an individual who had been screened for specific athletic potential. By the late 1970s the United States Olympic Committee had established their first Olympic Training Center in Colorado Springs to help put a scientific component into training athletes. By the mid to late 1990s coaches realized the importance of individualized training programs and began to develop them. Many professional athletes had their own conditioning coaches, sport psychologists, athletic trainers, sport nutritionists, and even massage therapists to help them with individual physical and mental preparation, injury management, nutrition, and recovery from training and competition.

The basic functioning of each physiological system is vital to the health and performance success of the athlete. A needs analysis for any sports conditioning program evaluates the demands of the sport, which include the range of metabolic requirements, the injury potential for different parts of the body, and the types of muscle actions or biomechanical characteristics involved in the sport (Fleck and Kraemer 1997). In sports medicine the first step is a thorough precompetition physical exam by the team physician to rule out potential pathologies and establish the fundamental health of the athlete. Documentation of prior injury is also important because part of the subsequent exercise prescription is designed to prevent both primary and secondary injuries (Hoffman, Sheldahl, and Kraemer 1998). It is vital that a comprehensive testing program be established to quantify the athlete's fitness levels (Kraemer and Fry 1995). From such testing, coaches and athletes can establish training goals, assess progress, and determine the effectiveness of each aspect of the program (e.g., strength, power, flexibility) at different phases of the program (see chapter 2).

SPORTS PERFORMANCE FACTORS

Many diverse factors have been considered important for sports fitness. However, the degree of reliance on each component is completely dependent on the specificity of each sport (swimming versus diving) or, in some cases, even within the sport (linemen versus running backs in football). Sports-fitness characteristics beyond physical size and inherent biological characteristics include power, strength, speed, agility, coordination, quickness, flexibility, local muscular endurance, and cardiovascular aerobic capacity and endurance.

Power

Power may be the most important factor in sports performance because the ability to produce force in a brief amount of time is vital to most sports skills, such as the vertical jump (Newton, Kraemer, and Häkkinen 1999). Also called *speed strength* by some, power plays a crucial role in all sports performance. In fact, the inability to maintain power output is considered by many to be representative of a state of fatigue.

Power output, although highly related to strength, especially at the higher levels of force, must be developed as a separate fitness component (Kraemer et al. 1995). This is especially important where development of acceleration is vital to the sport skill or rate of force development at the faster time points in the force-time curve (Fleck and Kraemer 1997). Although it may require an athlete 0.4 to 0.5 seconds to reach maximal force in performing a one-repetition maximum (1RM), the amount of time available to exert force in competition (e.g., for the forearm shiver in American football) may be as little as 0.1 second or less, thus making force capabilities after that time point irrelevant or at least unused.

Strength

The ability to produce maximal force is a classic performance ability of all athletes. Some athletes may depend on this characteristic more than others do (e.g., wrestlers versus distance runners). Strength is vital to power development at higher levels of force (moving heavier weights quickly) and provides the physiological stimuli needed for collateral development of other systems such as connective tissue. Strength development also engages motor units, which allow for the development of muscle hypertrophy. Preliminary data indicate that exercising with loads in the 3RM to 5RM range using multiple sets stimulates strength development and hypertrophy of all muscle fiber types because all are recruited by such training. However, such intensity must be periodized over the long-term training program. The development of strength is crucial for almost all sports for potentially different reasons. Distance runners, for example, may need to develop strength to offset the breakdown of tissue with high-volume, high-intensity mileage, whereas wrestlers' strength development benefits their ability to produce and sustain maximal force. Also, strength must be maintained during power development phases of training.

Speed

Speed has been called the defining difference in many sports. Many games are simply played faster as athletes progress to the next level of competition (Fry and Kraemer 1991). Speed in forward, backward, and lateral positions is important to many sports. With stops and starts, speed merges into the concept of agility. Speed is a vital attribute of strategy in many sports. Being able to move from point A to point B quickly allows the athletes to set up in the proper position for a sport skill (e.g., to hit the ball in tennis) or simply gives them a pure advantage in the competition (e.g., being able to break away to the goal in soccer).

Agility

The ability to stop and change direction quickly is an obvious example of a physical characteristic that provides a vital translation of speed in almost all sports. Few sports require speed in only a straight-line movement. Agility is a total-body phenomenon specific to the sports skill. Some sports also require the ability to move with a sports implement. For example, in one of our studies competitive tennis players showed greater agility when using a racket than without it, indicating that motor patterns are highly cued by the manipulation of the implement. Other sports such as football, racquetball, lacrosse, and basketball have interfaces with a sports implement or ball. Therefore, training agility using the implement may be vital for optimal transfer of the attribute to the actual sport competition.

Coordination

Coordination takes on many aspects of physical ability. Coordination can reflect how well joints manage the muscular firing patterns between or among them. Coordination can also indicate how well the athlete fires his or her motor-unit pattern for muscular force in relationship to the use of an implement such as a tennis racket or baseball bat. It can suggest how well an athlete times a jump to catch a ball or make a shot. Coordination is crucial in the hand-eye relationship needed in sports such as golf or baseball. Thus, coordinated movements in sports can be vital within the context of the sport.

Quickness

Quickness is a complex physical skill as well. Simplistically, quickness involves reaction time and movement time in response to a specific stimulus or set of stimuli. Anticipation is another dimension. The nature of the stimulus is one of the more intriguing questions in sport. What is it that an athlete responds to? Is it a touch? A look? A feel? The reaction to the stimuli within the sport context is the first cue needed for success. Only then does the ability to produce force quickly (power), which is based on the motor capability of the athlete, come into play. Fine motor movements such as a tennis player making a volley at the net and larger gross motor movements such as a running back making a cut in American football are different and may need to be trained differently within the sport context.

Flexibility

Flexibility, or the ability to move the joints in the needed range of motion demanded by the sport, is vital. For years some coaches and athletes feared that weight training would reduce flexibility and create "muscle-bound" athletes, but research has since shown that intelligent training, even with heavy weights, does not negatively affect flexibility.

Flexibility is highly variable among athletes, as are muscle stiffness and joint stiffness, and women are typically more flexible than men. Each athlete can have different levels of flexibility in various movements. Moreover, maximal flexibility is not vital in all sports because it is only necessary that the athlete perform the necessary sports skills with adequate range of motion. The golf swing is a good example of this. In some sports, flexibility in some movements is sacrificed to optimize the muscular support needed for the movement. For example, flexibility to touch elbow to opposite elbow in front of the body may be limited due to massive pectoral development needed for lifting heavy weights in the bench press. Thus, the amount of hypertrophy needed in different body parts and its effect on flexibility must be examined to prevent development of a physical barrier of muscle that would limit movement needed in the sport.

Weight training has been shown to improve flexibility, but specific flexibility training programs may also be needed to further enhance flexibility. In weight training, a full range of motion is typically used to enhance flexibility when exercising. It is vital to exercise both sides of a joint so as not to limit joint flexibility (Fleck and Kraemer 1997). Flexibility is an important component of any training program because it dictates movement ability for sports skills.

Athletes make diverse selections from among many types of stretching exercises. They typically stretch at the beginning and the end of a training session or workout. The benefits of stretching increase greatly, however, when the temperature of the joint is warmer than it would be at rest, making an active warm-up before stretching (e.g., jogging) important in a workout sequence.

Flexibility is important for athletic performance in several ways. Sometimes internal resistance within a joint may limit movement, and improving flexibility will increase the mobility of a joint. The bony structures of athletes vary and occasionally limit movement. Greater flexibility can improve athletic performance following injury. Muscle tissue that has been scarred because of an injury may not be elastic, thus limiting the mobility of an athlete and his or her ability to perform at maximum levels. Flexibility chronically increases the elasticity of muscle tissue and may contribute to increased athletic performance. Recent studies have raised a concern that stretching prior to some activities such as the vertical jump or isokinetic force production may in fact reduce force and power performance acutely. More study will be needed to clarify this finding and to determine the timeline of effects. Nevertheless, flexibility training is still important..

Local Muscular Endurance

Classically, local muscular endurance has been defined as the ability to perform repeated muscular actions. This can range from whole-body movements, a vertical jump for example, to single-joint movements such as repeated elbow flexion. Although the leg musculature of a marathon runner may be perceived to have a high level of fitness for local muscular endurance, many athletes are interested in the ability to perform repeated bouts of exercise at a relatively high power output (e.g., maximal vertical jumps in basketball). Because over 80 percent of competitive sports are dominated by anaerobic function, the ability to reproduce athletic movements at a relatively high percentage of maximal power output throughout a competition has become even more important. Conditioning the body to produce repetitive maximal efforts with little or no drop-off in performance has been the focus of many conditioning programs. In addition, the ability to perform repetitive bouts of exercise under stressful metabolic conditions such as high muscle-lactate concentrations has also become important to some sports (wrestling, for example). Thus, training for local muscular endurance is an important aspect of elite training programs (Kraemer 1997).

Cardiovascular Aerobic Capacity and Endurance

Development of a minimal level of cardiovascular fitness may be required for all sports. Obviously, some sports have greater reliance on aerobic energy sources supported by cardiovascular mechanisms. For example, endurance running relies more on aerobic energy than sprinting. But the concept of an aerobic base (i.e., minimal aerobic fitness level) does not mean all athletes need to perform distance running to achieve cardiovascular fitness. In fact, in some cases too much aerobic training can diminish the magnitude of gains in muscular power, speed, and strength (Fleck and Kraemer 1997; Kraemer et al. 1995). Therefore, other programs for cardiovascular training within the context of the sport, such as interval sprints for football players, may provide a more compatible training option.

The cardiovascular system is involved with a host of bodily functions (Fleck and Kraemer 1997). This includes delivery of oxygen and nutrients, removal of carbon dioxide and metabolic by-products from muscle and other tissues, transportation of compounds to the liver and other organs, assistance in regulation of body temperature, and transportation of hormones to their target tissues in the body. Thus, enhancement of the cardiovascular system increases the overall physiological function of the athlete. Cardiovascular conditioning is typically evaluated by the amount of oxygen that can be consumed—maximal oxygen consumption—or the efficiency of its use (e.g., running economy) during exercise.

In general, aerobic training results in an increase in the number of capillaries and mitochondria of activated muscle fibers (Kraemer, Fleck, and Evans 1996). The increase in the number of capillaries allows the blood to perfuse the muscle fibers more completely, delivering more oxygen and nutrients to each individual muscle fiber. The increase in the number of the mitochondria favorably enhances metabolic energy production from aerobic sources. Endurance training increases the ability of the muscle to use fat as a fuel and to rely less on carbohydrate energy while it reduces lactic acid and thus increases the lactate threshold. Preserving the carbohydrate stores in the liver and muscle provides the extra glucose needed during extended performance.

THE PHYSIOLOGY OF PERFORMANCE

Muscles are connected to tendons, which are connected to bones. The ability of the human body to move involves the stimulation of muscle in a specific manner. This in turn produces force, which ultimately causes the movement of the bone segments. Movement can be simple as in elbow flexion, which involves just one joint, or more complex as in a vertical jump, which involves a multijoint movement. Communication demands for muscles in multijoint movements are different from communication demands for single-joint movements. Thus, in a training program to optimize sports fitness, it is neccessary to train multijoint movements. The importance of training multijoint movements along with single-joint movements is based on this different pattern of neuromuscular activation and coordinated communication (Kraemer, Fleck, and Evans 1996).

A motor unit is the alpha motor neuron and its associated muscle fibers. When a motor unit is stimulated, all the muscle fibers in that motor unit are activated to contract. Motor units are recruited to produce a certain pattern of force—high force, power, speed, etc. The size principle is one of the primary concepts in neuromuscular activation (for review see Fleck and Kraemer 1997). In general, when only a small amount of force is required by a muscle, low-threshold motor units, which contain low numbers of fibers, small muscle fibers, or type I slow-twitch muscle fibers, are stimulated. As more force and power are needed, higher threshold motor units, which contain more muscle fibers, bigger fibers, or type II fast-twitch muscle fibers that can contract more forcefully and quickly, are recruited or stimulated. This means that for most activities lower threshold motor units are recruited before the higher ones, even when leading up to maximal voluntary recruitment of all available motor units. Exceptions to the size principle, in which lower threshold motor units are inhibited so that an athlete can jump more quickly to the use of higher threshold motor units, have been seen in well-practiced power and speed recruitment demands. Therefore it is clear that all sports skills have specific patterns of muscle recruitment of intact muscle to perform a skill. Unless one recruits a muscle fiber by activating its motor unit with an appropriate exercise demand, few training adaptations occur. Finally, some scientists believe that only so much of the total neuromuscular motor-unit pool can be voluntarily recruited. This means that all of the motor units cannot be fired or activated at the same time. It has been proposed that there is a "centrally mediated" safety range for muscle activation. Many training programs have tried to reduce the amount of inhibition to gain greater voluntary control of more motor units for maximal exertion (Kraemer and Koziris 1994).

The most important part of a training program is the pattern of recruitment of the motor units used in the activity. The principle of specificity states that carryover from a training activity to a sport is dependent on the similarity of the neuromuscular demands of the activity and the sport. Of course, many skills make up a sport. Therefore, a training program must address all of the various muscle actions used in the skills involved. It is possible to achieve 100 percent specificity only by performing the skills; overload of the muscles' actions in the context of the sports skills cannot accomplish this objective. It is also possible to overload the rate of force development, power, force characteristics, and so on using the basic biomechanical movements needed to train general body movements used in the sport. It is an oversimplification to say that it is necessary only to strengthen muscle and then practice the sport because that statement addresses only one component—strength—of muscular development. Many other biomechanical characteristics can be trained, as discussed earlier. Oversimplification of the way the neuromuscular system functions could lead to limited use of a variety of beneficial training tools—plyometrics, speed drills, power movements, strength training, flexibility training, and so on. Each of these components can augment the total integrated skill in a properly developed conditioning program.

The muscle fibers in the motor units that are activated are either type I (slow twitch) or type II (fast twitch) (Kraemer, Fleck, and Evans 1996). Within each muscle fiber a continuum of fiber types exists, reflecting different enzymatic and protein contents. For example, as an athlete stimulates a type IIB muscle fiber, it slowly shifts to a type IIAB and then to type IIA muscle fiber with faster contractile enzymes and stronger protein structures to tolerate higher use. In fact, with training, almost all type IIB muscle fibers can be converted to type IIA fiber types (Fleck and Kraemer 1997; Kraemer et al. 1995). Training affects many characteristics of a muscle fiber—amount of enzymes, number of mitochondria, number of capillaries, amount of glycogen, and so forth (for review see Kraemer, Fleck, and Evans 1996). The underlying changes in each muscle fiber depend on the specific type of exercise stimulus it receives. Although the subject is beyond the scope of this chapter, an understanding of the various types of adaptations that take place in response to different types of exercise training can help a coach understand subsequent changes in performance (Kraemer, Duncan, and Harman 1998; Kraemer, Fleck, and Evans 1996; Kraemer et al. 1995). High-power and high-force motor units use a different set of fibers than do the low-power motor units used in more aerobic activities. Unless significant energy substrates in muscle are lost, motor-unit activation attempts to recruit the type of fibers needed for the metabolic and force demands of the activity. For example, elite marathon runners have high percentages of type I fibers in their lower-body musculature because type II muscle fibers would not be optimal for force production. Type II fibers would produce more metabolic by-products such as lactic acid, which would be metabolically counterproductive to an elite performance in which higher lactate thresholds are optimal.

BASIC TRAINING PRINCIPLES

Many principles govern physical conditioning programs. As noted earlier, one important principle is that programs should be specific to the sport and should meet the individual needs of the athlete. A related principle that has played an important role in our understanding of physical conditioning is the SAID principle, the principle of specific adaptations to imposed demands. Both principles point to the importance of training for the specific sport. Nevertheless, each athlete will bring to the program a specific set of genetically based capabilities and physiological strategies. In turn, each sport favors specific biological strategies for success based on the rules of the game and its physiological and biomechanical demands (McCall et al. 1999). For example, it should be obvious that only those athletes with a specific set of inherent characteristics trained to the limits of their genetic potential will be on the starting line for the Olympic marathon or 100-meter sprint, will play center in the NBA, or will be on the lifting platform in the next Olympic Games. As performance demands go up—being a center in basketball in the NBA compared with playing center in high school—the number of physical, physiological, and biomechanical strategies for success will be reduced—you must be tall enough to play center in the NBA. In some team sports a greater number of strategies may exist to get the job done because of diversity in the various positions. Physical conditioning appears to improve inherent genetic basis (change in the phenotypic expression based on genotype you have) by about 15 to 45 percent depending on the specific characteristic (e.g., muscle-fiber size or heart size) being trained. This is different from a training improvement in a relative performance such as a vertical jump or strength; you may improve your 1RM by 100 percent as you train from an untrained state. It is a combination of inherent biological genetic factors that ultimately makes elite performance possible.

It is well known in sports that recruiting is vital to success. We often hear that an athlete picked his or her parents well. Thus, sports fitness is based on training what the athlete brings to the table. Sports skills and sports strategy also contribute to success in games or competitions and thereby help to reduce reliance on genetics. Finally, a host of other factors, from psychological factors to environmental conditions, can affect performance success. Sport is thus a dynamic scenario to prepare for, but physical conditioning is an essential element in the success formula for an athlete at any level.

Operationally defined by the exercise prescription, an exercise training program has several fundamental characteristics: *frequency* of exercise, *duration* of exercise, and *intensity* of exercise. Each of these variables is defined within the construct of the exercise modality (e.g., strength or aerobic) or program type (e.g., local muscular endurance weight-training program versus strength weight-training program). The frequency of exercise refers to the number of workouts per week and per day. Many training programs use workouts two or three times a day during certain phases of training to shorten the single workout and to increase the quality of exercise. This has been especially successful with resistance-training protocols.

In resistance exercise a single workout is described by the choice of exercises, the order of exercises, the amount of rest between sets and exercises, the number of sets for each exercise, and the intensity used (Fleck and Kraemer 1997; Kraemer and Harman 1998). The choice of exercises will affect many characteristics of muscle activation. Is a given exercise fixed form, involving a movement pattern that is fixed and balanced, or is it free form, using free weights that must be balanced with more use of the assistance muscles? Is it a single-joint or multijoint exercise? Is it an isometric, isokinetic, or "isotonic" exercise type? Being able to perform exercises and variations properly depends on having an in-depth understanding of equipment characteristics. The order of exercises affects the amount of fatigue and therefore the quality of the workout. The rest between the sets and exercises will dictate the degree of metabolic strain. Shorter rest periods (e.g., one minute) can produce higher lactate concentrations and require the use of lighter loads in subsequent sets if the athlete has not adapted to the dramatic disruption in the acid-base balance—the increase in hydrogen ions, decrease in pH, and increase in lactic acid. The number of sets will affect the volume of a particular exercise. Remember that an athlete need not perform the same number of sets of all exercises in a workout (Kraemer 1997).

The intensity of the exercise is typically defined as the amount of external resistance that the muscles must work against. Many studies have shown that a continuum of loading exists (Fleck and Kraemer 1997). Training adaptations for strength occur across all loads with the greatest changes taking place with loads in the 1RM to 10RM range. Local muscular endurance is enhanced with loading lighter than 15RM.

By using these five fundamental acute program variables—choice of exercises, order of exercise, amount of rest between sets and exercises, number of sets, and amount of resistance—it is possible to create many different types of resistance exercise workouts. The challenge is to plan how to change these variables over time to produce overload but not overtraining (Kraemer and Nindl 1998).

Overload is another basic concept that has been around since the inception of physical training. From ancient times when Milo would each day lift a growing young calf, demanding more from the muscle each day has been a basic principle of resistance training. A vital corollary to the concept of overload is the concept of training periodization. This type of sequencing, or periodizing, builds progressive overload in a training program while allowing needed variation in the training stimuli, along with rest and recovery, to allow the body to adapt positively to the exercise program. Positive adaptations in the physiological systems of the body influence the motor and biomechanical abilities of sports skills. Concomitant with this process of physical development is the psychological development needed to cope with the many demands in sports.

PERIODIZATION

Periodization has been one of the more important training theories related to sports conditioning over the past 30 years (Fleck and Kraemer 1997; Mateyev 1972; Medvedyev 1988; Stone, O'Bryant, and Garhammer 1981). Periodized training involves planned variation in the intensity of exercises and in the volume of a workout. Although periodization is typically used in resistance-training programs, any conditioning program can and should be periodized to provide variation in the exercise stimulus along with added rest and recovery.

There are a number of periodization schemes that can be used in resistance training (Polquin and King 1992; Willoughby 1993) for both larger- and smaller-muscle groups. A coach must consider the type of periodized program to use. Two basic types have been developed: linear and nonlinear periodized protocols for maximal strength development. Let's examine some of the basic differences between linear and nonlinear periodization when strength and power are the primary goals of a training program.

Linear Methods

Classic or linear periodization methods use a progressive increase in the intensity with small variations in each two- to four-week microcycle. For example, a classic four-cycle linear periodized program (four weeks for each cycle) may include the following:

Microcycle 1: 3 to 5 sets of 12 to 15RM
Microcycle 2: 4 to 5 sets of 8 to 12RM
Microcycle 3: 3 to 4 sets of 4 to 6RM
Microcycle 4: 3 to 5 sets of 1 to 3RM

Note the variation within each four-week microcycle due to the repetition range of each cycle. Still, the general trend for the 16-week program is a steady linear increase in intensity. Because of the straight-line increase in intensity, this program is an example of linear periodized training.

The volume of the training program will also vary in the classic program, starting with a higher initial volume and a lower intensity. As the intensity of the program increases, the volume gradually decreases. The drop-off in volume of exercise can become less pronounced as the training status of the athlete advances. In other words, advanced athletes with significant progression in their training can tolerate higher volumes of exercise during the heavy and very heavy microcycles. Breaking up workouts throughout the day facilitates this tolerance.

Note that it is important not to progress too quickly to training with high volumes using heavy weights. Too much too soon can lead to development of an overtraining syndrome (Kraemer and Nindl 1998), which can compromise progress for months. Although it takes a great deal of excessive work to produce an overtraining effect, highly motivated trainees can easily cross the line out of sheer desire to make gains and see progress in their training (Fry and Kraemer 1997; Kraemer and Nindl 1998). Therefore, it is important to monitor the stress of workouts for all exercises performed in a total conditioning program. Remember, exercises within a total program can interact to compromise other programs; for example, long-distance running can affect power development.

High-volume exercise in the early microcycles has been thought to promote the muscle hypertrophy needed to enhance strength in the later phases of training. Thus, the late cycles of training are linked to the early cycles of training. The cycles enhance one another because strength gains are related to size changes in the muscle. Programs that attempt to gain strength without muscle hypertrophy can be successful after initial increases in muscle size occur from the untrained state. This occurs as a function of the specific program used (e.g., loading, volume, etc.). In some cases, such as golf, the goal of continued hypertrophy of muscle is not important and could be counterproductive to skill development. In other words, not all athletes need to be big to be successful.

As the program progresses and the trainee begins to use heavier resistance, the increase in the intensity of the periodized program then starts to develop nervous system adaptations for enhanced motor-unit recruitment. Heavier weights demand that high-threshold motor units become involved in the force-production process. The increase in muscle protein in the muscles from the early cycle of training enhances the force production of the motor units. Here again, there is an integration of the different parts of the 16-week training program.

A 16-week program is called a mesocycle, and several mesocycles make up a yearlong training program, or macrocycle. Each mesocycle attempts to advance physical development toward the training goals. Thus, the theoretical basis for a linear method of periodization consists of the development of hypertrophy followed by the improvement of nerve function to produce optimal force in specific movements. This progression is repeated with each mesocycle to achieve progress in the training program. Linear periodization also provides rest and recovery.

Nonlinear Periodized Programs

More recently, the concept of nonlinear periodized training programs has been developed to maintain variation in the training stimulus (Polquin and King 1992). Nonlinear periodized training makes program implementation possible when competitive demands or other demands are intense. The nonlinear program allows for variation in the intensity and volume within each week over the course of the training program. Intensity and volume of training will vary within the week. An example of a week during a nonlinear periodized training program over a 16-week mesocycle would include the following:

> **Monday:** 4 sets of 12 to 15RM (or replace this with a power workout of 30% of 1RM)
>
> **Wednesday:** 4 sets of 8 to 10RM
>
> **Friday:** 3 to 4 sets of 4 to 6RM
>
> **Monday:** 4 to 5 sets of 1 to 3RM

This protocol uses a four-day rotation with one day of rest between workouts.

The variation in training is much greater within the week. Intensity spans over a range of 1RM to 15RM sets during the week's cycle. Training with this variation in intensity appears to be as effective as training using linear programs.

Unlike the linear programs, in nonlinear programs the athlete trains the different components of muscle size and strength, both the hypertrophy and the neural aspects of strength, within the same week. Thus, the athlete is addressing two different physiological adaptations within the same 7- to 10-day period of the 16-week mesocycle. This approach appears to be possible and may be more compatible with the schedules of many individuals, especially when competitions, travel, and other commitments make adhering to the traditional linear method difficult.

In this program, athletes simply rotate through the different protocols. The workout rotates between heavy, moderate, light, and power training sessions. If an athlete misses the Monday workout, the rotation order is just pushed forward, meaning that he or she performs the missed workout on the next workout day. For example, an athlete who misses the light 12 to 15RM workout (which provides rest for many motor units) scheduled for Monday would simply perform it on Wednesday and continue with the rotation sequence. In this way, none of the workout stimuli in the training program are missed. Rather than consisting of a set number of training weeks, a mesocycle in this program consists of a certain number of workouts (e.g., 48).

Both the linear and nonlinear program schedules appear to accomplish the same effect and are superior to constant training programs (Kraemer 1997; Willoughby 1993). Coaches can periodize a program by either training the hypertrophy component first and the neural strength component second in the linear method or by training both components within a 7- to 10-day period in the nonlinear method. The key to workout success is variation. Coaches can use different approaches over the year to provide adequate variation.

PERFORMANCE STRATEGIES

Each athlete brings to the specific sport competition a set of physiological and psychological strategies. A performance strategy includes the attributes that the athlete brings to the competition (e.g., body mass, height, muscle fiber type, and anxiety levels). Genetic inheritance, along with training, contributes to the status of the available strategies. How the athlete uses them or integrates them in a performance dictates the degree of success. Some attributes, such as height, cannot be trained. Each sport has a specific set of demands for success based on the characteristics and rules of the game or competition. The determinants of success in each sport have changed as rules have changed; for example, no blocking below the waist in American football has made taller linemen more effective. Athletes are continually bringing more capability to each sport; therefore, over the years the level of performance has increased. For example, men's 100-meter dash times on the elite level are typically below 10.0 seconds (Kraemer and Koziris 1994). This has made the strategies for success—such as the need for type II (fast-twitch) muscle fibers to be an elite sprinter—at the elite level of competition even more restrictive; you do not see athletes with a high percentage of type I (slow-twitch) muscle fibers running a 10-second 100-meter dash. The ability of the athlete to match physiological and psychological attributes to the demands of competition dictates success at all levels. As competitive demands (higher levels of competition) increase, so too do the demands on strategies.

In many sports, however, success can build on several attributes once the sports skills are solid. Most sports have complex demands. One athlete may succeed using one set of strategies while another athlete succeeds in the same sport using a different set. For example, in baseball one athlete may be tall, have large muscle mass in the upper and lower body, and be powerful. Another athlete might be short, have a lower muscle mass, and be extremely quick. Each can be a Hall of Fame baseball player but for different reasons: one for hitting home runs and hitting, and the other for fielding and hitting. Thus, baseball may allow many different strategies to be successful. Yet, we are just starting to understand what components explain the performances of elite competitors in many team sports. Nevertheless, an athlete must have a fundamental level of skill in any sport in order to engage physiological or psychological abilities (e.g., speed is not important in a hurdle race if you do not know how to negotiate a hurdle properly). At the elite level of sport, some attribute or some combination of attributes must provide a unique strategy to lift performance to the elite level. Integration of various capabilities may also be involved at the elite levels, thus making prediction of success in many sports difficult.

In a recent interview Tiger Woods alluded to the fact that golfers are now paying greater attention to their physical conditioning and are starting to train with weights. He stated that they are becoming better athletes with greater physical capabilities to use in their games. Nevertheless, the muscular development demands of a golfer are far different from those of a football player. Therefore, sport-specific, individualized programs must be used in conditioning. Even athletes with outstanding natural physical and psychological abilities in a sport can use physical conditioning to take those abilities to higher levels of performance. At the elite level, the prevention of injury and an enhanced ability to recover from small injuries contribute to success and a long career.

SUMMARY

The elite performances seen in sports today are a function of genetic inheritance, accomplished sports skills, psychological skills, and physical conditioning. In order to excel, the athlete should bring to his or her sport an entire strategy, which can be enhanced by physical conditioning and by establishing a solid fitness base for the sport. Thus the basis for elite performance in competition is not a single factor but a combination of many factors coming together. Ultimately, individualized, sport-specific strength and conditioning programs can enhance the fitness base for all athletes.

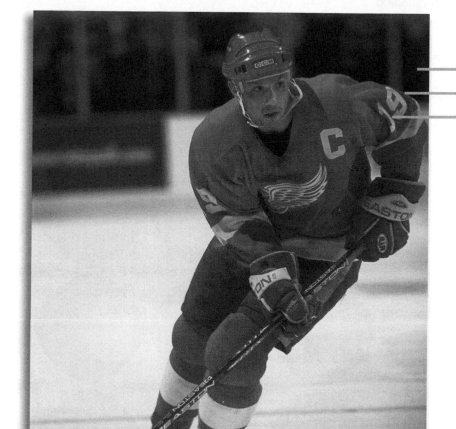

Baseline Sports-Fitness Testing

Gray Cook

*T*esting is used throughout athletics to document, assess, and predict sports performance. A review of the current literature reveals many interpretations of testing philosophy and methods. It is first necessary to define the intent of baseline testing and then develop a practical model for application. Miller and Keane (1997) define *base* as "the lowest part or foundation of anything." *Baseline* is defined as "an observation or value that represents the normal background level of measurable quality." The operative words in these two accepted definitions are *foundation*, the fundamental or essential components of a system or structure, and *quality*, a range, degree, or grade of excellence. Note that the word *quality* is used—not *quantity*. Most current testing methods are quantity based (time, distance, force, etc.), not quality based. The purpose of baseline testing is to demonstrate the fundamental building blocks of athleticism and preparedness for sport. Each building block should have specific relevance to athletics. The word *function* has become popular as a term to represent movements that are specific to a given activity. It is important to reconstruct testing using the terms *quality*, *foundation*, and *function* to represent accurately the purpose of baseline testing.

The goal of this chapter is to present a model that makes use of principles consistent with motor learning. Early testing practices focused on physiological energy systems and sport-specificity. This chapter will introduce functional movement patterns and motor control as key building blocks of performance. Examples of testing are presented; however the reader is encouraged to create new tests or to adapt conventional tests to fit within the proposed model.

CONSTRUCTING A TESTING MODEL

Baseline testing should ask three questions, regardless of the athlete's sport or position:

1. What is the status of fundamental or functional movement quality? Fundamental movement quality includes range of motion, balance, body control, and stability.

2. What is the status of fundamental or functional performance quantity? This describes functional movements, which are graded by time or distance. Examples of fundamental performance are the 40-yard sprint, the vertical leap, and so on. These movements should look at performance from a general viewpoint and not be sport specific; this will allow the comparison of all athletes before sport specificity is considered.

3. What is the status of sport-specific skills? This describes specific proficiency, ability, or dexterity with movements that define a sport and one of its positions. These tests will usually look at quantity and quality. A good example is pitching. A radar gun will measure speed (quantity), while the strike zone will measure accuracy (quality).

These considerations will improve problem solving by establishing a more refined breakdown of information. For the purposes of this chapter and to provide quick identification of performance problems, athletic movement will be observed in three categories:

1. Functional movement quality—basic fundamental movements that demonstrate full range of motion, body control, balance, and basic stability

2. Functional performance quantity—general, nonspecific performance demonstrating gross power, speed, endurance, and agility

3. Sport-specific skills—skills demonstrating sport-specific movement patterns

This chapter will not go into depth for sport-specific skill training because of the large volume of information concerning each sport. The focus will be on the first two categories because they are common to all sports.

If two athletes have poor 40-yard sprint times, and no fundamental assessment of movement quality has been conducted, then it must be assumed that both athletes are slow and need more speed training. If fundamental movement testing, however, reveals that athlete 1 has good flexibility, good core stability, and good balance and that athlete 2 does not, then the two athletes do not have the same problem. Athlete 1 has the fundamental building blocks but is not using them well for speed generation. Therefore, a speed-development program would be appropriate. Athlete 2 does not have the fundamental movement patterns necessary for speed development. Placing athlete 2 on a speed program will have some positive results but, as discussed later in this chapter, doing so would break a major rule about the neuromuscular system (see page 23 on functional movement). The test deduction and result for the two athletes is as follows:

Athlete 1: Basic speed (performance work) and plyometric work

Athlete 2: Basic mobility (fundamental movement work) and stability work progressing to speed and plyometric work

Focus is often placed only on the quantity (functional performance) aspect of movement and not the quality (foundation or functional movement). Those who develop conditioning programs commonly make two mistakes:

1. Placing minimal importance or emphasis on fundamental movement patterns

2. Confusing quality of movement and quantity of movement

Fundamental movement and the importance of quality will be examined in this chapter. A model called the performance pyramid, designed to help coaching and training staffs interpret baseline data, will be presented. The model will help coaches, trainers, and conditioning specialists develop a hierarchy of importance and an objective approach for managing athletes and teams. The first order of business is to identify the weakest link in movement through testing.

Roles of the Staff

The certified athletic trainer will be provided with data that is based in prevention, which facilitates better tracking of athletic function and movement efficiency. The trainer should identify and monitor any weak link, such as poor flexibility or muscle imbalances resulting from a previous injury or a poor training program. The trainer should be concerned with functional movement quality.

The same data will assist the conditioning specialist with performance-based problem solving for better prioritization of training. The strength coach must also focus on the weak link but more from a performance basis. The model will demonstrate a systematic progression designed to improve general performance. The conditioning specialist should be concerned with functional movement and functional performance.

Sports skill is the concern of the head coach and assistant coaches. It is their job, with the help of the certified athletic trainer and the conditioning specialist, to identify and understand the way in which the weak link will affect skill and sport-specific performance. A look at functional movement quality and functional performance quantity will help explain sport-specific skill data.

Baseline Testing Considerations

Baseline test data along with a sports medicine history (previous injuries) and sport-specific data (performance and skills) should be considered equally when setting goals. In case of injury the athletic trainer can use baseline measurements to guide and direct rehabilitation toward preinjury performance. The strength coach can use baseline data to direct the athlete's focus toward his or her weak link. Baseline testing must encompass a format that can both assist the strength and conditioning specialists and sports medicine team by predicting which athletes are predisposed to injury and provide performance tests that look at raw power, speed, agility, coordination, and endurance.

The appropriate time for baseline testing for sports is between the preparticipation physical (medical screen) and the sport-specific testing. Baseline testing should address general athleticism and physical preparedness. The testing should identify both attributes of and detriments to athletic performance and competition. The modern strength and conditioning program commonly employs baseline testing for athletes, but distinguishing between the athletes who test well (in the weight room and on the field) and those who perform well (in the competition arena) is often difficult. This means that current testing methods are sometimes poor predictors of true sports performance. Furthermore, no specific relationship has been drawn between an individual's performance-based test scores and the individual's tendency to sustain noncontact injuries—injuries that can be prevented because they result from tightness, weakness, poor coordination, and the compensatory strategies athletes use to perform in spite of these problems. Therefore, the athletic trainer has no reliable predictor of these unnecessary injuries. The trainer cannot be expected to prevent them unless a screening tool is implemented (Cook and Athletic Testing Services 1998).

THREE FORMATS FOR BASELINE TESTING

Baseline testing can be broken into three distinct formats. The first format looks at functional movement quality, the second at functional performance quantity, and the third at sport-specific skills.

Do not be surprised when highly skilled athletes do not test well for functional movement or functional performance. This should in no way diminish their skilled accomplishments. The fact that they are good attests to how well their neuromuscular systems have compensated for a particular weakness. But it is the responsibility of those in authority to expose limitations and forecast potential problems before they become reality. All athletes will ultimately make certain compensations. As they become more seasoned and specialized, their focus is usually on accomplishment (quantity), not functional movement and technique (quality). This is one reason why all great coaches stress skill fundamentals. Movement fundamentals should receive the same attention. The compensatory patterns are numerous and not readily detectable. It is better to identify the reasons for compensation through continual baseline testing.

The performance pyramid (figure 2.1) demonstrates how each level of baseline testing builds on the other. Consider the skills involved in throwing a baseball or softball:

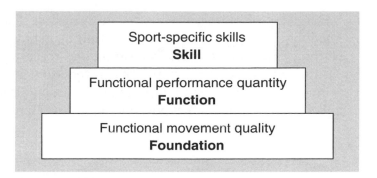

Figure 2.1   The performance pyramid shows how each level creates a stable base for the next.

1. The athlete must first possess good general mobility, especially in the shoulder region. Next, the athlete must have enough stability in the lower body to shift weight from one foot to the other to generate rotary movement while maintaining balance.

2. When the athlete adds speed and power to the weight shift, he or she is able to generate greater ball speed. The athlete will learn to transfer power from the hips to the trunk and from the trunk to the arm, a process known as kinetic linking.

3. Last, the athlete will learn control and skill. This will improve accuracy, conserve energy, and allow the athlete to become more relaxed and consistent.

One level creates a stable base for the next, and this sequence represents the way the brain prioritizes and processes movement information. Although this is an oversimplification of true motor learning, it will help the athlete understand that he or she must develop each level before moving to the next.

The first block (lowest) on the pyramid represents fundamental mobility and stability. Strength is not included because it is a subcomponent of stability measured only in force with no consideration control, time, or distance. The second block on the pyramid represents movement efficiency and productivity, including power, speed, agility, and endurance. The third block (highest) on the pyramid represents skill, movement timing, coordination, body control, muscle memory, motor learning, and consistency.

FUNCTIONAL MOVEMENT

Functional movement relates to fundamental mobility and stability, the building blocks for all other measurable physical fitness attributes. They represent the underlying quality of movement. Although these fundamental movement patterns are present in normal growth and development, the athlete can sometimes lose them when he or she focuses on only one aspect of human movement or performance.

Mobility

The term *mobility* represents much more than simple muscular flexibility as identified in a sit-and-reach test. It includes the way multiple body segments, such as the hips, pelvis, and trunk region, interact in functional situations. Individual assessment of one specific joint and muscle complex will not yield sufficient data to describe the athletic body in motion; sitting and reaching has limited functional application and little correlation with true functional movement. Mobility represents muscle flexibility, joint range of motion, and multisegmental interaction of the body parts in functional positions and movement patterns.

Stability

Stability, on the other hand, is not a representation of strength. It is more a representation of body control through strength, coordination, balance, and efficiency of movement. Stability can be divided into static and dynamic categories. Static stability is the maintenance of posture and balance. Dynamic stability is the production and control of movement and includes the following components:

- Mobility and flexibility
- Strength
- Coordination
- Local muscular endurance
- Cardiovascular fitness

Note that by definition dynamic stability cannot be optimal if mobility and flexibility are not optimal (because they are components of dynamic stability). Note also that strength is only *one* component of dynamic stability. To create efficient movement, all five components must work together. In the presence of normal mobility, the neuromuscular system will selectively use muscular contractions (isometric, eccentric, and concentric) to stabilize one body segment while creating motion in another body segment. This process is a result of timing and coordination and it explains why athletes with less than impressive weight-room statistics (isolated strength) can have impressive statistics in the vertical leap (power), medicine ball throw (power), and 40-yard dash (speed). These athletes demonstrate efficiency with maximal use of all segments in a unified and synergetic fashion to produce power, speed, and quickness. Raw force (strength) that the athlete cannot use efficiently demonstrates only the ability to move weight, not the body.

The foundations of mobility and stability are evident in human growth and development. The infant enters the world with unlimited mobility and selectively learns to stabilize first the core and then the extremities. Movement control and stability proceed in a head-to-toe progression (cephalo-caudal) as well as a core-to-extremity progression (proximal-distal). This simple law of the neuromuscular system produces a rule of thumb that should be the cornerstone in strength and conditioning programs:

Proximal stability (control) must precede distal mobility (movement).

This means that the athlete must train the muscles of the core and trunk adequately before focusing on the extremities. Therefore, movements like the bench press, although excellent for shoulder development and muscular hypertrophy for the upper extremities, will do little to train the core or educate the neuromuscular system about its role during upper-extremity patterns in a standing or functional posture. The simple push-up is more functional because it involves the core (if performed correctly). We must add a second rule to the first:

If a mobility problem exists it must be dealt with and rectified
before true stability can occur.

Training or testing on fixed-axis equipment in a seated or lying position often breaks both rules. Usually the region of questionable stability is compensating for the region of poor mobility. The knees, lower back (lumbar spine), and shoulders are good examples of areas that commonly develop poor stability. Before an attempt is made to stabilize these areas, the mobility of the ankles, hips, and upper back (thoracic spine) should be established. Testing functional movement allows the sports medicine and conditioning team to understand the interaction between mobility and stability. The combination of poor mobility and stability is the source of many common athletic problems. Athletes demonstrating poor functional movement patterns and poor mobility and stability should seek to regain these fundamental building blocks before focusing on other attributes of fitness such as strength, speed, power, and endurance. Innumerable unnecessary injuries have occurred because athletes have focused more on the quantity of their workout statistics (sets, reps, and weight) than the quality and technique of their movements. A common example is the squat. Many athletes will continue to lift greater amounts of weight with a poor-mobility (figure 2.2) squat even though they cannot perform a deep, full-range-of-motion squat with no weight at all (figure 2.3).

The most common mistake in sports conditioning today is training a movement pattern before achieving full range of motion and control in that movement. Poor technique and inadequate ankle and hip mobility will lead to poor posture and body mechanics during the conditioning session. The compensations that will occur because of a lack of mobility in the hips and ankles will not only create stress on the knees and spine but will also change the motor program for the squatting movement. These compensations will then become engrained into the central nervous system, adversely affecting timing, coordination, and

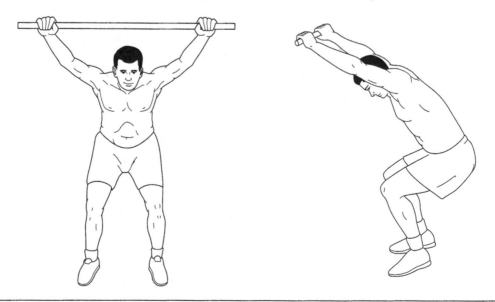

Figure 2.2 Poor-mobility squat.

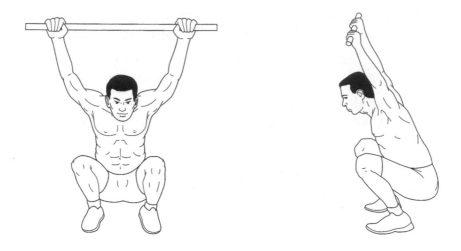

Figure 2.3   Full-mobility squat.

efficiency. Baseline testing must therefore always assess functional movement first to reveal *potential efficiency*. Once an athlete demonstrates functional movement through reliable and valid testing, performance testing can demonstrate *actual efficiency*.

When mobility and stability are poor, potential efficiency is poor, yielding less than optimal performance and a greater chance of injury during athletic conditioning and competition. Potential efficiency takes into account all aspects of human movement; it is not a predictor of any single performance parameter. An athlete may have poor mobility and stability and yet be an elite competitor in a given sport. This circumstance is becoming more prevalent as athletes specialize in one sport, and even one position, at an early age. If such an athlete is asked to perform another movement parameter or to change technique, he or she will have fewer movement options from which to choose. The highly specific movement patterns will cause imbalances by overdeveloping some areas and neglecting others, as well as increasing the potential for injury. Efficient rehabilitation in the event of an injury is also reduced because the system is already compensating in one form or another. Mobility and stability provide a buffer zone that allows adaptability of movement patterns.

FUNCTIONAL MOVEMENT SCREEN

The functional movement screen (FMS) was developed in an attempt to quantify movement quality and fulfill the first requirement of baseline testing (mobility and stability assessment). The screen uses seven movements that represent the mobility and stability milestones in human growth and development—squatting, stepping, lunging, reaching, striding or kicking, and two movements that require trunk stability for anterior-posterior stress (pushing) and rotary stress (segmental stabilization). These movements have been placed in a format that is cost effective, time efficient, reproducible, and representative of the basic foundation for human movement. The functional movement screen assigns a specific score to each athlete. Each sport and position will require a minimum level and optimum level of baseline function. Over time, a movement screen database will reveal how certain injuries correlate with functional movement rankings, which can serve as predictors for the sports medicine team. The screen assists coaches, athletic trainers, and strength coaches in communicating with one another by providing common ground for discussing an athlete's functional status and future potential.

Scoring

The scoring criteria for the test are quite simple. If the athlete is able to produce the required movement without any of the common compensations described, he or she receives a score of 3. If the athlete reproduces the movement but has one or more of the common compensations or any difficulty, the athlete scores a 2. If the athlete is unable to reproduce the movement as described, the athlete receives a score of 1. If pain is present during the test, regardless of the athlete's performance, he or she receives a 0 for that particular movement. A perfect score for all 7 movements is 21.

Interpretation

Interpretation of this scoring system is done on a priority basis. Any 0 scores will be considered first by the team physician and athletic trainer, who will conduct a sports medicine evaluation of the painful site considering the movement pattern that produced the pain. Next, the score of 1 demonstrates that an athlete does not have a functional base of mobility and stability and is therefore probably experiencing microtrauma, poor efficiency, and poor technique with common athletic movements (even if performance seems adequate). This score may also indicate a relatively higher degree of stress during normal activities because a basic movement pattern is absent. A sports medicine professional should specifically evaluate the flexibility and strength of the areas in question (even though the athlete reports no pain). A score of 2 demonstrates areas of priority in conditioning and flexibility. It is advisable that the athletic trainer, strength coach, and sport coach work together to develop complementary exercise, conditioning, and sport-specific training programs around these areas of limitation. A score of 3 demonstrates appropriate or optimal mobility and stability for a particular movement pattern; screening is still periodically necessary to check for common imbalances acquired in training. Five of the seven screens are performed on the left and right sides of the body, allowing for comparison. If testing on one side of the body produces a lower score, then that is the score given for the test.

Besides the seven movement screens, three clearing screens have been added. The clearing screens are for the shoulder and lumbar spine areas (which can sometimes go undetected in routine movement screening). Research and literature reviews have shown that these areas hide potential problems unless specifically addressed. The clearing screens are scored as pass or fail for pain. A 0 score is assigned to the movement screen when pain occurs regardless of the previous score. An impingement clearing screen is added to the shoulder exam. An individual who scores 3 on shoulder mobility but has a positive impingement screen is given a 0. This simple addition to the shoulder movement screen will pick up potential shoulder problems. A spine-flexion clearing screen and a spine-extension clearing screen are added to each of the trunk-stability tests to look at passive spine range of motion in an unloaded position (Cook and Athletic Testing Services 1998).

Deep Squat

Purpose

The deep squat assesses bilateral, symmetrical, and functional mobility of the hips, knees, and ankles. The dowel held overhead assesses bilateral, symmetrical functional mobility of the shoulders as well as the thoracic spine.

Description

1. The athlete places the feet slightly farther than shoulder-width apart and places the hands on the dowel so as to form a 90-degree angle at the elbows with the dowel overhead.

2. The athlete presses the dowel overhead with the shoulders flexed and abducted and with the elbows extended, then descends slowly into a squat position with the heels on the floor, the head and chest facing forward, and the dowel maximally pressed overhead.

3. The athlete is allowed up to three chances to perform the test.

4. If the athlete does not achieve the criteria for a score of 3, he or she then performs the test with a 2 × 6 board under the heels.

3 POINTS

- Upper torso is parallel with tibia or toward vertical.
- Femur is below horizontal.
- Knees are aligned over feet.
- Dowel is aligned over feet.

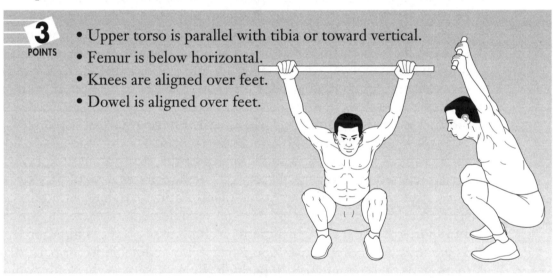

2 POINTS

- Upper torso is parallel with tibia or toward vertical.
- Femur is below horizontal.
- Knees are not aligned over feet.
- Dowel is aligned over feet.

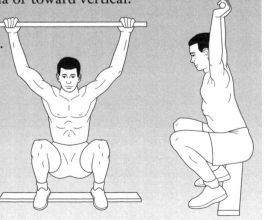

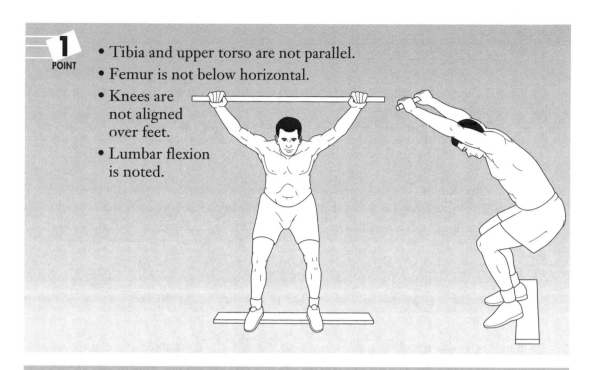

1 POINT
- Tibia and upper torso are not parallel.
- Femur is not below horizontal.
- Knees are not aligned over feet.
- Lumbar flexion is noted.

0 POINTS

The athlete will receive a score of 0 if pain is associated with any portion of this test. A medical professional should perform a thorough evaluation of the painful area.

Clinical Implications for the Deep Squat

The ability to perform the deep squat requires closed kinetic-chain dorsiflexion of the ankles, flexion of the knees and hips, and extension of the thoracic spine, as well as flexion and abduction of the shoulders.

Poor performance on this test can be the result of several factors. Limited mobility in the upper torso can be attributed to poor glenohumeral or thoracic-spine mobility. Limited mobility in the lower extremity including poor closed kinetic-chain dorsiflexion of the ankle or poor flexion of the hip may also cause poor test performance.

When an athlete achieves a score less than 3, the limiting factor must be identified. Clinical documentation of these limitations can be obtained by using standard goniometric measurements.

Previous testing has indicated that when an athlete achieves a score of 2, minor limitations most often exist with either closed kinetic-chain dorsiflexion of the ankle or extension of the thoracic spine. When an athlete achieves a score of 1 or 0, gross limitations may exist with the motions mentioned above as well as flexion of the hip.

Hurdle Step

Purpose

The hurdle step assesses bilateral functional mobility and stability of the hips, knees, and ankles.

Description

1. The athlete places the feet together and aligns the toes directly beneath the hurdle.
2. The hurdle is adjusted to the height of the athlete's tibial tuberosity, and the dowel is positioned across the athlete's shoulders below the neck.
3. The athlete slowly steps over the hurdle and touches the heel to the floor while keeping the stance leg in an extended position. Weight should remain on the stance leg.
4. The athlete then slowly returns to the starting position.
5. The athlete is allowed up to three chances to perform the test.
6. Have the athlete perform the test again, using the opposite leg. If testing produces a lower score for one leg, record the lower score.

3 POINTS

- Hips, knees, and ankles remain aligned in the sagittal plane.
- Minimal to no movement is noted in lumbar spine.
- Dowel and hurdle remain parallel.

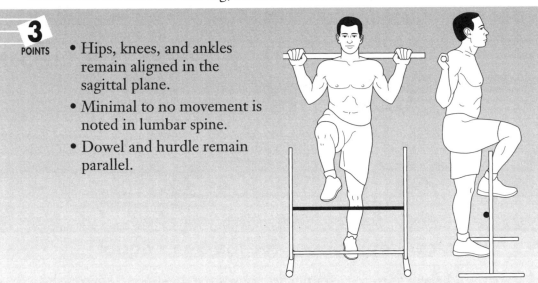

2 POINTS

- Alignment lost between hips, knees, and ankles.
- Movement is noted in lumbar spine.
- Dowel and hurdle do not remain parallel.

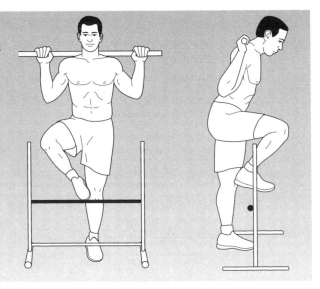

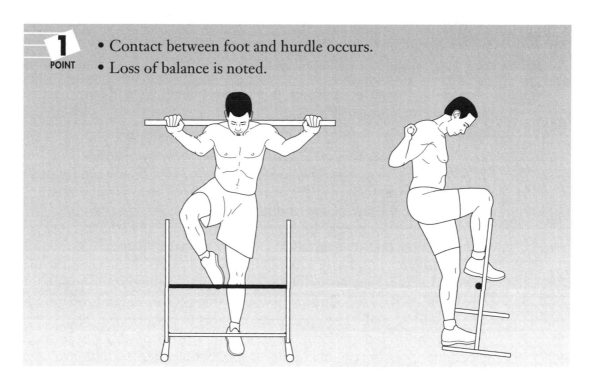

1
POINT

- Contact between foot and hurdle occurs.
- Loss of balance is noted.

0
POINTS

The athlete will receive a score of 0 if pain is associated with any portion of this test. A member of the sports medicine staff should perform a thorough evaluation of the painful area.

Clinical Implications for the Hurdle Step

Performing the hurdle step test requires stance-leg stability of the ankle, knee, and hip as well as maximal closed kinetic-chain extension of the hip. The hurdle step also requires step-leg open kinetic-chain dorsiflexion of the ankle and flexion of the knee and hip. In addition, the athlete must display adequate balance because the test imposes a need for dynamic stability.

Poor performance on this test can be the result of several factors. It may simply be due to poor stability of the stance leg or poor mobility of the step leg. Imposing maximal hip flexion of one leg while maintaining apparent hip extension of the opposite leg requires the athlete to demonstrate relative bilateral, asymmetric hip mobility.

When an athlete achieves a score less than 3, the limiting factor must be identified. Clinical documentation of these limitations can be obtained by using standard goniometric measurements of the joints as well as muscular flexibility tests such as the Thomas test or Kendall's test for hip flexor tightness (see Cook and Athletic Testing Services 1998).

Previous testing has indicated that when an athlete achieves a score of 2, minor limitations most often exist with ankle dorsiflexion or hip flexion with the step leg. When an athlete scores a 1 or 0, relative asymmetric hip mobility may exist secondary to an anterior tilted pelvis.

In-Line Lunge

Purpose

The in-line lunge assesses hip mobility and stability, quadriceps flexibility, and ankle and knee stability.

Description

1. The tester measures the length of the tibia with a yardstick.
2. The athlete places one foot on the end of a 2 × 6 board and holds the dowel behind the back, with the right arm up and the left arm down, so that it is touching the head, thoracic spine, and sacrum.
3. The tester then places the yardstick at the end of the athlete's toes and makes a mark on the board equal to the length of the tibial height.
4. The athlete takes a step with the left leg and places the heel on the mark, then lowers the back knee enough to touch the board behind the front foot. The feet should be on the same line and pointing straight throughout the movement.
5. The athlete is allowed up to three chances to perform the test.
6. Have the athlete perform the test again, with arms and legs in the opposite positions. If testing produces a lower score with either the left or the right leg in front, record the lower score.

3 POINTS

- Minimal to no torso movement is noted.
- Feet remain in sagittal plane on the 2 × 6.
- Knee touches the 2 × 6 behind heel of front foot.

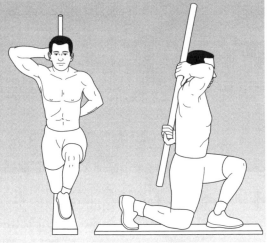

2 POINTS

- Movement is noted in torso.
- Feet do not remain in sagittal plane.
- Knee does not touch behind heel of front foot.

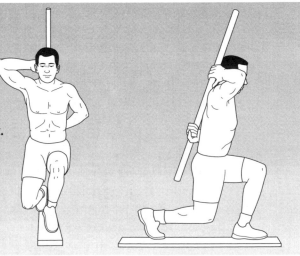

1 POINT

• Loss of balance is noted.

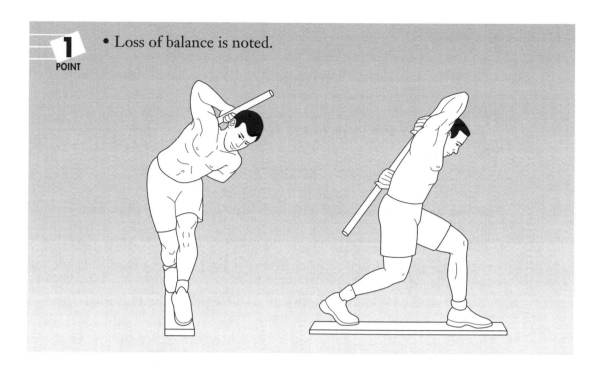

0 POINTS

The athlete will receive a score of 0 if pain is associated with any portion of this test. A member of the sports medicine staff should perform a thorough evaluation of the painful area.

Clinical Implications for the In-Line Lunge

The ability to perform the in-line lunge test requires stance-leg stability of the ankle, knee, and hip as well as apparent closed kinetic-chain hip abduction. The in-line lunge also requires step-leg mobility of hip adduction, ankle dorsiflexion, and rectus femoris flexibility. The athlete must also display adequate balance because the test imposes lateral stress.

Poor performance in this test can be the result of several factors. First, hip mobility may be inadequate in either the stance leg or the step leg. Second, the stance-leg knee or ankle may not have the required stability as the athlete performs the lunge. Finally, an imbalance between relative adductor weakness and abductor tightness in one or both hips may cause poor test performance.

When an athlete achieves a score less than 3, the limiting factor must be identified. Clinical documentation of these limitations can be obtained by using standard goniometric measurements of the joints as well as muscular flexibility tests such as the Thomas test and the Ober test (see Cook and Athletic Testing Services 1998).

Shoulder Mobility

Purpose

The shoulder mobility screen assesses bilateral shoulder range of motion, combining internal rotation with adduction and external rotation with abduction. It also requires normal scapular mobility and thoracic spine extension.

Description

1. The tester determines the athlete's hand length by measuring the distance from the distal wrist crease to the tip of the third digit.

2. The athlete makes a fist with each hand, placing the thumb inside the fist, and assumes a maximally adducted and internally rotated position with one shoulder and an abducted and externally rotated position with the other. In one movement the athlete places the hands on the back. During the test the hands should remain clenched.

3. The tester then measures the distance between the two fists.

4. Have the athlete perform the test again, with arms and hands in the opposite positions. If testing produces a lower score with either the left or the right arm up, record the lower score.

3 POINTS
- Fists are within one hand length.

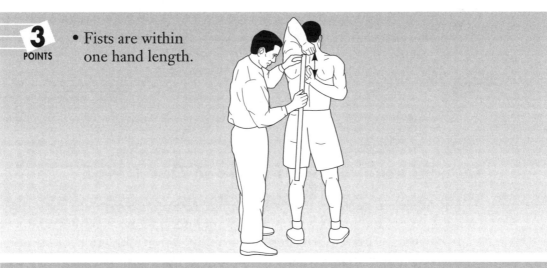

2 POINTS
- Fists are within one and a half hand lengths.

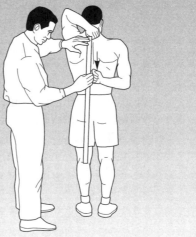

POINT

- Fists are not within one and a half hand lengths.

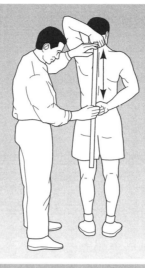

POINTS

The athlete will receive a score of 0 if pain is associated with any portion of this test or if pain is noted during the shoulder stability screen. A member of the sports medicine staff should perform a thorough evaluation of the painful area.

Shoulder Stability Screen

A shoulder stability screen should be performed even if the athlete scores a 3. The athlete places his or her right hand on the opposite shoulder and then attempts to point the right elbow upward. If the athlete experiences pain or is unable to perform this movement, a score of 0 will be given for the shoulder mobility test and the shoulder should be evaluated more thoroughly. This screen should be performed bilaterally.

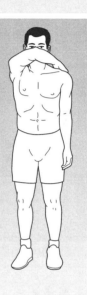

Clinical Implications for Shoulder Mobility

The ability to perform the shoulder mobility test requires shoulder mobility in a combination of motions including abduction–external rotation and adduction—internal rotation. It also requires scapular and thoracic spine mobility.

Poor performance during this test can be the result of several causes, one of which is the widely accepted explanation that increased external rotation is gained at the expense of internal rotation in overhead-throwing athletes. Excessive development and shortening of the pectoralis minor or latissimus dorsi muscles can cause postural alterations of forward or rounded shoulders. Finally, a scapulothoracic dysfunction may be present, resulting in decreased glenohumeral mobility secondary to poor scapulothoracic mobility or stability.

When an athlete achieves a score less than 3, the limiting factor must be identified. Clinical documentation of these limitations can be obtained by using standard goniometric measurements as well as Kendall's test for pectoralis minor and latissimus dorsi tightness (see Cook and Athletic Testing Services 1998).

Previous testing has indicated that when an athlete achieves a score of 2, minor postural changes or shortening of isolated axiohumeral or scapulohumeral muscles exists. When an athlete scores a 1 or 0, a scapulothoracic dysfunction may exist.

Active Straight-Leg Raise

Purpose

The active straight-leg raise assesses active hamstring and gastroc-soleus flexibility while maintaining a stable pelvis and active extension of the opposite leg.

Description

1. The athlete assumes the starting position by lying supine with arms at the sides, palms up, and head flat on the floor; a 2 × 6 board is placed under the knees.
2. The tester identifies the athlete's anterior superior iliac spine (ASIS) and the jointline of the knee (usually midpatella).
3. The athlete lifts the test leg with a dorsiflexed ankle and an extended knee. During the test the opposite knee should remain in contact with the board, and the lower back and head should remain flat on the floor.
4. Once the athlete has achieved the correct position, the tester aligns a dowel through the medial malleolus of the athlete's test leg perpendicular to the floor.
5. Have the athlete perform the test again, raising the opposite leg. If testing produces a lower score for raising either the left or the right leg, record the lower score.

3 POINTS
- Dowel resides between midthigh and ASIS.

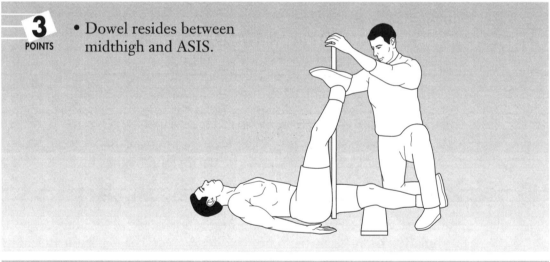

2 POINTS
- Dowel resides between midthigh and the jointline.

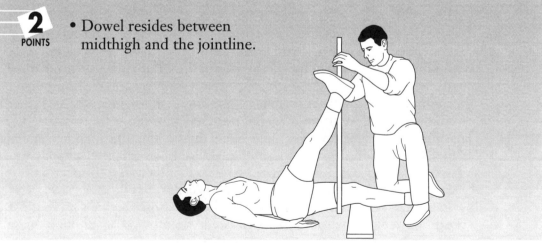

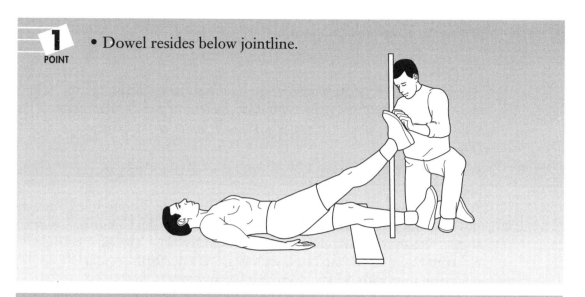

1 POINT
• Dowel resides below jointline.

0 POINTS
The athlete will receive a score of 0 if pain is associated with any portion of this test. A member of the sports medicine staff should perform a thorough evaluation of the painful area.

Clinical Implications for the Active Straight-Leg Raise

The ability to perform the active straight-leg raise test requires functional hamstring flexibility, the flexibility that is available during training and competition. This is different from passive flexibility, which is more commonly assessed. The athlete is also required to demonstrate adequate hip mobility of the opposite leg as well as lower-abdominal stability.

Poor performance during this test can be the result of several factors. First, the athlete may have poor functional hamstring flexibility. Second, the athlete may have inadequate mobility of the opposite hip stemming from iliopsoas tightness associated with an anteriorly tilted pelvis. If this limitation is gross, true active hamstring flexibility will not be realized. A combination of both factors will produce relative bilateral, asymmetric hip mobility. Like the hurdle step test, the active straight-leg raise test reveals relative hip mobility; however, this test is more specific to the limitations imposed by the muscles of the hamstrings and the iliopsoas.

When an athlete achieves a score less than 3, the limiting factor must be identified. Clinical documentation of these limitations can be obtained by Kendall's sit-and-reach test as well as the 90-90 straight-leg raise test for hamstring flexibility. The Thomas test can be used to identify iliopsoas flexibility (see Cook and Athletic Testing Services 1998).

Trunk-Stability Push-Up

Purpose

The trunk-stability push-up assesses trunk stability in the sagittal plane while a symmetrical upper-extremity motion is performed. Scapular stability is assessed indirectly.

Description

1. The athlete assumes a prone position with the hands spaced shoulder-width apart.
2. The athlete places the hands so that the thumbs are alignbed with the top of the head and fully extends the knees. The female athlete should lower the hands so that the thumbs are aligned with the chin.
3. From the appropriate position, the athlete performs one push-up, lifting the body as a unit with no lag in the lumbar spine.
4. The male athlete who cannot perform a push-up from the standard starting position lowers the hands so that the thumbs are aligned with the chin and then performs a push-up. If the female athlete cannot perform a push-up from this position, she lowers the hands so that the thumbs are aligned with the clavicle and performs a push-up.

3 POINTS
- Males perform one repetition with thumbs aligned with the top of the head.
- Females perform one repetition with thumbs aligned with the chin.

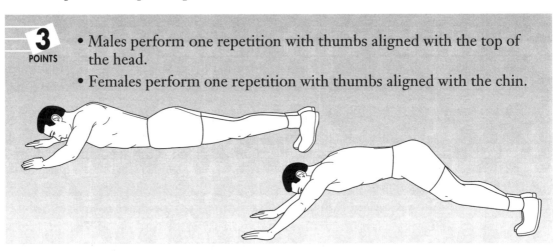

2 POINTS
- Males perform one repetition with thumbs aligned with the top of the head.
- Females perform one repetition with thumbs aligned with the chin.

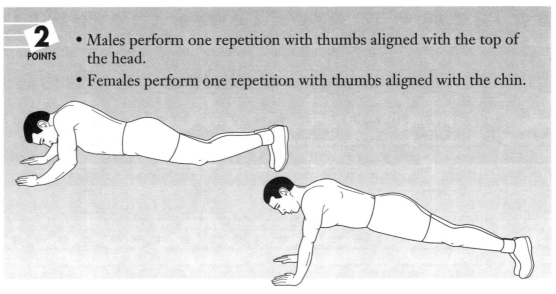

1
POINT

- Males are unable to perform one repetition in modified position.
- Females are unable to perform one repetition in modified position.

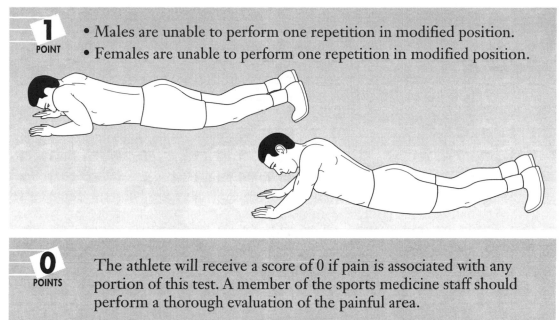

0
POINTS

The athlete will receive a score of 0 if pain is associated with any portion of this test. A member of the sports medicine staff should perform a thorough evaluation of the painful area.

Lumbar Extension

Lumbar extension should also be cleared after this screen, even if a score of 3 is given. Performing a press-up in the push-up position will clear spinal extension. If pain is noted during the lumbar extension, a score of 0 will be given for the trunk-stability push-up.

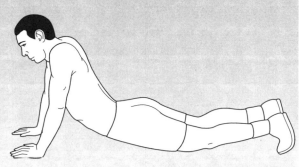

Clinical Implications for the Trunk-Stability Push-Up

The ability to perform the trunk-stability push-up requires trunk stability in the sagittal plane during a symmetric upper-extremity movement. Many functional activities in sports require the trunk stabilizers to transfer force symmetrically from the upper extremities to the lower extremities and vice versa. Movements such as rebounding in basketball, overhead blocking in volleyball, or pass blocking in football are common examples of this type of energy transfer. If the trunk does not have adequate stability during these activities, kinetic energy will be dispersed, leading to poor functional performance as well as increased potential for injury.

Poor performance during this test can be attributed simply to poor stability of the trunk stabilizers. When an athlete achieves a score less than 3, the limiting factor must be identified. Clinical documentation of these limitations can be obtained by using Kendall's test for upper- and lower-abdominal strength (see Cook and Athletic Testing Services 1998).

Rotary Stability

Purpose

The rotary-stability screen assesses multiplanar trunk stability during a combined upper- and lower-extremity motion.

Description

1. The athlete assumes a quadruped position with the shoulders at 90 degrees relative to the upper torso and the hips and knees at 90 degrees relative to the lower torso; the ankles remain dorsiflexed.

2. A 2 × 6 board is placed between the knees and hands so that the knees and hands are in contact with the board.

3. The athlete flexes the shoulder and extends the same-side hip and knee. The athlete raises the leg and hand just enough to clear the floor by approximately six inches. The lifted elbow, hand, and knee should all remain in line with the board. The torso should remain in the same plane as the board.

4. The athlete then flexes the same-side shoulder and knee (left-left) enough for the elbow and knee to touch.

5. The athlete is allowed up to three chances to perform the test.

6. If the athlete does not attain a score of 3, he or she performs the drill in a diagonal pattern, using the opposite-side shoulder and hip (left-right).

7. Have the athlete perform the test again, with arms and legs in the opposite positions. If testing produces a lower score with either the left or the right arm elevated, record the lower score.

3 POINTS
• Athlete performs one correct repetition while keeping torso parallel to the board and elbow and knee in line with the board.

2 POINTS
• Athlete performs one correct diagonal, flexion, and extension lift while maintaining torso parallel to board and floor.

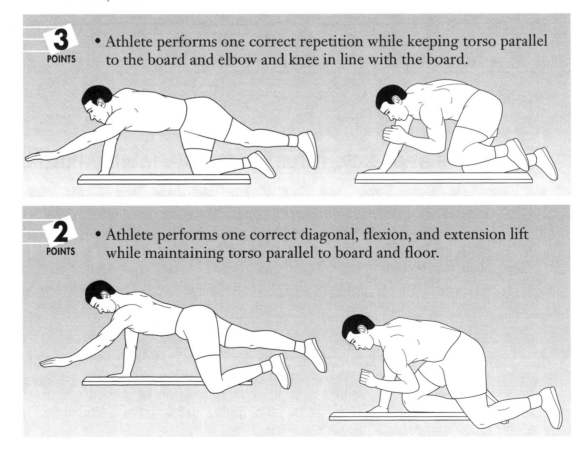

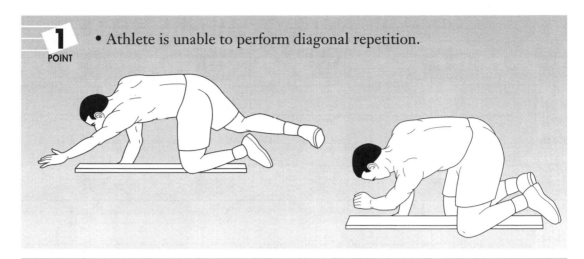

 • Athlete is unable to perform diagonal repetition.

0 POINTS The athlete will receive a score of 0 if pain is associated with any portion of this test or if pain is noted during lumbar flexion. A medical professional should perform a thorough evaluation of the painful area.

Lumbar Flexion

Lumbar flexion should be cleared after this screen, even if a score of 3 is given. To clear spinal flexion, the individual assumes a quadruped position, rocks back, and takes the buttocks to the heels and the chest to the thighs. The hands should remain in front of the body, reaching out as far as possible; feet and toes should be plantar flexed. If pain occurs, a 0 is given.

Clinical Implications for Rotary Stability

The ability to perform the rotary-stability test requires trunk stability in both sagittal and transverse planes during asymmetric upper- and lower-extremity movement. Many functional activities in sports require the trunk stabilizers to transfer force asymmetrically from the lower extremities to the upper extremities and vice versa. Running and exploding out of a down stance in football and track are common examples of this type of energy transfer. If the trunk does not have adequate stability during these activities, kinetic energy will be dispersed, leading to poor functional performance as well as increased potential for injury.

Poor performance during this test can be attributed simply to poor asymmetric stability of the trunk stabilizers. When an athlete achieves a score less than 3, the limiting factor must be identified. Clinical documentation of these limitations can be obtained by using Kendall's test for upper- and lower-abdominal strength.

FUNCTIONAL MOVEMENT SCREEN™ SCORING SHEET

Name: _____ School: _____

Age: _____ Height: _____ Weight: _____ ☐ Male ☐ Female

Address: _____ Phone: _____

City: _____ State: _____ Zip: _____

Sport: _____

Position: _____

Hand dominance: L R   Leg dominance: L R   Eye dominance: L R

Previous injuries: _____

_____

_____

_____

_____

Previous score: _____

Test and score   Comments

Deep squat	3 2 1 0	_____
Hurdle step	3 2 1 0	_____
In-line lunge	3 2 1 0	_____
Shoulder mobility	3 2 1 0	_____
Active straight-leg raise	3 2 1 0	_____
Trunk-stability push-up	3 2 1 0	_____
Rotary stability	3 2 1 0	_____

Total: _____

Tester or group: _____

FUNCTIONAL PERFORMANCE TESTING

Functional performance is a representation of actual efficiency through specific testing of gross performance (power, speed, etc.). The athlete can be ranked and monitored by comparison with normative data. Functional performance data bridge the gap between foundation movements and skill. Foundation testing will identify basic human movement patterns. Functional performance testing will help assess the way the athlete generates, transfers, and controls power.

Performance testing for athleticism must assess and quantify the way the athlete uses his or her body in forceful, explosive movements without being biased toward a particular skill or activity. To look at the way the human body works as a functional unit to produce movement, tests are commonly done for three primary movements: jumping, throwing, and running.

The jumping test involves a vertical jump and tests for explosion. The characteristics of jumping include the following:

- Upper-body pulling movement
- Lower-body extension movements
- Trunk transfer of energy from upper body to lower body
- Trunk extension stability
- Top to bottom coordination

The throwing test involves a medicine ball chest pass and tests for propulsion. The characteristics of throwing include the following:

- Upper-body pushing movement
- Lower-body stability
- Trunk transfer of energy from lower body to upper body
- Trunk flexion stability
- Bottom-up coordination

The running test involves a 40-yard sprint and tests for locomotion. The characteristics of running include the following:

- Upper-body and lower-body countermovement
- Transfer of energy from upper body to the trunk and from one leg to the other
- Trunk rotary stability
- Simultaneous coordination of upper body and lower body

Each test relies heavily on sound motor programming—the way the brain and body interact. The three tests also represent kinetic linking—the timing and sequencing of each specific movement to complement the next.

Vertical Jump

The vertical jump is commonly considered the true test of human power because the force of gravity affects the body of each athlete equally. An athlete who has the ability to summon the strength of the body in a quick, coordinated, and balanced fashion will accelerate past the pull of gravity and achieve greater height than an athlete who does not have equal ability, regardless of size. The role of the upper body in jumping is considerable. The difference between good jumpers and great jumpers is usually the ability of the upper body to contribute with forceful movements of the arms and dynamic stabilization of the trunk. Jumping must also be considered a top-down recruitment activity because the upper body and trunk are loaded before the lower extremities. Testing the vertical jump is quick and efficient, and numerous standards are available for sex, age, and sport specificity. Right and left differences can be measured in special cases by performing a single-leg vertical jump. The landing should still be on two legs to avoid unnecessary stress. Differences between left and right should not be greater than 15 percent.

Standing Medicine Ball Chest Pass

In this test, instead of propelling the body against gravity, the athlete propels another object. The goal is not to look at sport-specific throwing movements in this test; rather, it is to look at general athleticism and the ability to produce power from a bottom-up transition. Throwing a medicine ball from a standing chest pass position (without a step) will allow the tester to identify power and coordination generated in a bottom-up fashion. The athlete must load the legs and trunk and maintain stability before achieving any vigorous movement of the upper body to propel the medicine ball. Unlike the vertical leap, which looks at extension dynamic stability (with respect to the trunk), a chest pass with a medicine ball looks at flexion dynamic stability (with respect to the trunk). The vertical leap is body relative, meaning that gravity treats all bodies equally. But the medicine ball throw is not body relative if a standardized-weight ball is used because that requires each athlete to propel a different percentage of body weight. The standing medicine ball chest pass can be performed without this bias by making a simple calculation; a medicine ball of approximately 2 percent of the

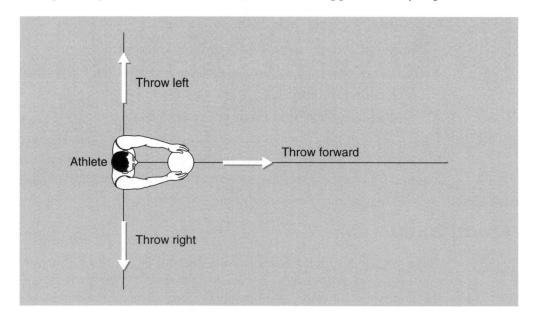

thrower's body weight provides a standard for all athletes with a similar amount of resistance to the throwing movement, thus allowing valid comparison of data. Using the same stance, differences between the right and left can be tested. The athlete should twist and throw left and then right. Compare the differences, using the 15 percent rule as a standard.

40-Yard Sprint

The third test is the 40-yard sprint. This test has come under criticism in the past because it is not sport specific. Most field and court sports have minimal opportunity for an all-out linear run for 40 yards. In many sports, however, large amounts of data have been collected on the 40-yard dash. Therefore, convenient comparison can be made about general athleticism for all field and court sports. Moreover, 40-yard dash speed represents the efficiency of the body. It allows the athlete to demonstrate the ability to store energy, using the plyometric abilities of each leg in propulsion. It illustrates mobility in the hips and legs through stride length, and it displays coordination through stride frequency. Last, it indicates the ability of the torso to provide dynamic stability and redirect the power generated in one leg directly to the other leg with minimal loss and maximum efficiency. Therefore, the sprint test does more than measure simple sprint speed; it allows the athlete to demonstrate efficiency, coordination, energy storage, and momentum management.

If time, space, and equipment allow, the 120-yard sprint presents an interesting way to understand athletic speed. The 120-yard dash is even less sport specific than the 40-yard dash, but it provides the strength and conditioning specialist with unique criteria when analyzing deficits in running. Running is a base movement for almost all sports. Distances shorter than 40 yards may be more specific, but they require electronic timers for true accuracy. By looking at the 120-yard dash, the tester can observe three unique and specific 40-yard sprints. The first 40-yard dash displays the athlete's ability to start and accumulate speed through acceleration. The second 40-yard dash measures the athlete's ability to maintain speed through efficient body mechanics. The last 40-yard dash demonstrates the athlete's speed endurance and ability to maintain efficiency, technique, and momentum as fatigue mounts. The 120-yard dash thus offers data to analyze quickness, speed, and speed endurance. It is easy to see how a problem with quickness could greatly affect all field and court sports. Field and court sports also require running and plyometrics as primary methods of conditioning. Problems with speed and speed endurance will affect training and reduce the benefits of conditioning. Athletes with such problems will not be able to improve running form or plyometric performance because fatigue will set in before adequate training can occur.

Other Functional Performance Considerations

In summary, the three tests represent basic movements for general athleticism and measure motor programming and efficiency. They look at two forms of power as well as linear speed. The tester can conduct the three primary tests quickly and efficiently, permitting their use throughout the year to monitor changes in performance. Other tests for general athletic performance consider anaerobic power, agility and body control, and aerobic power. These tests are more involved and take more time.

Anaerobic Power Tests

- Line drill for basketball (preferable for court sports)
- 300-yard shuttle run (preferable for field sports)

Agility and Body Control Tests

- T-test
- Edgren side step

Aerobic Power Tests

- 2-mile run
- 12-minute run
- 3-minute step test

SPORT-SPECIFIC SKILLS

Skill movements vary from sport to sport, but most coaches prefer sport-specific skills assessment and even position-specific assessment. It is, of course, important to use a test that is reliable and valid. Radar guns compute the speed of baseball pitches and tennis serves, and electronic timers measure baserunning and pass rushing. Most sports skills are assessed from a quantitative, not qualitative, perspective. Until recently, the eyes of coaches were the only quality standard. Current advances in movement analysis have linked photography and computers to bring greater objectivity to sports-skills analysis. Options for the future will be discussed later. For now make sure that analysis is objective and has qualitative parameters (accuracy, consistency, adaptability, etc.) as well as quantitative parameters (time, distance, etc.). Books dedicated to a single sport cover sport-specific skills testing in detail.

USING TEST DATA

Once data is collected, an individual performance pyramid can be constructed for each athlete (see figure 2.4, a-c). Figure 2.4a represents the athlete with poor mobility and stability scores but good functional performance and skill. This common situation represents a majority of athletes in field and court sports. Note that the foundation does not support the functional and skill activities. Injury potential is greater because the athlete's performance exceeds his or her mobility and stability. The athlete has the potential to produce greater momentum and power than he or she can potentially control. The athlete should first work on mobility and stability not only to broaden the movement foundation but also to improve efficiency and functional performance.

Figure 2.4b represents the athlete who is highly specialized and is skilled at one aspect of a position or sport but does not possess general athleticism. This individual does not test well but is an excellent competitor. He or she has invested a large amount of time honing sports skills but will now need to focus on the foundation base and functional base to see a significant change in performance.

Figure 2.4c represents an athlete who has good mobility and stability but poor function. This individual will benefit greatly by focusing on functional performance deficits. This individual is ready for all the benefits that periodization, plyometrics, interval training, and sport-specific conditioning can offer. He or she possesses the basic framework and foundation movements to start functional training. This athlete will need supervision because he or she may demonstrate poor technique. The individual may also have less energy-storing capability than the athlete in figure 2.4a. Therefore, supervision is needed with explosive and ballistic training.

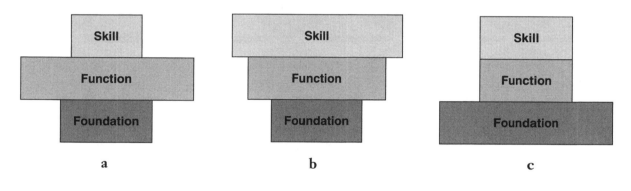

Figure 2.4 Individual performance pyramids.

Constructing a team performance pyramid is also beneficial in identifying team attributes and detriments compared with other teams or previous teams. Doing so creates a philosophy and methodology for the athletic trainer and strength and conditioning professional. Pyramids act as a compass to direct individual athletes and teams to the areas of greatest weakness. Historically, a distinguishing characteristic of a good athlete versus an elite athlete has been a focus on his or her weaknesses, rather than strengths. Good athletes focus on their strengths, maximizing potential benefits while ignoring, covering up, and compensating for weaknesses. Elite athletes confront their weaknesses and focus on them in their conditioning programs. These athletes will enter competition with the physiological and psychological advantages that come from knowing that they have confronted and rectified their weakest links. Because athletes don't always intuitively adopt such a mindset, the coaching and training staff must use baseline testing to expose the weakest link and direct the progression of the training program. Follow-up testing can validate the rehabilitation or conditioning techniques employed. Testing also serves as a continuous monitor to expose other potential weak links that commonly arise as athletes become more specialized and experienced.

SUMMARY

Technology will continue to progress, but human movement will always obey neuromuscular, biomechanical, and physical laws. Therefore, the conditioning specialist must focus on the job, not the tool. Technology (testing tools) should always be subservient to an objective testing philosophy based on sound principles.

The performance pyramid illustrates an athlete's functional strengths and weaknesses. This simple diagram is an effective teaching tool for athletes and coaches alike. Athletes must be continually reminded that reaching the top of the pyramid is possible only after building a good foundation. This simple pyramid demonstrates the necessary priority and progression of baseline testing and analysis to develop high-performance sports conditioning.

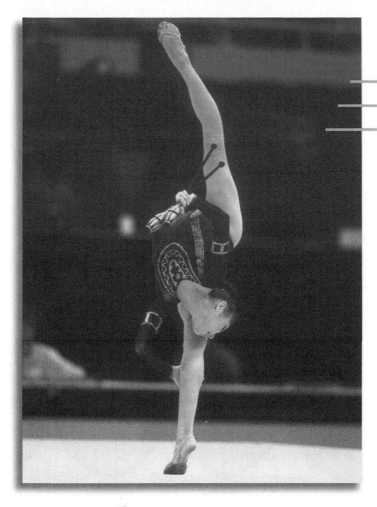

Performance Flexibility

Nikos Apostolopoulos

*T*his chapter looks at the importance of flexibility to performance. Unlike strength, speed, and other motor abilities, flexibility belongs not to the causative factors of movement but to the morpho-functional properties; that is, it helps govern motion. In fact, flexibility helps determine the efficiency of the athlete's other physical abilities. Besides governing simple contraction and relaxation, the motor system carries out the additional task of coordination within muscle groups. Other duties include technique development and skill acquisition. Proprioceptors in the muscles, tendons, and joints, which sense muscle length, tension, and joint angle, are critical in providing information to the motor system. Therefore, flexibility enhances the development of coordination and technique and the ability of the proprioceptors to receive stimuli.

Flexibility training must be viewed as a workout in itself, not a token warm-up or warm-down. For the greatest benefit, flexibility training should begin in the childhood or teenage years and continue throughout life. Proper flexibility training can moderate, or even delay for many years, the deterioration of range of motion that occurs with age.

In the world of sport, athletes and coaches always seek better and newer methods to increase the athlete's potential. The benefits of flexibility extend to athletes of all ages and abilities, whether elite, professional, or amateur. The goal of training is to achieve good performance in competition. The more directly training is aimed at preparing the athlete for a particular sport, the more effective it will be. An understanding of the principles of flexibility provides the tools to design individual stretching programs.

Training and competition expose the body to a tremendous volume and intensity of exercise. These constant demands result in great wear and tear and possibly even injury. To prevent injury, the athlete must maintain structuro-functional integrity of the musculoskeletal system. Different muscle groups should exert symmetrically balanced forces on the skeletal elements, and individual muscular forces themselves should be correctly balanced and aligned. Proper development of flexibility produces a balanced system, restores muscles, and maintains key physiological processes. Proper integration of the musculoskeletal system is essential for a qualitatively and quantitatively well-executed movement. Therefore, performance flexibility is actually balanced flexibility.

ANATOMY OF INJURY

The anatomical structures that relate to flexibility are muscles, tendons, ligaments, and bone (see figure 3.1). Muscle by nature is elastic, whereas tendons and ligaments are inelastic. Skeletal muscle cells (sarcoplasms) are contiguous with tendon fibrils. There is no continuity between the muscle cells and the tendon fibrils, from the origin and insertion ends of the musculotendon system to the bone (Ippolito, Perugia, and Postacchini 1986). Tendons are much stronger than the muscles that act on them. The maximal tensile strength of muscle (its resistance to pull) is approximately 77 to 80 pounds per square inch, whereas tendons can resist 8,600 to 18,000 pounds per square inch (Hollinshead and Jenkins 1981, as shown in figure 3.2). This enables a large muscle to act through a small tendon. Therefore, it is almost physically impossible for an injury to result from a tendon tearing in the middle. When an injury does happen, it occurs either in the muscle fiber near the junction between muscle and tendon, or where the tendon connects to the bone.

When the athlete performs a stretch and feels the muscles burning or senses an extreme pull in the muscles, that is a strain. A form of stretching that exemplifies strain is the isometric contraction phase of a proprioceptive neuromuscular facilitation (PNF) stretch. A strain results in microtears of the muscle near the muscle-tendon junction. Microtears are microinjuries. The body responds to these tears by releasing collagen in the area, resulting in the development of scar tissue. As scar tissue ages it contracts, further tightening the surrounding tissues. These microtears, unlike those that occur in the postlifting and pregrowth repair process during muscular hypertrophy, are located in an area of transition

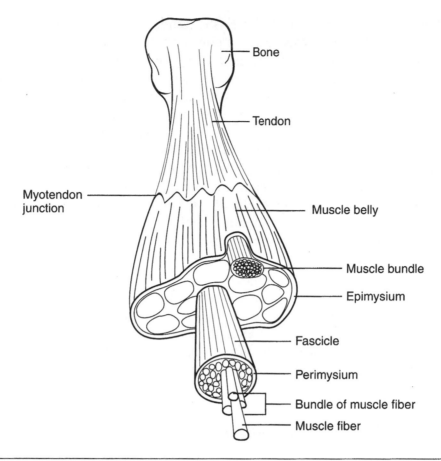

Figure 3.1 Arrangement of muscular tissue, tendon, and bone.

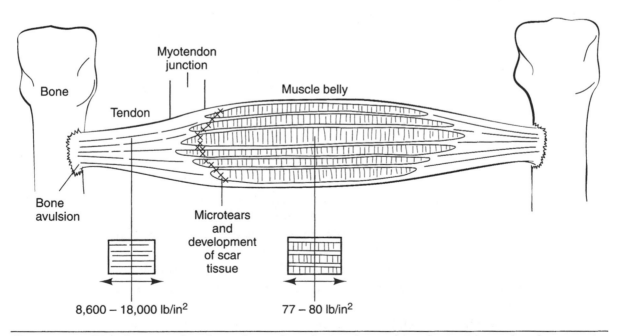

Figure 3.2 Tensile strengths of muscles and tendons; microtears and scar tissue related to a strain.

between elastic (muscle) and inelastic (tendon) tissue. In contrast to the middle of the muscle belly, this area has poor circulation, which is further diminished with the development of scar tissue. Therefore, the repair process is slower.

As these microtears increase in number and size, they progress into an acute injury. The injury causes muscles or muscle groups to shift and compensate for inadequate function of a weak muscle or muscle group. Muscle imbalance begins to develop as the body strives to minimize pain, protect the injury, and retain maximum function. If the athlete does not deliberately try to repattern these natural shifts during the acute phase, the injury progresses to the chronic phase. The constant avoidance of pain results in the alteration of motor patterns, manifested by a physical decrease in the range of motion around the joint. If the individual does not resume normal activity, this altered motor pattern and its related suboptimal function will continue.

Short-duration strain similar to the tension developed during the 6- to 10-second isometric contraction phase of a PNF stretch can result in microtears. As alluded to earlier, the constant repetition of such tension will predispose the athlete to, and possibly result in, an injury. Proper flexibility training takes into account the different stresses and strains of the connective tissues. A well-designed program will help increase flexibility in the inelastic tissues (ligaments and tendons), break down scar tissue, and decrease the chance of injuries caused by strains.

PRINCIPLES OF PERFORMANCE FLEXIBILITY

It is possible to improve the elasticity of normally inelastic connective tissue without deformation or tearing. The flexibility of all the links that compose the locomotor system should be trained to the maximum range allowed by the joint structure. The type of movement is determined by the shape and contact of the joint surfaces as well as the elasticity and strength of the ligaments, tendons, and muscle. Overdevelopment of the elasticity of connective tissues may result in an irreversible deformation of joints, ligaments, and tendons. This will directly and adversely affect motor abilities.

When an individual does flexibility training properly, maintaining the integrity of the connective tissue and muscle, he or she can develop a flexibility reserve. This reserve enhances performance, allowing the athlete to execute movement without excessive tension. The reserve also decreases the resistance of the extended muscles and serves as a safeguard against injury.

Flexibility developed through static stretching and micro-Stretching® (a technique I developed) is more beneficial than flexibility attained through other forms of stretching (passive-active, ballistic, active assisted, and PNF). Done at low intensity, static stretching and micro-Stretching develop the flexibility reserve, decrease the influence of hypertrophy and other muscular changes during the development of strength, and decrease muscle tension, thereby increasing circulation and neural conductivity. This decrease in muscle tension also assists in decreasing muscle tone and aids the removal of metabolic wastes (i.e., lactic acid).

Like all forms of training, performance flexibility training adheres to certain principles of frequency, duration, and intensity. Table 3.1 summarizes these principles.

Table 3.1   Principles of Performance Flexibility Training

Training principle	Application of training principle
Frequency	Once or twice per day Three times per muscle group per session
Intensity	30–40% of maximum stretch (100% = pain)
Duration	Each stretch should be held for approximately 60 seconds

Frequency

As suggested by Tudor Bompa, an athlete must stretch at least twice per day to improve flexibility (Bompa 1983). The athlete must stretch each muscle group at least three times per session. Repetition is important. In both infancy and adulthood, we learn movements and improve skills through repetition. Repeated stimulation of the central nervous system integrates the new physical pattern, turning it into an automatic response.

With the ongoing development of flexibility, perceptual skills improve. The tendons and muscles become more elastic, increasing the sensitivity of the joint receptors and thereby processing more information. The athlete senses more accurately the significance of a physical stimulus and, in turn, effects a more suitable motor response.

Intensity

Performance flexibility stretching is always done at a low intensity level (approximately 30 to 40 percent of perceived exertion). At this level, stretching increases the pliancy of the connective and muscle tissues. Low-intensity stretching can be referred to as micro-Stretching. The influence of micro-Stretching, like that of microinjuries, occurs at the cellular level. Unlike a strain, micro-Stretching results in minimal activation of the specialized receptor tissues of the muscle and tendon (the muscle spindle fibers and the Golgi tendon organ). The muscle spindle senses muscle lengthening, whereas the Golgi tendon organ senses tension.

Micro-Stretching helps damaged tissue recover and regenerate and aids in the breakdown of scar tissue. If there is a lot of scar tissue between the muscle and tendon, micro-Stretching can bypass the specialized receptor tissues, which would be activated by a strain.

While stretching, it is critical to avoid strain or pain, which would result in the activation or constant maintenance of a subconscious protective loop. The body maintains this loop to respond to an injury. Its activation results in the development and reinforcement of muscle imbalances and a further decrease in the range of motion around a joint.

With low-intensity stretching, an athlete is able to recover from injury, decrease the muscle tone affected by connective tissue (i.e., fascia), regenerate connective tissue (i.e., tendons, ligaments, and muscles), and reestablish and repattern the musculoskeletal system.

Duration

The optimum length of time to hold a stretch is approximately 60 seconds. It normally takes about 30 seconds for a stretch to progress from the middle of the muscle belly to the tendons. Thus a token 10- to 15-second stretch may be beneficial to the muscle but will have minimal influence on the ligaments, tendons, and fascia that are largely responsible for range of motion and flexibility.

At the Serapis Stretch Therapy Clinic I have found that individuals who hold a stretch longer than 90 seconds often complain of feeling tighter. The Golgi tendon organ is the cause for this. Prolonged low-intensity stretching of a muscle causes it to lengthen slightly beyond its normal resting length, which is sufficient to trigger a slight increase in tension. This increase stimulates the Golgi tendon organ to react, thereby triggering the muscle to contract. Because this increase in tightness may cause some microtears, a stretch should not be held longer than 60 seconds.

FLEXIBILITY FOR SPORTS

All athletes benefit from performance flexibility. Whether competing as an individual or on a team, an athlete with a balanced muscular system devoid of compensational shifts will perform better. The notion of 30 percent exertion may be foreign to athletes who identify with the "no pain, no gain" philosophy. Stretching at this intensity, however, helps the athlete develop power and remain injury free. No sport can be singled out as benefiting the most from flexibility.

Quality of movement, whether judged or not, is affected by flexibility. When athletes have command of their flexibility, they are able to perform exercise or events more strongly, quickly, and expressively.

Strength, speed, and endurance are qualities of every sport. Performance flexibility determines how proficiently and efficiently the athlete can apply them. Flexibility in endurance and power sports is fundamental for high motor economy. Flexibility aids in the development of conditioning and coordination. An athlete with flexibility generates acceleration over a greater range of motion, thereby increasing speed. Flexibility is the rate-determining factor. It governs movement.

STRETCHING EXERCISES

The human body occupies many positions in sports, all of which fall into three general categories: standing, sitting, or lying. All positions involve the coordination of many muscles or muscle groups. A properly designed flexibility routine enhances the interaction of the muscles.

The suggested flexibility routine is based on two principles. The first principle, discussed earlier in this chapter, comprises frequency, intensity, and duration. The second principle concerns stability, balance, and control (SBC—a principle developed at the Serapis Stretch Therapy Clinic). To observe this principle, position the body in a manner that isolates a muscle group, thereby allowing the rest of the body to relax. This can be accomplished by using a floor, wall, chair, or any other base of support. Isolation helps decrease the metabolic cost to the body. Adherence to both principles facilitates micro-Stretching.

The stretches selected follow a specific kinetic order. Morphologically, there is no value in doing a lower-body stretch followed by an upper-body stretch. The orderly progression is useful because each stretch leads into another. This flow imprints itself on the neural system. The intention is to make the stretches second nature. The perceived flow of the stretches is facilitated through the fascial communications of the muscles. (Note that each stretch should be performed at 30 percent of perceived exertion.)

Posterior Lower Leg

For a tight calf muscle the athlete should do the following:

1. Sit in a chair with feet flat on the floor and shoulder-width apart.
2. Place a 3- to 5-inch book on the floor.
3. Place the ball of one foot on the book, making sure the heel is on the floor.
4. Position the lower leg to create a light stretch in the calf region.
5. Hold the stretch for 60 seconds, then repeat with the other leg.
6. Do three repetitions per leg.

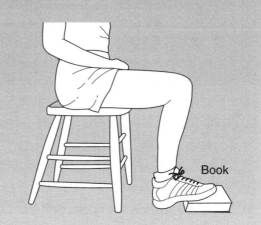

Book

For a moderately tight calf muscle the athlete should do the following:

1. Stand with feet 12 to 18 inches from a wall. Face the wall and place both hands on the wall for support.
2. Keep the pelvis squared and the feet shoulder-width apart.
3. Bend one knee slightly toward the wall and bend the back knee slightly, keeping both heels down.
4. Hold a light stretch for 60 seconds, then repeat with the other leg.
5. Do three repetitions per leg. Alternate to the other leg.

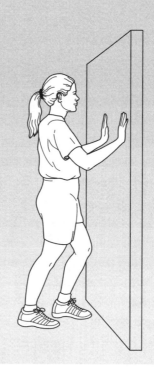

Anterior Lower Leg

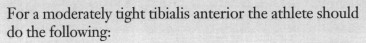

For a tight tibialis anterior the athlete should do the following:

1. Sit in a chair and cross one leg over the other so that the ankle of the crossed leg rests on the outside edge of the knee of the anchor leg.
2. Grab the top of the foot at the outside of the crossed leg.
3. Pull the foot toward the body.
4. Hold the stretch for 60 seconds, then repeat with the other leg.
5. Do three repetitions per leg.

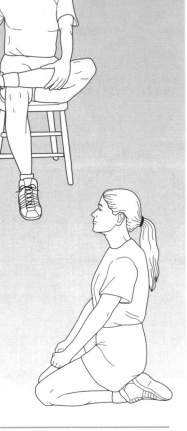

For a moderately tight tibialis anterior the athlete should do the following:

1. Sit on the floor with the front of the lower legs touching the floor and the heels of the feet touching the buttocks.
2. Position the legs shoulder-width apart.
3. If the stretch is a little too much, put a pillow between the buttocks and the back of the lower legs.
4. Hold the stretch for 60 seconds.
5. Repeat the stretch three times with a 60-second break between stretches.

Gluteal Region

The athlete should do the following:

1. Lie on the floor on the back in front of a wall. Place a pillow under the head.
2. Place the legs against the wall with the knees flexed at 90 degrees.
3. Keep the hips and pelvis on the floor.
4. Position the legs shoulder-width apart.
5. Cross one leg over the other, placing the ankle of the crossed leg just past the knee of the leg that is against the wall.
6. Feel the sensation of the stretch in the buttock region of the crossed leg.
7. Hold the stretch for 60 seconds, then repeat with the other leg.
8. Do three repetitions per leg.

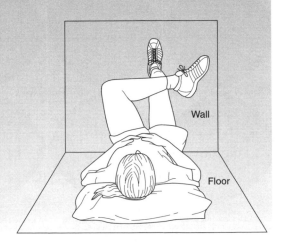

Posterior Thigh Region

The athlete should do the following:

1. Lie on the floor in front of a door jamb and place a pillow under the head.
2. Keep the hips and pelvis squared and on the floor.
3. Place the leg to be stretched up against the wall.
4. Do not force the knee straight; doing so may cause pain behind the knee.
5. Lace the other leg through the door jamb. If you have discomfort in the front of the leg that you put through the door jamb, place a pillow under the knee to alleviate the discomfort.
6. Hold the stretch for 60 seconds, then repeat with the other leg.
7. Do three repetitions per leg.

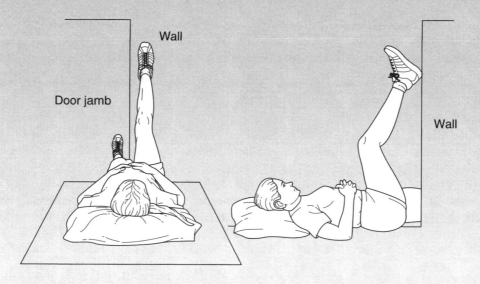

Medial Thigh Region

The athlete should do the following:

1. Sit on the floor with the back up against a wall and bring the soles of the feet together.
2. Keep the back straight.
3. Do not force the knees down.
4. Feel the stretch sensation in the groin area.
5. Hold the stretch for 60 seconds, then release the stretch for 60 seconds.
6. Repeat three times.

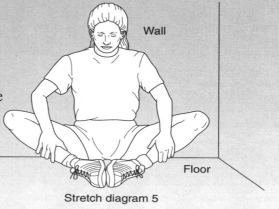

Stretch diagram 5

Lateral Thigh Region

The athlete should do the following:

1. Lie flat on the back on the floor and a place a pillow under the head.
2. Keep the hips and pelvis squared on the floor and the legs shoulder-width apart.
3. Bring one knee up toward the stomach.
4. Place the foot on top of the anchor leg, just above the knee.
5. Try to move the stretching leg to a position that forms a 90-degree angle to the body, keeping the pelvis and hips flat on the floor.
6. Using the hand opposite the leg that is being stretched, gently pull the knee over the anchor leg.
7. Do not force the stretch. Hold the stretch for 60 seconds, then repeat with the other leg.
8. Do three repetitions per leg.

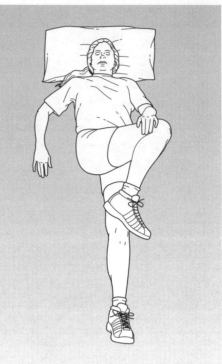

Anterior Thigh Region

The athlete should do the following:

1. Kneel on the floor with the knees shoulder-width apart and the pelvis and hips squared.
2. Raise one leg off the ground and extend it in front of the body.
3. Lower the body into the stretch, bending the extended knee to form a 90-degree angle.
4. Feel the stretch in the hip opposite the extended leg.
5. Keep the back straight, not bent or hunched over.
6. Hold the stretch for 60 seconds, then repeat with the other leg.
7. Do three repetitions per leg.

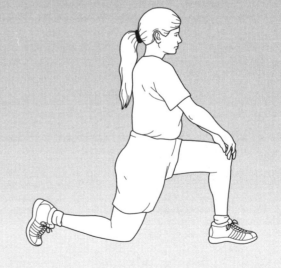

Lower-Back Region

The athlete should do the following:

1. Lie flat on the back on the floor and place a pillow under the head.

2. Bring both knees up toward the chest until the knees are bent at a 90-degree angle.

3. Keep both shoulders on the floor while bringing both knees over to one side to rest on the floor. Be sure to keep both knees at 90 degrees.

4. Hold the stretch for 60 seconds before straightening the legs and repeating on the opposite side.

5. Do three repetitions on each side.

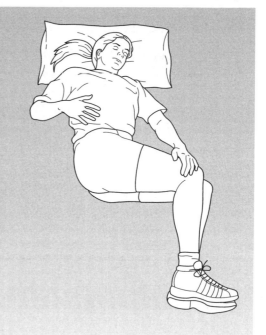

Midback Region

The athlete should do the following:

1. Sit on the floor with the upper body nearly vertical. Bend one knee and place it outside the straight anchor leg.

2. Place the elbow opposite the bent leg on the outside of the bent knee. Place the hand of the anchor arm on the floor for support.

3. Push the arm with the elbow on the knee into the bent leg to produce a twisting movement of the upper body away from the bent leg.

4. Turn the head in the direction opposite the bent leg.

5. Hold the stretch for 60 seconds, then repeat with the other leg.

6. Do three repetitions per leg.

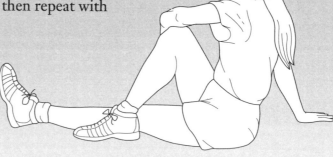

Upper-Back Region

The athlete should do the following:

1. Sit in a chair with the shoulders squared and relaxed.
2. Slowly and gently bring one arm across the front of the body by pulling the elbow with the opposite hand.
3. Try to keep the lower back and upper body straight.
4. Keep the feet planted firmly on the floor.
5. Hold the stretch for 60 seconds, then repeat with the other arm.
6. Do three repetitions with each arm.

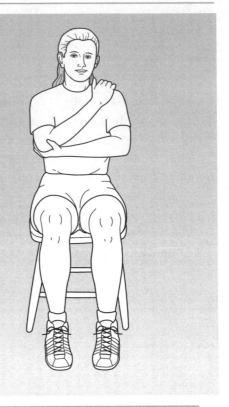

Chest and Anterior Shoulder Region

The athlete should do the following:

1. Stand erect with the right side of the body toward a door frame and the feet shoulder-width apart.
2. Extend the right arm straight out to the side such that the hand is at about rib-cage or waist height.
3. Rotate the forearm and grasp the edge of the door frame with the palm of the hand and the fingers.
4. Turn the upper body to the left.
5. Hold the stretch for 60 seconds, then release slowly.
6. Repeat with the other arm.
7. Do three repetitions per arm.

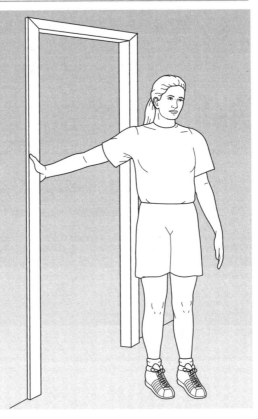

Neck Region

The athlete should do the following:

1. Sit in a chair with the shoulders and pelvis squared.
2. Extend one arm to the side of a chair and grasp the edge of the chair.
3. Keep the head back and the ears aligned with the shoulders.
4. Gently lean away with the neck from the hand grasping the chair.
5. Slightly turn the neck away from the hand grasping the chair and drop the head toward the chest.
6. Hold the stretch for 60 seconds, then repeat with the other arm.
7. Do three repetitions per arm.

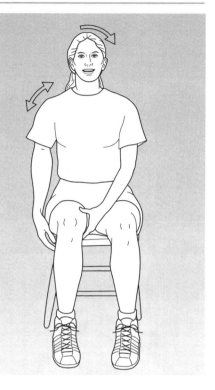

SUMMARY

Performance flexibility is balanced flexibility and is best developed through the technique of micro-Stretching and the principle of stability, balance, and control. The concepts presented in this chapter enable coaches and athletes to develop an effective flexibility program. By using 30 to 40 percent perceived exertion, the athlete performs a proper stretch without strain, thus decreasing the development of scar tissue and microinjuries. The holding of a stretch for 60 seconds helps repattern the connective tissue system and ultimately the muscle groups. Repetition of the stretch reinforces the imprint on the neuromuscular system.

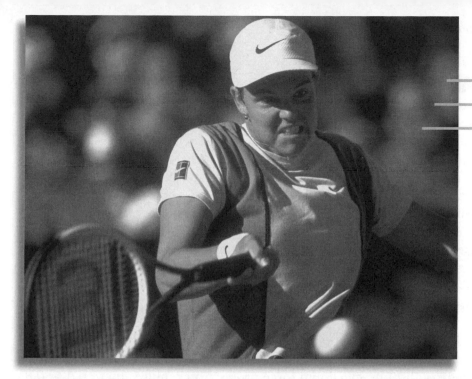

Muscular Strength and Stamina

Steven Scott Plisk

*T*he need for strength and endurance in sports is now generally accepted. Despite the potential for direct transfer to performance enhancement and injury prevention, however, their role is often perceived as indirect or foundational. Indeed, strength is often thought to be independent from or incompatible with movement velocity, when in fact the latter is a result of explosive force application. Realization of this fact is crucial to achieving optimal training effects.

Technical precision and speed of execution are fundamental goals of any athletic movement, and, of course, the two are interrelated. Sports performance is determined by the ability to properly execute skills and assignments at a planned effort level. Training tasks should therefore be selected and prioritized according to how well they target the coordinative, biomechanical, and bioenergetic demands of competition.

In general, maximum strength training and speed-strength training should be conducted with limited work volumes and minimal metabolic stress; doing so maximizes the quality of learning and training effects. Methods designed to increase muscle bulk (hypertrophy) as well as strength, which require greater intensity of training, are an exception. Likewise, strength-endurance training usually involves fatiguing workloads and greater overall volume. As part of the overall sports-preparation process, specialized strength training should be planned and implemented according to sound principles to optimize the athlete's performance capabilities.

MOVEMENT MECHANICS

Effective strength training begins with a working knowledge of basic movement mechanics, especially aspects such as rate of force development (RFD) and impulse, stretch-shortening cycle (SSC) and reactive ability, power, and the role of each of these qualities in "endurance" sports versus "power" sports. The operative concept in each case is *speed strength*—that is, the ability to develop forces rapidly or at high velocity. Collectively, this section illustrates that evaluation of an athlete's explosive and reactive strength capabilities is the starting point for planning the preparation process. Fortunately, such tests are relatively simple to administer and interpret.

Rate of Force Development and Impulse

The brief execution times of most athletic tasks require a high RFD. For example, force is applied for 0.1 to 0.2 seconds during the ground-support phase of running, whereas absolute maximum force production requires up to 0.6 to 0.8 seconds. Even in nonballistic locomotion such as cycling, rowing, skating, or swimming, performance is usually determined by the ability to generate force quickly and thereby achieve a critical impulse output (defined as the change in momentum resulting from a force, measured as the product of force and time; see figure 4.1).

The practical implication of this is that amplitude, direction, and rate of force application are equally significant when performing functional tasks. As will be discussed in more detail in the section "Exercise Prioritization and Substitution" on page 67 the issue is one of specificity to competitive demands. Thus, a basic objective of training is to improve RFD, effectively moving the force-time curve

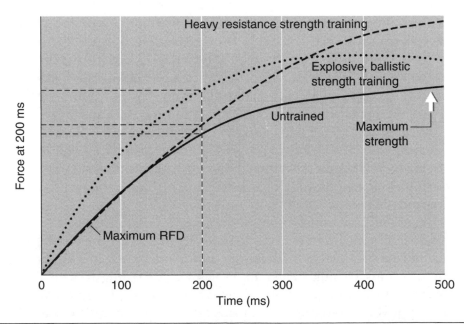

Figure 4.1   Isometric force as a function of time, indicating maximum strength, rate of force development, and force at 0.2 seconds for untrained, heavy-resistance trained, and explosive-ballistic trained subjects. Impulse is represented by the area under each curve and is increased by improving RFD.

up and to the left, thereby generating greater impulse during the limited time (and distance) in which force is applied. Furthermore, the significance of this parameter is not limited to biomechanics. According to the *impulse-timing hypothesis*, the force-time relationship is a central component in motor programming and has important implications for motor control and learning.

Stretch-Shortening Cycle and Reactive Ability

Many functional movements involve springlike muscle-tendon actions and are ballistic in nature, even when initiated from a static position. The action begins with a preparatory countermovement in which the involved muscles are rapidly and forcibly lengthened, or "stretch loaded," and immediately shortened in a reactive or elastic manner. This eccentric-concentric coupling phenomenon— referred to as the stretch-shortening cycle (SSC)—is especially prevalent in sports involving running, jumping, and rapid changes in speed and direction. SSC actions exploit motoneural reflexes as well as intrinsic qualities of the muscle-tendon complex, and their performance is a distinct capability that is independent of maximum strength in elite athletes. Training for such sports should therefore progressively include plyometric methods besides basic heavy-resistance movements, as will be discussed in the section "Training Methods" (page 74).

It is important to distinguish the concept of reactive ability from that of reaction time. The former is a characteristic of speed strength exhibited in SSC actions that can be improved through reactive-explosive training. In contrast, the latter is a relatively untrainable quality that correlates poorly with movement action time or performance in many brief explosive events. For example, an elite sprinter's auditory reaction time typically ranges from 0.12 to 0.18 seconds but is not significantly related to his or her 100-meter results. Other factors such as acceleration, speed endurance, and (to a lesser extent) maximum speed are more closely associated with overall sprint times. Reaction time is, however, an important determinant of performance in quick-timing tasks (e.g., a batter hitting a baseball) and defensive types of stimulus-response actions (e.g., a goaltender making a save).

Power

Power is the rate of doing work, or the product of force and velocity. The peak levels of force and power absorbed by the tissues while they are actively lengthening are often greater than those produced while they are shortening (see figure 4.2). If not adequately addressed in training, these forces can be the cause of so-called noncontact injury, technical inefficiency, or outright nonathleticism. Thus, in addition to improving concentric power production capability, the demands of SSC movements dictate two more training objectives: (1) to develop the eccentric strength needed to tolerate extreme power absorption while explosively braking during the initial lengthening action, and (2) to develop the reactive strength needed to recoil rapidly into the subsequent shortening action.

Figure 4.2 also illustrates that achievable velocity depends on the load to be overcome and that the role of strength in determining movement speed or acceleration in any task therefore increases with resistance. In terrestrial movement this resistance usually includes the athlete's body mass and possibly his or her equipment or opponent. In comparison, despite the fact that aquatic locomotion is not weight

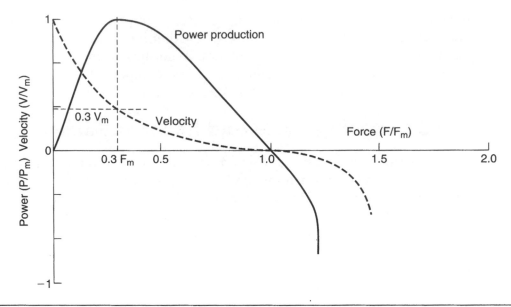

Figure 4.2   Power production and absorption as a function of force and velocity in concentric and eccentric muscle actions. Maximum concentric power (Pm) occurs at ~30% of maxumum force (Fm) and velocity (Vm). Note that the greatest force and power is produced during explosive eccentric actions.

bearing, consider the challenge presented by hydraulic resistance—in other words, energy cost as a function of drag. Indeed, it is difficult to find examples of sports that do not require power and high-speed force output to accelerate rapidly, decelerate rapidly, or achieve high velocities quickly. These capabilities are determined primarily by the athlete's percentage of type II fast-twitch motor units, and, of course, his or her ability to activate them optimally. In contrast, isometric, or low-velocity, strength is a function of muscle cross-sectional area (i.e., the number of active sarcomeres in parallel). Once the athlete has achieved the upper limit for specific muscle tension (40 to 45 newtons per centimeter^2 in trained athletes), hypertrophy is required—especially in type II fibers—to increase force and speed production further.

Endurance Versus Power Sports

It is generally accepted that these speed-strength capabilities are important in "power" sports (those involving explosive running, jumping, and changes in speed or direction), but many believe that their role in "endurance" activities is minor. The ability to apply force rapidly and accelerate one's body mass is important in most athletics. Prolonged activities often involve a series of brief, explosive spikes in power output, and therefore one should not simplistically classify such activities as submaximal endurance events. The task-specific importance of an athlete's speed-strength capabilities should be critically evaluated on a mechanical basis rather than categorically assigned based on physiological factors.

SYSTEMS VERSUS COMPONENTS

In general, structural movements such as multijoint weight-bearing exercises have a systemic effect that reaches far beyond the muscle fibers used in their execution. Muscles act—and should be targeted—in functional task groups rather than in isolation. This is one reason athletes should emphasize powerlifting and weightlifting-style movements, and compound exercises in general in their training. Furthermore, such movements are a potent means of activating the neuromuscular and neuroendocrine systems, which in turn regulate every system in the body. Thus, there are several reasons why strength-training programs should be based on free-weight movements rather than isolated muscle movements.

1. *Power.* The greater the effort and acceleration with a given weight, the greater the power development and subsequent training effect. Power output during Olympic-style weightlifting is the highest ever documented and comparable to the theoretical maximum for a human. For example, lifters execute the explosive jump-and-pull or dip-and-drive actions of these movements in 0.2 to 0.3 seconds. Peak power production is 4 to 5 times that of the deadlift or squat and 11 to 15 times that of the bench press.

2. *Motor coordination.* Skillful movements have a motor-control learning effect that carries over to the following coordinative abilities:

   - Orientation and differentiation
   - Reactiveness, rhythm, and balance
   - Combinatory and adaptive abilities

3. *Systemic effect.* The greater the exertion in the big lifts, the higher the production of endogenous hormones and the greater the activity and number of tissue receptors, which in turn stimulate overall muscle mass and strength to a greater degree. These guidelines are not definitive, and it is likely that no ideal workload protocol exists for either effect. However, a sound training strategy must account for and exploit basic adaptive mechanisms:

   - Moderate weights with high reps and high-intensity endurance activities in general tend to maximize the somatotropin response.
   - Heavy weights with low reps and brief maximal efforts in general tend to maximize the testosterone response.

The sound of clanking iron invokes no magic. Certain machines, such as a hip sled or cable-pulley system, serve useful roles. But multijoint free-weight training has an advantage that cams, levers, and linear bearings will never match. It requires—and develops—functional strength and has excellent transfer to athleticism and explosiveness.

EXERCISE PRIORITIZATION AND SUBSTITUTION

In terms of specificity, training tasks should be selected and prioritized according to their dynamic correspondence with the demands of the activity. Their basic biomechanics, but not necessarily their outward appearance, should be specific to the biomechanics occurring in competition. The rate and time of peak force production (impulse, see figure 4.1) and dynamics of effort (power, as shown in figure 4.2) are especially important criteria in explosive athletic movements. Other practical considerations include amplitude and direction of movement, accentuated region of force application, and regime of muscular work. This concept is analogous to the motor-learning principle of practice specificity with respect to sensorimotor processing and contextual effects on acquisition, retention, and transfer. Although these may appear to be commonsense statements, it is difficult to overstate their importance because failure to address them in training can result in limited transfer to competitive performance.

Classifications

Basic exercises are straightforward. There is little need to substitute other movements or supplement them with all sorts of assistance exercises intended to target the muscles differently. This is not a concrete rule, however, and some prudent alternatives are offered below. Long-term variety is often best achieved by adjusting the workload for a limited number of functional movements rather than attempting to include every possible exercise. Pages 69 to 73 provide exercises that are commonly applied in sports training.

In this light, strength-training exercises can be classified into three categories:

1. Primary, or "structural"—multijoint, weight bearing (e.g., Olympic-style lifts, squats, dead lifts)
2. Secondary, or "supplemental"—multijoint, non-weight bearing (e.g., upper-body pressing or pulling exercises)
3. Tertiary, or "isolation"—single-joint, non-weight bearing

Primary exercises are inherently functional movements that by definition yield the most profound results. Those further down the continuum have lesser effects and are technically simpler. The examples cited above for each category are certainly not comprehensive, and it is not difficult to find hybrid movements. For example, Olympic-style weightlifting movements represent a special case of primary exercises that are semiballistic in nature, with explosive impulse and power as the fundamental objectives.

The lunge and step-up each meet the criteria for a primary exercise, whereas machine exercises such as a hip sled or leg press arguably do not, despite the fact that they may involve similar muscle mass and exertion. The latter may be viable options during extremely intensive workloads or when the athlete's trunk cannot safely support the weight required to train the legs in movements such as the squat or dead lift (as discussed on page 71).

The chin-up, pull-up, dip, push-up, and related exercises can be considered multijoint weight-bearing movements, placing them in the primary category according to this scheme. But they often receive less emphasis than the traditional upper-body exercises mentioned above. Furthermore, they usually do not involve the same muscle mass or resistance used in other primary movements, making it difficult to justify placing them in the same group. Overall, however, they may deserve greater consideration than "standard" upper-body movements.

Additional examples could be cited, but the point is that this classification scheme is not an attempt to label certain movements as good or bad. It is simply a place to start making rational decisions about selecting and prioritizing them. As with all aspects of a program, use principles rather than preferences as a guide. Perhaps most important, training effect takes precedence over strength demonstration. The objective is to choose the most effective movements and execute them in the most beneficial way.

Weightlifting Variations

Although using sound movement mechanics is imperative, it may not always be necessary to perform the classical lifts as they are done in competition. For example, the Olympic-style movements can often be adapted or modified for the sake of simplicity.

In any case, the athlete should observe the following safety guidelines:

1. Use bumper plates and an eight-foot-by-eight-foot platform that is clear of loose plates, obstacles, and people. Do not have anyone attempt to spot you.

2. Technique, especially position and quickness, always has priority over weight.

3. Be prepared to miss a rep. If you lose control of the bar or can't complete a rep for any reason, quickly get out from underneath and let it drop. Do not try to save it on the way down.

   - Use the barbell's downward momentum to move out of the way. Keep your grip and push yourself away from the bar as it falls.
   - Stay between the plates; this does not mean that you remain under the barbell but that you move backward or forward (not sideways) to escape.

Power Clean

In terms of training effect, it makes little difference if the athlete starts from the floor or the hang position or whether he or she catches the bar. In fact, one way to teach these exercises to a novice athlete is to have him or her perform a high pull from the hang position, where the bar does not descend below knee level at the start of the movement and is not caught at its completion. Once the athlete masters this movement, he or she can progress into a power pull from the floor, the hang clean, and finally the power clean.

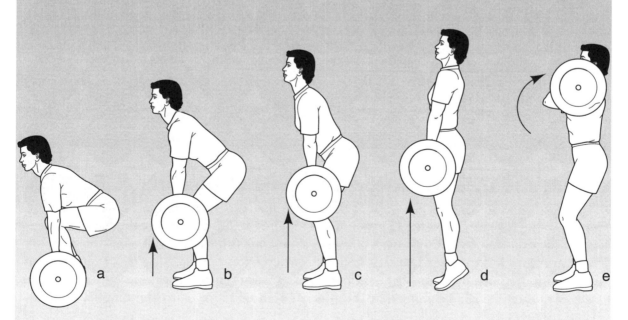

Snatch

A similar progression can be used in teaching the snatch. In either case, the success of each rep can be gauged by the athlete's ability to get into the "power position" (with the bar just above the knees) and use the hips and legs to get action on the bar, jumping and pulling explosively enough to separate his or her feet from the platform.

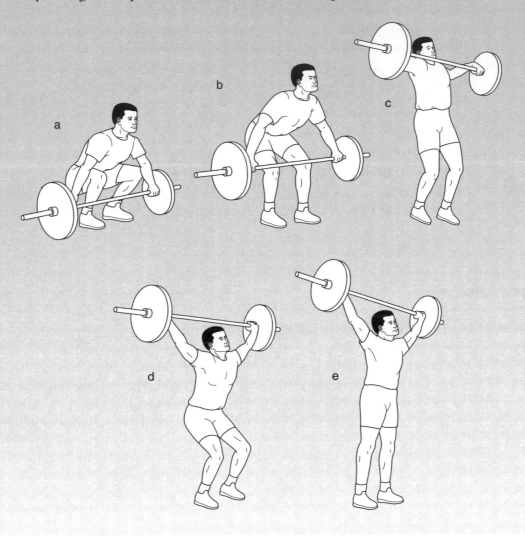

Jerk

Again, in terms of training effect it makes little difference if the athlete performs a split when catching the bar overhead. Once the athlete masters the basic mechanics of this lift, however, the split can improve an experienced athlete's ability to manage the bar by achieving a lower receiving position than is otherwise possible (unless he or she has the mobility to drop into a full overhead squat). A simple progression for teaching this exercise is to begin with the push press or push jerk before progressing into the jerk. In either case, the success of each rep can be gauged by the athlete's ability to dip (six to eight inches or about

10 percent of body height), drive through the "power position," and use the hips and legs to get action on the bar, jumping and pushing explosively enough to separate his or her feet from the platform.

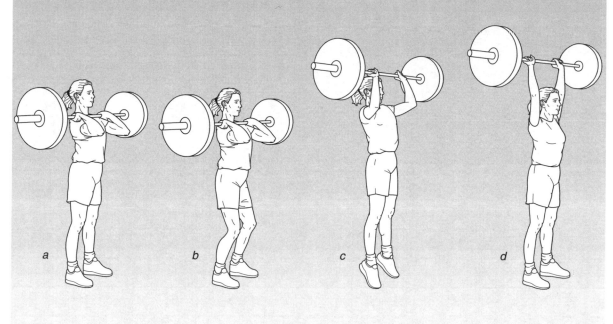

a   b   c   d

Powerlifting Variations

This discussion will address some adjunct considerations for safely and effectively performing the conventional squat and dead lift. These guidelines apply generally to both movements because of their gross similarities. Although technique checklists are presented, this section is not intended to present a complete overview of their execution.

Squat and Dead Lift

Optimal range of motion in the squat or dead lift does not cause the trunk to lean excessively forward or cause the athlete to feel unusual pain (to be distinguished from the discomfort of exertion). Many athletes can safely achieve the classic parallel-depth position with heavy weights, but some cannot. Those who do not compete in the sports of powerlifting or weightlifting should consider several points when pursuing an optimal training effect.

First, flexibility is an element of any functional movement. Active or passive mobility is intrinsic to every skill or technique, no matter how simple or complex. As discussed in chapter 3, the athlete should develop flexibility to optimal levels because functional strength is applied through a movement path (that is, a range of motion), and because an athlete's neuromuscular system generates peak power and operates most efficiently when explosively stretch loaded and recoiled.

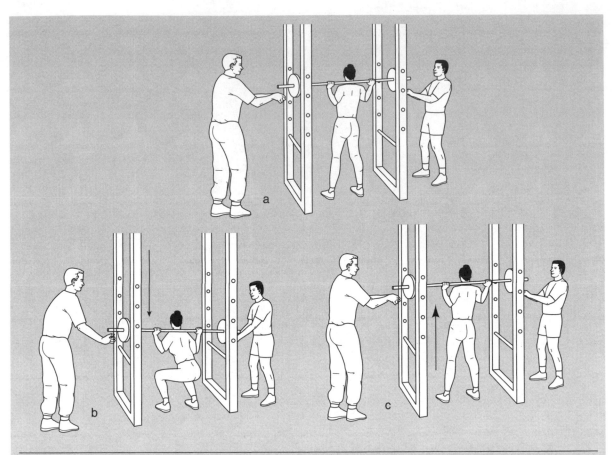

Squat

Second, achievable depth depends on the resistance being used. Even athletes who cannot get parallel with limit weights often can (and generally should, unless otherwise contra-indicated) do so during submaximal or warm-up reps. Thus, the inability to achieve a predetermined depth with heavy weight does not necessarily mean that it cannot be done at all.

Third, contrived methods of keeping the hips in line with the center of gravity, moving the knees in front of it, or otherwise altering the normal execution of these movements (e.g., by elevating the heels) are counterproductive and potentially injurious. The athlete can best achieve a stable base and balanced position by positioning the hips, the stronger and more stable structure, behind the center of gravity to receive most of the torque and driving through a "full foot" that is flat on the floor, with weight distributed between the heel and forefoot.

Fourth, and most important, the names of these (or any) movements are not as important as what they are intended to do. Function should dictate form. Multijoint exercises provide an opportunity to overload the major structures of the body by putting the "power zone" (i.e., the hips) in an optimal position to transmit the largest force. It follows then that to maximize torque at the hips, the athlete should move them as far behind the center of gravity as possible, while flexing as far as leverage and body position allow. Squatting or dead-lifting depth is therefore secondary to position. The key to a beneficial training effect is to move the hips back while sitting to an optimal depth, not necessarily to aim for any predetermined thigh angle. Depending on the athlete's body proportions, maximal torque may occur at or below an angle of 90 degrees at the hip or knee, with the midline of the thigh above the parallel position. In the squat, it is interesting to note the effect of bar placement. The powerlifter's low-bar position usually allows the hips to move farther backward than does the weightlifter's high-bar position, although this varies with individual body proportions and mechanics.

In summary, the effort required to overcome a given resistance obviously increases with depth. Beyond a certain point, however, this is the result of a loss in leverage rather than a gain in torque, in turn bringing stress-strain relationships into question. This does not imply that athletes should abandon parallel depth or universally adopt the half squat. The latter can be effective for those whose mechanics or flexibility do not permit them to safely get their thighs parallel according to the criteria presented above. The salient point is that the standardized depth established decades ago to judge powerlifting competitions may not be appropriate in all circumstances. "Full range of motion" should be critically evaluated for each situation rather than simplistically accepted as an absolute rule.

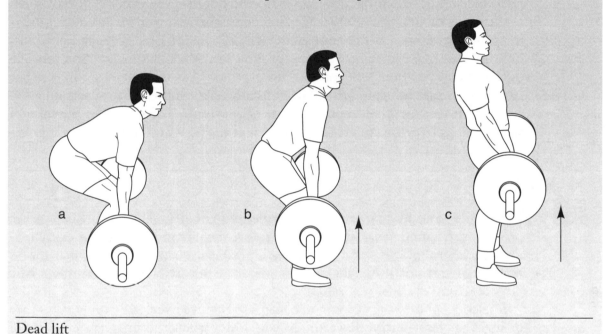

Dead lift

Alternatives

With the obvious exception of the competitive lifter, an advanced athlete may develop to the point where it is no longer judicious for the trunk to support the heaviest weights that the hips and legs are capable of moving. This observation is not intended to dissuade athletes from performing heavy structural movements. Indeed, one of the most effective ways to strengthen a healthy trunk is to load it in a fixed position while the lower body does the work, transferring force through the segments of the body. Likewise, lack of torso strength is an underlying cause of many so-called back problems. But it is important to realize that the human spine is a tower that was originally designed as a bridge. One should therefore consider its limitations and corresponding training options when approaching advanced levels of strength.

One recommendation is to view the primary exercises as a family of ground-based movements that are interchangeable. It is a simple matter of whether the weight is supported across the shoulders or suspended from them. If an athlete is better able to handle heavy squat weights by substituting the conventional dead lift in its place, that may be appropriate because the two movements are more similar than they are different. Furthermore, if the athlete has difficulty maintaining good posture when dead lifting from a static bottom position, it may be appropriate to set the bar up on blocks or racks and descend into each rep from an upright position. In this way, the athlete can combine the best features of each movement to achieve an optimal training effect.

Many athletes reach a point where they simply cannot maintain a flat back when venturing into very heavy squats or dead lifts. The trunk must then be unloaded or supported to train the hips and legs to their limit. One option is to introduce other structural movements that do not load the trunk as heavily, such as the lunge or step-up. Another is to include assistive hip and trunk strengthening movements such as the glute-ham raise, Romanian or stiff-legged dead lift, or trunk-reverse extension into the program to work the major structures in different combinations while unloading the torso. An additional option is to use barbell exercises for submaximal weights and perform the heaviest sets on a hip sled, leg press, or other apparatus that supports the torso. When pursuing a specific objective, the athlete should consider the pros and cons of various alternatives.

Balance

Imbalances are a leading cause of nonathleticism, injury, and chronic orthopedic problems. A sound program should therefore include movements for every major muscle group. It is possible to make big gains in strength and see little or no functional transfer if certain movements are neglected, allowing antagonistic muscle-group deficits to develop.

The concept of using power and control to achieve overload largely takes care of itself (at least during lower-body workouts) when the program consists of athletic free-weight movements. A useful rule of thumb is to include a "pulling," or flexion, exercise for every "pushing," or extension, exercise so that each movement plane is worked equally in both directions. In the case of lower-body training, exercises such as the glute-ham raise, abdominal-trunk flexion, and various isolation exercises can largely balance out primary movements. But this becomes more challenging with upper-body training because of the mobility of the shoulder girdle and the resulting need to offset traditional pressing exercises. High-low cable stacks and various free-body exercises are valuable here.

TRAINING METHODS

A hierarchy of training methods for specialized strength development is illustrated in table 4.1. This classification scheme is largely a matter of practicality and includes some overlap. The key to applying these methods lies in their skillful combination rather than exclusive or disproportionate use of any one of them.

Table 4.1 Classical Training Methods for Specialized Strength Development

Purpose	Method	Intensity	Action speed	Volume	Density
Maximal strength	Brief maximal efforts	75–100%	Slow to explosive	15–25 reps/session at 95–100% 20–40 reps/session at 90–95% 70–110 reps/session at 75–80% 8 or fewer reps/set for low-skill movements 3 or fewer reps/set for high-skill movements	Full (up to 8 minutes) recovery between sets
	Repeated submaximal efforts (hypertrophy) between sessions	80–90%	Slow to explosive	5–10 sets per exercise reps to exhaustion each set 24–48 hours	1–4 minutes recovery between sets;
	Combination methods				
Strength endurance	Extensive interval	30–40%	Brisk, continuous	3–6 sets per exercise 20–30 reps per set	Less than 5 minutes recovery between sets
	Intensive interval	50–60%	Explosive	3–6 sets per exercise 20–45 seconds duration per set (rep count irrelevant)	1–3 minutes of recovery between sets
Speed strength	Submaximal accelerative efforts (power; RFD)	30–85%	Explosive, maximal	3–7 sets per exercise 1–3 reps per set at 85% 3–5 reps per set at 80–85% 5–8 reps per set at 70–80% 8–15 reps per set under 70%	2–8 minutes of recovery between sets; daily sessions
	Reactive ballistic efforts (SSC)		Explosive, maximal		
	Contrast methods		Explosive, maximal		

Sources: Aján and Baroga 1988; Fleck and Kraemer 1987; Hartmann and Tünnemann 1989; Lyttle 1994; Schmidtbleicher 1985a; Siff and Verkhoshansky 1999; Stone and O'Bryant 1987; Zatsiorsky 1992.

Maximum Strength

Developing maximal strength is best achieved with two methods: brief maximal efforts and repeated submaximal efforts.

Brief Maximal Efforts

Brief maximal efforts improve intra- and intermuscular coordination and to minimize neuromuscular inhibition. Although this method activates a relatively narrow corridor of motor units, it recruits high-threshold (and quickly fatigable) motor units at their greatest discharge frequency and synchronicity. It is useful for advanced athletes but generally inappropriate for novices. This method tends to improve RFD and the ability to accelerate heavy loads but has minimal hypertrophic effect (which can be advantageous in certain situations).

Repeated Submaximal Efforts

Repeated submaximal efforts are usually applied with various intermediate intensities and a traditional "repetition maximum" approach. It is an effective means of developing basic strength and muscle mass in novice athletes, as well as maintaining them in advanced athletes. Although it can also be useful in improving high-intensity endurance performance, this response is dissociated from, and often diluted by, its hypertrophic effect. This method targets a relatively large population of motor units and tends not to improve RFD or high-resistance acceleration ability (at least in highly qualified athletes). Furthermore, advanced athletes should limit its use because of the high work volumes associated with it.

Strength Endurance

Extensive and intensive intervals are intended to improve endurance capacity during prolonged low-intensity and brief high-intensity workloads, respectively, and to improve subsequent recovery ability. Both approaches, especially extensive intervals, involve comparatively large work volumes. Intensive intervals at first may appear similar to the method of repeated submaximal efforts, but this method tends not to yield the same hypertrophic effect. In fact, the use of these methods can be considered a variation of the metabolic conditioning discussed in chapter 10.

Speed Strength

Speed strength can be improved through reactive-ballistic efforts, submaximal accelerative efforts, or contrast methods that maximize the effects of each.

Reactive-Ballistic Efforts

As previously mentioned, springlike movements involving SSC actions are characteristic of many sports activities. Ballistic plyometric drills are intended to develop the athlete's reactive-explosive strength (refer to the section "Movement Mechanics" on page 64 as well as chapter 5) by exploiting two phenomena: neuromuscular reflex potentiation and musculotendinous elastic energy recovery. Acute training responses include increased mechanical efficiency and overall "working effect" (e.g., power, impulse), whereas chronic responses involve up-regulation of muscle stiffness and motoneural activation. The basic classification scheme for SSC actions is the following:

- Long-response—ground contact greater than 0.25 seconds, large angular displacement (e.g., sprint start and acceleration, squat and countermovement jump)
- Short-response—ground contact less than 0.25 seconds, small angular displacement (e.g., maximal sprint velocity, high jump, and long jump)

This scheme is useful in selecting plyometric drills to improve specific performance qualities. For example, long-response training tasks would have the greatest transfer to the sprint start and initial acceleration, whereas short-response tasks would have the greatest transfer to top-speed performance.

Submaximal Accelerative Efforts

Inherently impulsive movements such as Olympic-style lifts, plyometrics, and other reactive-ballistic actions are not the only methods for developing speed strength. However, the role of acceleration and RFD in nonballistic tasks is often misunderstood or neglected. These factors are especially important for athletes and are fundamental to force production even when executing basic structural exercises. Indeed, note that explosive movement intent is recommended for most of the training methods itemized in table 4.1. It is a simple matter of understanding the fundamental nature of force and of addressing practical considera-tions about task and workload.

As is the case with reactive-ballistic efforts, the method of submaximal accelerative efforts is inferred from a basic physical law. Force is the product of mass and acceleration ($F = m \times a$). Simply put, because the forces acting on an object are proportional to its acceleration, the athlete must accelerate that object, regardless of weight, to the limit of his or her ability to generate maximum force. As mentioned previously, successful execution of most functional tasks requires rapid force application. Nonballistic movements, including traditional strength-training exercises, are no exception. Thus, in all cases, range of motion can be considered an acceleration path. The only distinction is whether the athlete accelerates the object through the sticking region or through the entire movement to project it ballistically.

At first glance, this law may seem to imply that there is no force without motion or vice versa. But this is not necessarily the case. For example, because gravity is expressed as an acceleration constant (about 9.8 meters per second^2), a vertical force of about 980 newtons (kilograms $\times$ meters per second^2) is required to hold a 100-kilogram barbell in place statically. Despite the apparent simplicity of this fact, the inability or unwillingness to grasp its functional significance is an underlying cause of many nonsensical training methods. It is a foundational principle for all motion. When considering that any movement is essentially an act of defying gravity, which itself is an accelerative force, the central issue becomes this: what is being moved, and how fast?

Simply stated, the athlete should move the object through an optimal acceleration path within a certain time to maximize impulse production and subsequent training effect. Olympic-style weightlifting is an iron game that is close to the high-speed end of the spectrum, whereas powerlifting is relatively nearer the low-speed end. Regardless of whether these movements are performed in training or competition, the salient point is the same for each: Peak force and motoneural activity (relative to one's capabilities) are generated only by accelerating the load maximally through the "power position" or "sticking region." Aside from the obvious fact that an athlete can move light weights more rapidly than heavy ones and that some tasks are inherently ballistic whereas others are not, this has two other fundamental implications:

1. *The intent to move explosively can be more important than actual velocity achieved.* Full volitional effort (i.e., a deliberate attempt to accelerate the resistance maximally even if it is too heavy to move rapidly) yields the greatest neuromuscular activation and subsequent adaptive response. Submaximal force production and neuromuscular activation—which, by definition, are precisely what occurs when one does not accelerate a given resistance to the limits of one's ability—simply don't make sense as a viable or productive means of training.

2. *Rate, direction, and amplitude of force production are equally important (and trainable).* Their brief application in certain parts of the movement is more important than sustained application over the movement's full distance or duration. Some athletes and coaches mistakenly believe that RFD is relevant during ballistic tasks but not in basic exercises when the weight is not projected; however, this notion needs to be revised.

It is important to understand that high-speed movements are not the only way to activate and train fast-twitch muscle fibers. Motor units exist in a spectrum and are progressively recruited as power output increases. Given the range of force-velocity combinations possible in any movement, it is not surprising that the neuromuscular system activates motor units as well as muscles in functional task groups. Furthermore, force production is a matter of not only motor-unit recruitment but also coordination and synchronization. The higher centers of the neuromuscular system that govern this process are as plastic as the muscle fibers themselves. Adaptation is a function of activation, and maximal effort at a given resistance is the means of achieving it. Indeed, adaptive tissue remodeling may be an up-regulation response to innervation signals more than a simple cellular repair process (when a fast-twitch motor nerve is grafted onto a slow-twitch muscle fiber, the properties of that fiber reverse themselves).

Practically speaking, a wide range of workload intensities and volumes can be justifiably recommended. Despite all these options, the effectiveness of a strength-training program will be limited if an athlete approaches it exclusively in terms of weights and reps while ignoring the accelerative quality of force. Likewise, it is a mistake to assume that full activation automatically occurs whenever the bar is moving or that the last rep of a set triggers the desired training effect. These are particularly costly errors for those who abbreviate work volume to the point where they cannot afford anything less than extreme emphasis on training quality. The solution is to maximize force output and neuromuscular activity on each repetition by accelerating through the sticking region at full power, regardless of resistance or rep count.

Some individuals have misunderstood the method of submaximal accelerative efforts to mean that they should accelerate light weights through the entire range of motion without releasing them (i.e., "speed reps"). Such movements have been shown to be futile because more effort is spent decelerating the bar for self-protection than accelerating it for beneficial force or power production. Although eccentric muscle actions are intrinsic to functional tasks, in training they are generally appropriate for performing controlled "negatives" (e.g., during non-ballistic exercises) or preparatory countermovements (e.g., during ballistic movements) rather than terminal braking motions.

In practical terms, it is important to consider how acceleration interacts with the sticking region, defined as the part of the movement path where leverage and resistance interact to create the greatest difficulty in moving or controlling the bar. Using the squat or dead lift as an example, the sticking point resides about 30 degrees above the parallel position. As with many multijoint exercises, the sticking point is a small portion of the movement but may occupy a relatively larger segment (perhaps up to a third or a half) of the time required to execute, fatigue or 1RM attempts notwithstanding. Because maximal effort is not required elsewhere in the movement path, the peak force generated in this region is the primary reason for performing these exercises in training. Arguably, the lesser forces applied elsewhere in the range of motion are secondary.

The relevant point is that brief, rapid force application is characteristic of a wider range of activities than is often believed. The practical implication of this concept is straightforward and presents a radical departure from the so-called time-under-tension theory as well as other purposefully slow training methods. An example of how to apply the method of submaximal accelerative efforts when performing basic movements such as the squat or dead lift follows (note that this approach can be adapted to other compound exercises as well):

1. Sit at a controlled speed into an optimal position; do not free fall into the descent.

2. Immediately accelerate out of the hole and through the sticking region as powerfully as possible with good form.

3. Be careful to throttle down at the top of each rep so the bar doesn't jump off your shoulders or out of your grip.

Two other practical issues apply to this method: deceleration at the end of the movement path and possible breakdown of technique. Consider that it is not easy to move even moderately heavy weight rapidly despite a deliberate attempt to do so. Furthermore, as the athlete backs off from maximal acceleration toward the top of the ascent, gravity will decelerate the vertical velocity of the bar. In any case, if it is still moving upward by virtue of its momentum upon reaching full extension, two possibilities exist:

• The athlete is accelerating the weight beyond the sticking point and should adjust his or her effort during the latter third to half of each rep to avoid "jamming" it at the top.

• The chosen resistance is so light that the athlete would do better by performing a ballistic exercise with equipment designed to be launched explosively.

The athlete need not sacrifice technique for impulse or power, although form often does degrade to some extent during very heavy, slow lifts. If athletes were incapable of achieving a reasonable degree of technical precision whenever they accelerated above first or second gear, it would be impossible to execute simple acts of running, jumping, throwing, and other functional tasks. This is not to suggest that barbells and dumbbells are to be yanked on and hurled recklessly around the weight room. The point is simply that anyone with enough common sense and motor coordination to perform basic exercises properly should be able to maintain control when applying this method. If anything, it allows the athlete to stay in the groove through the sticking region where the bar otherwise tends to drift off course.

Contrast Methods

This approach is intended to exploit the aftereffect of preceding work to increase the efficacy of subsequent work in a single training session. An example would be to "complex" explosive-reactive efforts with brief maximal efforts to activate the athlete's neuromuscular system in alternating but complementary ways. This advanced strategy capitalizes on the acute residual effect of certain work regimes in much the same way that cyclic, long-term workload variation improves adaptive responses by exploiting their cumulative and delayed effects. The athlete should conduct this method with optimal rest intervals and minimal fatigue. It is generally inappropriate for novice athletes.

PROGRAM DESIGN

To optimize the athlete's performance capabilities, the sports-preparation process must be planned and implemented according to sound principles (as discussed in chapters 12 and 13). For specialized strength development, the athlete should rationally manipulate the following variables:

- Action speed—the intent to accelerate or achieve high velocity with a given load as a means of manipulating power or impulse production
- Exercise order—the sequence in which a set of exercises is performed
- Density—the amount of work performed in a set or training session
- Frequency—the number of training sessions performed in a given time period (e.g., day or week)
- Intensity—the effort with which a repetition is executed (usually characterized by resistance but more accurately associated with impulse or power output)
- Recovery—the time interval between sets
- Repetition—the execution of a specific workload assignment or movement technique
- Series—a group of sets and recovery intervals
- Set—a group of repetitions
- Volume—the amount of work performed in a given training session or time period (usually characterized by repetitions but more accurately associated with the product of resistance and distance moved per repetition)

These parameters are useful in quantifying training and in most cases can be adapted or directly applied to speed, agility, and speed-endurance development.

To be useful in practice, however, they must be accompanied by qualitative guidelines regarding movement mechanics and planned variation in training objectives.

SUMMARY

Specialized strength training offers the athlete tremendous potential to improve performance capability and minimize risk of injury. Principle-based planning and implementation of the preparation process are the keys. They require a working knowledge of physiological and biomechanical bases of maximum strength, speed-strength, and strength-endurance development.

In conclusion, the following practical implications can be recommended:

1. *Explosive force application is the basis of strength training for sports.* Functional strength is expressed in terms of acceleration, execution time, or velocity—especially in athletics. Training tactics that disregard this fact are fundamentally unsound. Moving through an acceleration path and applying rapid or high-speed force is the name of the game.

2. *Emphasize big basic movements that have the greatest training effects.* Use equipment that challenges the athlete to control, direct, or stabilize it. Muscles act in functional task groups and must be targeted by force transmission through (rather than isolation within) the body's kinetic chain. Multijoint free-weight movements are superior in this regard.

3. *Distinguish between specificity and simulation.* Select and prioritize training tasks according to the coordinative, biomechanical, and bioenergetic demands of competition.

4. *Balance the need for specificity versus variability.* Maintain stability in the program by sticking with a basic exercise menu rather than trying to include every possible movement. Achieve variation by cycling workloads on a periodic three- to four-week basis to summate training effects and avoid accommodation problems.

5. *Quality of effort, not quantity, is the bottom line.* Although it is necessary to do enough work to get a training effect, the athlete reaches a threshold of diminishing returns above which effort is diluted and recoverability and adaptability are compromised. Fitness and fatigue are a trade-off beyond a certain point. In general, athletes achieve optimal results by maximizing the quality of effort within a prescribed amount of work.

6. *Effort and recovery are interdependent.* Workload intensity, frequency, and volume are interrelated and cannot be changed arbitrarily. They must be adjusted together; this occurs automatically with a sound plan. A training program is only as good as the athlete's ability to recover from and adapt to it!

7. *Fitness qualities are means toward an end, not ends in themselves.* The goal is to develop the athlete's performance capabilities and skills and thereby couple effort with execution. Power, flexibility, agility, speed, and endurance combined with motor coordination are the elements of athleticism. Each is trainable, but the athlete must train them collectively because they are parts of a larger whole. None is a separate entity, nor is one more important than another. Train athleticism, not muscles!

8. *Most important, skillful tasks are the basis of sports training.* Learning how to perform them requires the services of a qualified strength and conditioning coach. If simply counting reps and sets were the answer, anyone could do it. As in all aspects of coaching or teaching, attention must be directed toward what the athlete is doing and how he or she is doing it—not just how much the athlete does. Skilled training requires skilled coaching. Without it, a strength-training program will fall far short of its potential.

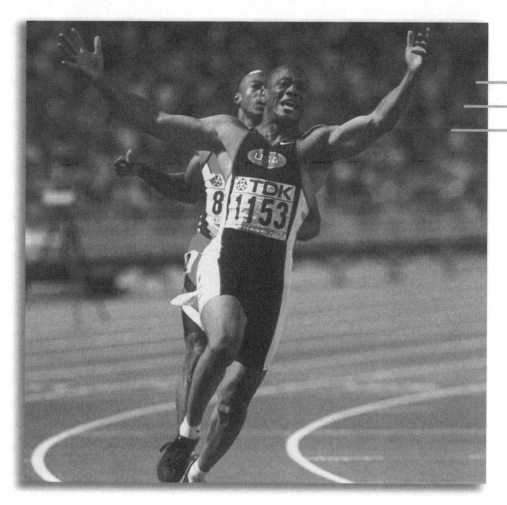

Explosive Power

Donald A. Chu

Every mathematical formula used to calculate power demonstrates that this quality of movement is a function of time. Power is the product of work × time, or force × distance × time, or force × velocity (distance × time). Thus, the common denominator for the development of power in sports activities is based on applying speed to the desired movement or specific sports situation.

Speed in the development of force is crucial to success in sports activity. Abilities such as running fast, jumping high, and throwing far and fast are all related to the ability to develop and impart forces quickly. All athletes seek to be their best, but they may not understand that they must develop those abilities over time and choose appropriate means for doing so. Even those who possess the physical characteristics that others only wish they had must develop and refine their abilities if they want to be at the top of their game. This chapter explains how to go about accomplishing this goal.

Whenever speed of movement is increased, a subsequent increase occurs in the "stress" and "strain" on soft tissues. Stress can be defined as the rate at which forces are applied to and absorbed by the body. Strain has to do with the ability of the body to absorb these forces and recover from them. Terms associated with power development—explosive, reactive, quick—all define the ability of the individual to overcome the inertia of the body or outside object and place it in motion. To do this, the athlete must defeat Newton's law of inertia, which states that a body at rest tends to remain at rest. To overcome inertia effectively and repeatedly, he or she must have a method of dealing with the stresses and strains of training. In other words, the coaching cliché "training to train" holds great truth. Coaches and athletes should be aware that training for power is the icing on the cake, not the cake itself. Training for power is the end of a progression of athletic development.

TYPES OF MUSCLE FIBERS

Genetics partly determines potential for speed of movement. Those who have muscle dominated by fast-twitch (type II) fibers have the potential to develop speed of movement by exerting forces more rapidly than those whose fiber make-up is predominantly slow twitch (type I). Maximizing genetic potential requires an understanding that three subclassifications of type II fibers—namely IIA, IIAB, and IIB—can be influenced to act like fast-twitch fibers if subjected to forms of training designed to develop power.

Muscle fibers will always fire in the same sequence: type I, II, IIA, IIAB, IIB. The way in which these fibers are recruited is related to the effort required to overcome an external resistance. This means that maximal effort in resistance training, plyometrics, and speed work will be required to develop power.

TRAINING PROGRESSION

The ability to demonstrate explosive power movements must come from development in a progression of physical qualities, as shown below.

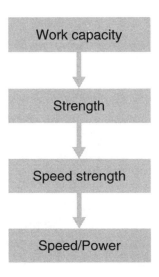

Work Capacity Training

The most basic level of training is referred to as "work capacity." This can be thought of as the "training to train" phase, or the preparation phase. In the young athlete (11 to 13 years of age) or in the untrained older athlete, this phase could last as long as 8 to 12 weeks. This phase consists of developing several physical qualities, including the following: (1) core strength, (2) joint mobility, (3) strength endurance, (4) anaerobic capacity, (5) body composition, and (6) aerobic capacity.

- Core strength refers to the individual's ability to stabilize joints as well as the trunk. This is the foundation of ability to develop power in movement. The body must be connected, and core strength is what accomplishes this.
- Joint mobility refers to normal ranges of motion available within and between joints, including both flexibility of muscles and extensibility of connective tissue.
- Strength endurance is the ability to sustain muscle force production at a high level over a period of time.
- Anaerobic capacity is the ability to withstand repeated efforts of short-term activity (up to 90 seconds) at a near maximal or maximal effort.
- Body composition relates to the efficiency of the body to perform physical activity. Training at this stage of development affects the relationship of muscle to fat mass.
- Although the ability to develop power is anaerobic in nature and will improve most by using anaerobic training methods, aerobic capacity is important for recovery between exercises and training sessions. But the power athlete should not use aerobic training as a dominant form of training. It should be an adjunct form of physical development that takes place during the warm-up or cool-down. The athlete can also train the aerobic system during off-season training periods.

Strength Training

Developing strength is the next stage of development on the road to becoming an explosive athlete. Strength comes in many forms and is more complex than the mere development of force tension within a muscle. For example, within the scheme of physical development are several classifications:

- Maximal strength refers to the maximum amount of weight that an individual can lift at any one time.
- Relative strength refers to the ability to work against one's body weight.
- Static strength is the ability to hold or stabilize a position.
- Eccentric strength, or "yielding" strength, is the ability of a muscle to develop force while it is lengthening. This form of strength is essential to success in power tasks such as jumping, cutting, or changing direction.

Speed-Strength Training

Next in the progression of developments is a crucial aspect of athletic development—speed strength—the foundation of power development. This area of development tends to be less familiar to the athlete. To make the transition from the weight room to the field, the athlete must make a shift in thinking about how to train. The components of this form of training are the development of (1) starting strength, (2) explosive strength, and (3) reactive-elastic strength.

- Starting strength is the ability to exert maximal forces instantly.
- Explosive strength refers to the rate at which the athlete develops force.
- Reactive-elastic strength is the coupling of eccentric strength with concentric strength. It can be measured in the time it takes (e.g., 0.25 seconds or less) to reverse direction from an eccentric, or braking, contraction to a concentric, or accelerating, contraction.

Here the exercise regimen shifts to more dynamic, uniquely designed forms of exercise. If an athlete trains only for maximal force development, he or she will be capable of developing great amounts of force tension but will create no change in the rate of force development. This athlete will exhibit great strength in the weight room but will not display the same prowess on the field. This circumstance is probably what led many coaches in the past to decry the use of resistance training by their athletes, noting the athletes' lack of improvement in their play within the sport after becoming bulkier and stronger.

It is here that activities must begin to adhere to the SAID (specific adaptation to imposed demands) principle, which means that training must become more mechanically and velocity specific. The training drills or exercises must begin to relate closely to the demands of the sport or event itself. Medicine ball and plyometric drills are examples of sport-specific forms of training under the SAID principle.

Speed or Power Training

The final level of training for athletes in their quest for optimal performances is speed training. This form of training improves the ability to move the body or body part through a range of motion in the least amount of time possible. The components of speed development include the following.

- Acceleration—the rate at which speed of movement increases.
- Absolute speed—the highest velocity (distance ÷ time) reached during the activity.
- Speed endurance—the ability to repeat high-quality efforts of movement without suffering a drastic decrement in performance.
- Specific speed—the ability to demonstrate speed in a specific movement pattern on the track, field, or court.

The road to explosive power may be longer than the athlete originally expected. Many characteristics of the athlete and his or her activity influence the progress made in training for this quality. Gender, age, training background, genetics, and sports activity are all considerations. The lesson to be learned in reaching for the skills that define the elite athlete is that becoming an explosive athlete is not always easy. The athlete must learn patience in order to achieve success in physical development. Without a substantial strength base, proper instruction, and careful planning, many sections on the road to success can be rocky.

TRAINING PROGRAMS FOR EXPLOSIVE POWER

Once the athlete has gone through the preparation, or "training-to-train," phase and begins to consider which exercises to adapt as part of a training program, he or she should remember that *progression* is the operative word. My training approach consists of performing these exercises as part of the total program. The training cycle (phase or stage) will dictate the volume and intensity of the exercises. I prefer to develop training programs that include plyometric drills, weight training, and speed work, often all on the same day. This method takes advantage of the fact that the nervous system is in a progressive state of arousal after performing each type of exercise. The athlete can thus enjoy the advantage of having the exercises maximally affect the body. This does not mean that the athlete gives a high-volume effort in all three types of exercise. When the volume is increased or emphasized in one area, such as speed work, the volume of effort in the others, plyometrics and lifting, should be reduced. Thus the athlete does not overtrain or become overly fatigued.

My philosophy on training for explosive power is that athletes best develop it by focusing on multijoint, ballistic weightlifting exercises such as cleans, snatches, push presses, and various forms of jump squats. The purpose of these types of lifts is to teach the athlete to initiate force with maximal effort against a maximum or near maximum resistance.

Once the athlete has learned the skills associated with these exercises and can adapt them into a training program, the next step is to add plyometric training. Plyometric training is designed to teach the muscular system of the athlete to develop maximal forces over a brief period.

Plyometric exercises depend on the quality of movement, not the quantity of exercises, to accomplish speed-strength characteristics. Exercises can be of a general nature, designed to work on start speed, acceleration, or absolute speed. Alternatively, exercises can be adapted to sport-specific movements or skills.

The final ingredient in the process of developing the explosive athlete is speed training. For sports performed on courts and fields, coaches and trainers speak of sprint training, which should be an important element in the development of any athlete. It is usually thought of as a means of conditioning the athlete in a cardiovascular sense. In fact, sprint training should be part of the total development of the neuromuscular system. The volume of sprint training need not exceed a total distance of 300 to 600 meters (subdivided into shorter sprints) in a single workout.

Combining various aspects of speed training (lifting, plyometrics, and sprinting) is known as "complex" training. This is an excellent short-term method for improving power and speed, but it cannot be the mainstay of the development program. Conducted for too long in the training year, complex training would overtrain the athlete, causing him or her to be unable to make significant gains. By alternating methods of exercise, an athlete can draw nearer his or her peak in the periodization or training scheme. A complex training cycle four to six weeks long will generally yield the best results. The section that follows centers on plyometric drills because weightlifting and sprinting are covered in chapters 4 and 9 of this book.

Tuck Jump

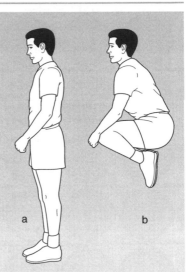

Focus
Calves, thighs, and hips

Procedure
1. The athlete stands with the feet shoulder-width apart and the body in a vertical position with no bend at the waist (a).
2. The athlete jumps up, brings the knees as close to the chest as possible, and briefly grasps the knees with the hands before letting the feet return to the floor (b).
3. He or she lands in a vertical position and repeats the jump immediately for the prescribed number of repetitions.

Key Points
The athlete should strive for hang time. The jump should combine an explosive movement from the ground with bringing the knees quickly to the chest. This will help develop the hip flexor speed that is so necessary for the drive phase of running and sprinting.

Backward Medicine Ball Throw

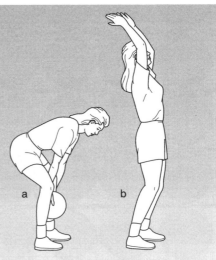

Focus
Calves, thighs, hips, lower back, and shoulders

Procedure
1. The athlete stands with the feet shoulder-width apart and holds a medicine ball in the hands in front of the body.
2. The athlete drops down into a squat position (a) and uses the hips and thighs to explode up and throw the ball over the head in a backward motion (b).

Key Points
Encourage the athlete to throw with maximum effort on each trial. If the athlete is throwing against a wall, he or she should try to knock the wall down! The athlete should always use the hips and legs to bend, never the lower back only.

Overhead Medicine Ball Throw

Focus

Calves, thighs, hips, abdominals, and shoulders

Procedure

1. The athlete stands with the feet shoulder-width apart while holding a medicine ball overhead.

2. The athlete takes a step forward with either foot and brings the ball behind the head.

3. He or she arches the back and brings the ball forward while generating force from the ground (feet) through the legs, hips, abdominals, and finally through the chest and arms.

4. The athlete throws the ball forward using the whole body to generate force.

Key Points

One of the hardest things to teach young athletes is the art of incorporating all their force in a single effort. This drill offers the opportunity to do just that. The athlete must push against the ground to develop a maximal effort, and that force must travel up the kinetic chain and finally through the hands to the ball to achieve maximal distance and effort.

Large-Amplitude Squat Jump

Focus

Calves, thighs, and hips

Procedure

1. The athlete assumes a thigh-parallel squat position with the hands behind the head.

2. The athlete jumps forward with a submaximal effort by extending the legs, lands with the knees flexed at 30 to 40 degrees, and eccentrically drops into the thigh-parallel position again.

3. From here, the athlete immediately moves forward again for the prescribed number of repetitions.

Key Points

The athlete should simulate a ball bouncing across a surface. Each jump should be controlled in both the descent (eccentric, or lowering) phase and the ascent (concentric, or raising) phase.

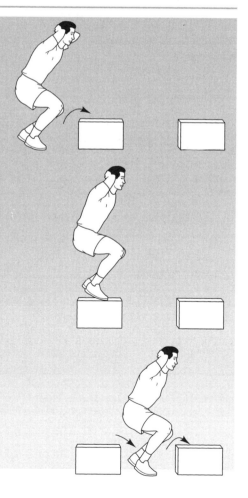

Wave Squat Jump

Focus

Calves, thighs, and hips

Procedure

1. The athlete stands with the feet shoulder-width apart and a weight of not more than 60 percent of estimated or measured 1RM (repetition maximum) across the shoulders.
2. The athlete jumps forward using submaximal, but progressive, efforts on each jump. He or she continues forward for three small jumps.
3. On the final effort, the athlete explodes up as quickly as possible, attempting to drive into full extension of the body.

Key Points

The athlete should keep the weight close to the shoulders while performing this exercise, not letting it get away from the body. If the bar does come away, it can create bruises. The athlete should try to keep each of the submaximal jumps on a progressive plane until the final effort, which should be close to maximal.

Standing Long Jump

Focus

Calves, thighs, hips, and shoulders

Procedure

1. The athlete stands with the feet shoulder-width apart in the ready position.
2. The athlete uses a big arm swing in the direction of shoulder extension, performs a counter-movement (flex) of the knees, and explodes forward and out as far as possible.

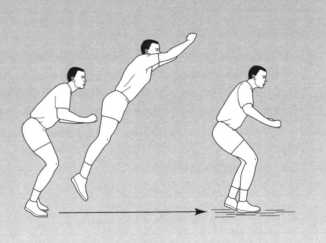

Key Points

Prepare the athlete to absorb the impact of landing. Depending on the surface, teach him or her to flex the knees and control the landing with eccentric muscular control.

Hurdle (Barrier) Jump

Focus
Calves, thighs, hips, and shoulders

Procedure

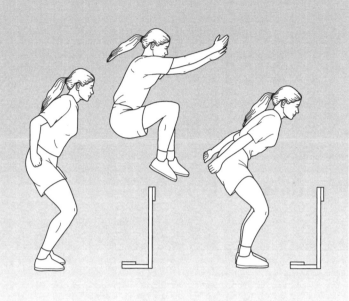

1. Place three to five hurdles or barriers approximately three feet apart. The athlete stands in front of the first hurdle in the ready position with the feet shoulder-width apart.

2. The athlete jumps forward over the barriers with the feet together. Movement comes from the hips and knees. The body should be vertical and straight. The knees should not move apart nor should the feet go to either side. The athlete should use a double-arm swing to maintain balance and gain height.

Key Points
Make sure that the landing between barriers is brief. Emphasize spending as short a time as possible on the ground. As the barriers become easier to clear, do not be afraid to progress to higher heights. Use the time spent on the ground to gauge whether the height of the barrier is too much for the athlete.

Long Vertical Hurdle Jump

Focus
Calves, thighs, hips, and shoulders

Procedure

1. Place five or six hurdles or barriers approximately six feet or farther apart. The athlete stands approximately six or seven feet from the first hurdle in the ready position with the feet shoulder-width apart.

2. The athlete performs a linear jump (standing long jump) to within 18 inches of the barrier and immediately transfers to a vertical jump to clear the barrier.

3. Upon landing, the athlete repeats this procedure to clear the prescribed number of barriers.

Change-of-Direction Hurdle Jump

Focus
Calves, thighs, and hips

Procedure
1. Set up hurdles or barriers on a series of diagonals or in a square or hexagonal pattern. The athlete stands in the ready position with the feet shoulder-width apart in front of the first hurdle.
2. The athlete jumps over the first barrier and continues to follow a preset pattern of jumps, for example, three times around the hexagon.

Variation
A variation is to set a time limit for the athlete to clear all the hurdles.

Standing Triple Jump

Focus
Calves, thighs, hips, and shoulders

Procedure
1. The athlete starts from a two-footed stance with the feet shoulder-width apart. The arm swing is done with straight arms from the shoulder joints to maximize the force contribution.
2. Action—The athlete explodes off both legs and lands on one foot (hop phase; a).
3. Using the swing of the arms to help move the body forward, the athlete steps out with the opposite leg and lands on that foot (step phase; b).
4. Finally, the athlete takes off and performs a "hanging long jump" before landing on both feet (jump phase; c).

Variation
A variation of this drill is to use a rocker step and let the athlete begin the hop phase with a single-foot takeoff.

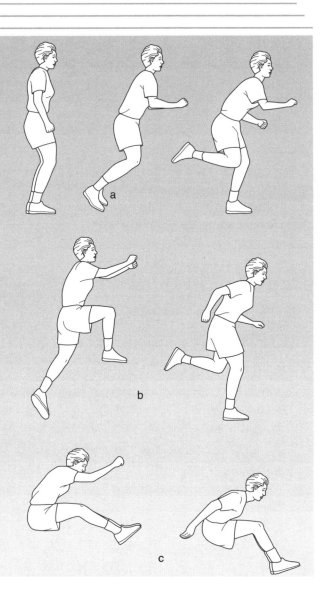

Single-Leg Bound

Focus

Calves, thighs, and hips

Procedure

1. The athlete begins from a rolling start to develop momentum because he or she will be performing this drill over a prescribed distance, usually 20 to 30 meters.

2. Establish a takeoff mark 2 to 4 meters beyond the actual starting line. The athlete hits this spot and executes repeated single-leg hops, attempting to cover as much ground as possible. The athlete should sacrifice vertical height to maximize and maintain speed across the ground.

3. After the athlete covers the distance, allow him or her to walk back for full recovery before performing the next repetition.

Alternate Bound

Focus

Calves, thighs, hips, and shoulders

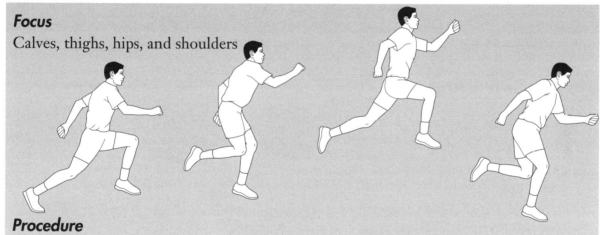

Procedure

1. The athlete begins from a rolling start. The distance covered in this drill may start at 30 meters and eventually progress to as far as 100 meters for each repetition.

2. Establish a takeoff mark 2 to 4 meters beyond the actual starting line. The athlete hits this spot and proceeds to use a series of exaggerated running strides to develop force against the ground. The arm action can be single or double depending on the athlete and his or her skill level.

Key Points

The athlete must be urged to focus on pushing against the ground from landing through takeoff. Immediately after takeoff, the athlete should attempt to maintain hang time. The result will be a glide or float pattern to each stride. This action should have an aesthetic quality, with the athlete attempting to make it look effortless yet demonstrating great power at takeoff.

Combination Bound

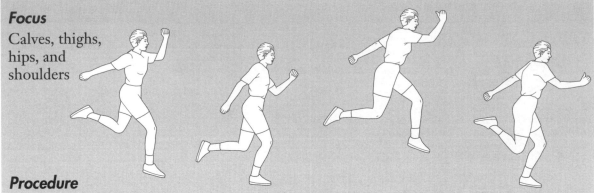

Focus

Calves, thighs, hips, and shoulders

Procedure

1. The athlete starts in the same position as in alternate bounds. The drill is virtually the same as alternate bounding except that it includes a double-hop phase.

2. The athlete takes off and uses a left-left-right foot pattern followed by a right-right-left foot pattern (shown), repeating this sequence for a prescribed distance, usually 40 to 60 meters.

Key Points

Remind the athlete that after the first sequence (left-left-right) he or she should be mentally ready to hop immediately from the landing foot (right) to begin the next sequence (right-right-left). Note that all the bounding drills involve complex movement skills and will take some time to perfect. Do not worry if the athlete does not look particularly graceful in the beginning. Skill will improve with time and repeated efforts.

Repeat Rim Jump

Focus

Calves, thighs, and hips

Procedure

1. The athlete stands with the feet shoulder-width apart in the ready position with a target slightly in front and above. This target may be a mark on a wall, hanging object, net, or basket. The athlete holds the arms in the most common position for his or her sport. For example, the volleyball player hoping to improve blocking ability may have a ready position with the hands up by the shoulders and palms facing the net.

2. On command the athlete performs a series of vertical jumps, aiming to touch the target.

3. Perform this drill for no more than six repetitions to avoid undue fatigue and maintain maximal efforts.

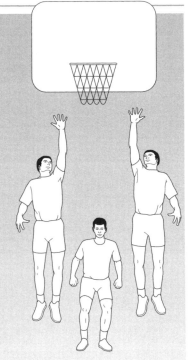

Key Points

Do not let the athlete settle to more than 20 to 25 degrees of knee flexion. Remember that you are teaching the athlete to be quick off the ground.

Depth Jump

Focus

Calves, thighs, and hips

Procedure

1. The athlete assumes a standing position, with the knees slightly flexed and the toes at the edge of a platform or box of a prescribed height.

2. The athlete steps out from the edge of the box and drops to the ground, using the landing impact as the stimulus to reverse the descent and jump vertically as high as possible. The athlete must give maximal effort with each repetition lest the drill become simply one of the athlete absorbing the impact of landing.

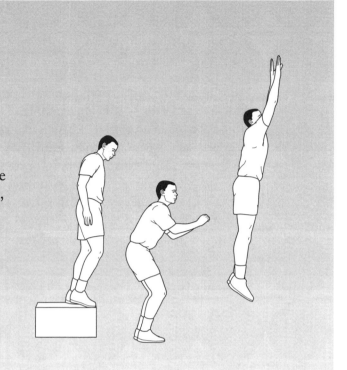

Key Points

The coach must be careful not to overwhelm the athlete with the height of the platform. If the athlete cannot reverse direction quickly after making contact with the ground, the benefits of performing this exercise disappear. Most young athletes can benefit from using a 12- to 18-inch platform to improve their ability to generate vertical velocity.

POWER IN SPORTS

Tudor Bompa describes power in sport activities as "acyclic" (jumping or throwing events in the field events) and "cyclic" (sprinting, speed skating, and cycling). Each form of activity has a slightly different priority in a training program.

The acyclic athlete is concerned with a single maximal effort in an event. Although the athlete might perform the event several times during the competition, time is usually available for full recovery between events. The high-jump event in track and field and the vault in gymnastics are two examples of such sporting competition. The force and rate of acceleration become major priorities for these events. In these situations, maximal strength should always be a goal of training, but speed of movement is crucial as well. Training should incorporate rapid movement of lighter loads. Power as a result of training, technique, and execution is imperative for success in these activities. Acyclic sports that require power include the following:

• Shot put, discus, hammer throws

• Line positions (football)

• Olympic weightlifting

- High, long, and triple jumps
- Javelin throw
- Gymnastics
- Volleyball
- Diving

Cyclic events require frequency of performance for success. The role of a running back in football is an example. Despite the need for start strength and a rapid rate of acceleration, a touch of speed endurance is necessary to guarantee a fourth-quarter performance similar to the first-quarter effort. Bompa cites the need to employ lighter (30 to 50 percent of 1RM) loads performed dynamically with long (five-minute) recovery periods between sets during the strength-training phase. He also advocates using relaxation techniques to teach the athlete how to employ contraction-relaxation states during muscle use when performing. Cyclic sports that require power include the following:

- Downhill skiing
- Ice hockey
- Speed skating
- Skill positions (football)
- Sprinting (athletics)
- Rugby
- Basketball
- Boxing
- Lacrosse
- Water polo
- Cycling
- Sprint events (swimming)
- Martial arts
- Rowing
- Soccer
- Figure skating
- Synchronized swimming
- Fencing

The form of power that is required may vary from sport to sport. To say that one exercise, or one way of doing all exercises, will be effective is risky at best. Athletes will find it better to develop a power training program on the theory of specificity, particularly during the competitive phase, making sure the program meets the needs analysis conducted by the strength and conditioning specialist.

The nature of the athlete, playing time, position, body mass, limb length, and technical ability are confounding factors. What we can say is that all sports require the athlete to exhibit the physical quality known as power to achieve any degree of success.

SUMMARY

In summary, the ability to exhibit power in sports often depends on how quickly the athlete can develop maximal force within the neuromuscular system. Power, or the ability to develop that characteristic, is the result of a developmental chain. Like any other chain, the athletic chain of development is only as strong as its weakest link. Therefore, when attempting to become an explosive athlete, it is important to consider the total spectrum of athletic development.

Ballistic lifting, which includes Olympic lifts (cleans and snatches) and various accessory or related movements, is one of the foundations of developing power. Strength alone will not accomplish the ability to be explosive. The athlete must learn to combine the ability to develop force with speed of movement. These lifts are movement and speed specific for developing explosive power.

Plyometric exercises or drills are another fundamental aspect of developing power. The athlete can use these exercises for both general and specific skill development. Plyometrics are not to be performed in great volume (repetitions). The athlete should focus on quality of movement, allowing the neuromuscular system to adapt to a stimulus that challenges the body to perform.

Finally, sprint training or speed-of-movement drills are not only a training method but also a means for assessing improvement in explosive power. Improvement in sprinting speed is a result of the body becoming more reactive, which is one indication that the athlete has accomplished his or her goal.

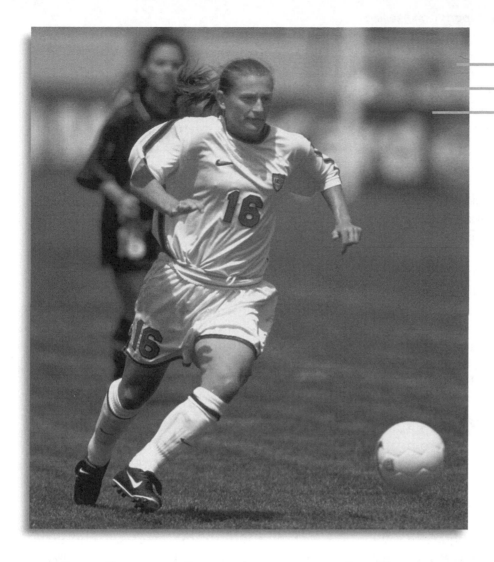

Lightning Quickness

Peter Twist

Lightning quickness is best described as the first gear of speed. While the third, fourth, and fifth gears of speed are evident during linear acceleration and ultimately measured as the velocity at the top end, the foundation for successful offensive and defensive tactics is an athlete's ability to initiate skilled movements more quickly than his or her opponents.

Lightning quickness is undoubtedly the strongest discriminator between star major pro players and stalled minor pro players. Analysis of game-breaking plays reveals that an explosive tactic created most of them. The quickest athlete will always dominate team sports that involve one-on-one confrontations and individual sports whose strategies follow a read-react-and-explode pattern.

In team sports, players must cooperate with their teammates, quickly moving into position to receive passes, drawing opponents away from the play, or blocking opponents. Each athlete moves in accordance with the rest of the play, adjusting positioning to meet changes in offensive and defensive strategies, such as a ball turnover or an opponent cutting toward the net or end zone. The most consistent contributor to successfully meeting these demands is lightning quickness.

Quickness allows small athletes to prosper in a big man's game and gives large-mass players another way to improve their game. Both need the skills to perform complex maneuvers explosively. Extend your arms straight out to your sides—quickness is often executed within this distance. Successful shooting, passing, serving, spiking, rallying, rebounding, face-offs, throw-ins, and handoffs are all fueled by quickness. Moreover, unsuccessful attempts fall back on quickness, because quickness affords young players room for error while they refine their decision making, positioning, and coverage.

Quickness is even critical to bodychecking, tackling, and blocking. First, the player must read the play, react, and move quickly into the correct position. Then the athlete must quickly drop the center of gravity before instantaneously driving upward toward the target to execute and win the collision.

BIOMECHANICAL CONSIDERATIONS

The weight transfer is just one of many movements in the sports quickness paradigm. From a biomechanical perspective, the 100-meter sprint provides a poor model for teaching sports acceleration. Practicing sprinting in a straight line may serve some bioenergetic conditioning purpose, but it has limited utility for sports that require the athlete to execute stop and start movements, lateral movements, backward movements, and turns and pivots while concurrently strategizing, reading the play, and coordinating skill execution with sports equipment. The mechanical demands of sports quickness are multidirectional and rely much more on eccentric power, dynamic balance, proprioception, and balanced flexibility.

Although quickness is often summarized as an explosive start, it can be drawn upon in many other situations. A common movement is crossover first-step explosion, such as when reacting and exploding from a stationary position, crossing over, pushing off the inside crossover leg, and lunging to return a serve with a backhand stroke. Defenders face the demand of controlling their high speed to stop on a dime and explode laterally to contain an opponent. Likewise, offensive players will cut, turn, and zigzag to evade a defender.

In these ways, lightning quickness is a learned skill that contributes to sports technique, individual tactics, and team systems. Each individual tactic relies on a series of quick biomechanical adjustments, such as the sequence of backpedaling, cutting into a power shuffle, and then jumping forward to control a turnover.

Because most team systems are dynamic, game-specific quickness is also used in transit to change velocity rapidly. For example, full-out speed is easy for a defender to handle because it is predictable. Similar speed, proper positioning, and smart angles provide the defender with all the tools he or she needs. But if the offensive player can instantaneously adjust speed, rapidly alternating between decelerating and accelerating, the defender is challenged to read and react to each maneuver. The ability to change speed quickly while already moving fast is a deceptive tactic that proves effective in throwing off a defender. Being able to shift from fourth gear to second gear and jump right back up to fifth in the blink of an eye is one of the most dangerous offensive tools.

The mechanics of quickness start with a good power position, athletic position, or ready position. During movement, the feet remain close to the ground with more horizontal displacement than vertical. During the first two or three strides, 85 percent (or more) of time is spent supported by one leg. Furthermore, directional change relies on independent leg action or weight transfer from one leg to the other. From there, quickness is manifested in many ways: forward, backward, and sideways stopping; forward, sideways, sideways crossover, and backward starting; reacting into lateral movement, cutting, turning, and spinning; backpedaling; crossing over; lunging; and controlled falling (to block a shot or dive for a ball). All these actions have unique mechanical demands. For many skills such as passing, throwing, and shooting, athletes must have effective rotational quickness.

ANATOMICAL AND PHYSIOLOGICAL CONSIDERATIONS

One of the most common sports actions, the stop-and-start, harnesses the natural system of the body for explosive force production. The underlying anatomy and muscle physiology of quickness includes sensory receptors in the muscle spindle and musculotendinous junction. The series elastic element, myotatic stretch reflex, and intrafusil muscle fibers are worth noting for their contribution to the powerful force-production process.

The stopping action loads the muscle under tension during the eccentric prestretch. This produces stored elastic (potential) energy that may increase the contractile speed of the agonist muscle during the concentric phase to produce a more explosive start. The keys to this equation are the rate of the stretch and the ability to minimize the time from ground contact to initiating the reversal of movement. Most books on plyometrics define this as the amortization phase. Because amortization has more to do with negotiating a mortgage than developing quickness and tends to confuse those new to the theory behind plyometrics, let's bury that unsuitable term forever. We will simply refer to this process as the countermovement.

During a stop, the legs are loaded with potential elastic energy when the muscles are forced to lengthen (stretch) to absorb and control the stop. If the countermovement time is too long, which means there is a slow stop or a pause at the bottom because of inadequate strength and power to reverse the movement immediately, the elastic energy is lost as heat. If the countermovement time is short, the elastic energy will contribute to a more explosive concentric contraction. So one essential goal of quickness practice is to eliminate, or more realistically minimize, the pause that happens between the end of the eccentric phase and the beginning of the concentric (coupling time) phase of movement. Drills targeting the stop-and-start will always involve a rapid countermovement and minimal coupling time, both of which are vital to producing quickness.

The myotatic stretch reflex is the "stretch receptor" in the muscle spindle. The muscle is made up of extrafusal (EF) fibers that contract or elongate under external tension to produce movement. The muscle also includes intrafusal (IF) muscle fibers, which serve as the chaperones of the EF fibers, providing feedback on the magnitude and rate of muscle lengthening as a protective mechanism. When the EF fibers elongate, the IF fibers stretch. If this stretch is rapid, the sensory neurons of the IF fibers send a message directly to the spinal cord, which in response delivers a command to inhibit the agonist muscle and concentrically contract the stretched muscle.

During a rapid stop, the quadriceps are stretched and loaded eccentrically. This produces potential elastic energy, and the sensory receptors of the IF fibers detect the rate of stretch and send a message directly to the spinal cord and back to achieve a protective concentric contraction. If the eccentric stretch is slow, the stretch receptor sends no message and no elastic energy is produced. Likewise, if the athlete lacks the strength to minimize the pause between stopping and initiating the start, the elastic energy is lost as heat and the receptor signal ceases. The countermovement rate must be rapid and the coupling time short to generate the command for explosive contraction and to harness the elastic energy as kinetic energy. Moreover, the strength to brake abruptly and decelerate rapidly simply trims down the absolute time getting from point A to point B in and of itself. For these reasons, improved stopping is the key to improved quickness!

For explosive quickness, first coach players how to stop more effectively rather than keying in on starting. Use drills that are designed to improve and accelerate braking capability to help stimulate the natural joint and muscle sensors. The stop-start action, eccentric-concentric sequence, countermovement, and center-of-gravity shift are drawn on to produce the maximal force in the shortest time.

NEUROMUSCULAR CONSIDERATIONS

To improve quickness, training must focus on the neuromuscular system. Practice drills must be structured scientifically in order for the muscles to learn to fire more quickly and to allow the brain to rehearse specific movement patterns at high speeds. Nervous-system training produces stored motor patterns of explosive complex movements. Improvement is not a physical adaptation that requires overload but a neuromuscular adaptation that requires explosive and precise movement patterns with perfect technique. This kind of training increases the ability of the brain to turn on the machine more quickly. Nervous-system training results in an increased firing rate of motor neurons, selective and maximal recruitment of fast-twitch fibers, quicker reactions, and more explosive force production.

Neurophysiological synchronization is needed to control and fire the appropriate muscle fibers in proper sequence to achieve the desired movement. This is critical given that many of the muscles contributing to sport-specific quickness are relatively small (lateral and medial rotators, adductors, and abductors) and not powerful enough for explosive contraction. Only through the summation of these smaller groups can the athlete achieve the desired movement pattern and velocity.

BIOENERGETIC CONSIDERATIONS

Synchronization is less than optimal when fatigue and lactate accumulation impede performance. So, from a bioenergetics perspective, quickness is improved exclusively with the adenosine triphosphate-phosphocreatine (ATP) energy system (thus through anaerobic training), and training is prescribed accordingly. In the game environment, however, explosive actions are often needed when the athlete is already in a fatigued state. At the end of a match, during a prolonged shift, or in overtime, the successful athlete will still be able to mobilize motor units to coordinate explosive skills under fatigue. This too is a learned ability.

DEVELOPING QUICKNESS

Coaches should evaluate athletes and then build the prequickness foundation. At all ages and levels, introduce quickness drill technique by incorporating the movements into dynamic warm-ups and agility drills. This affords athletes an opportunity to understand and rehearse the technique at casual speeds and provides the coach an opportunity to detect strength or flexibility imbalances that hamper technique execution.

At this stage, the athlete's readiness for quickness training can be assessed with a simple athleticism test. When the player performs a simple lateral stop-and-start drill, does he or she land evenly with both feet at the same time? Is the footprint consistent, or does the athlete land at different places throughout the drill? Athletes who fail this test must spend more time building their quickness foundation.

Coaches must teach and train quickness as a skill, not some genetic gift or elusive component that magically develops through standard anaerobic lactate-tolerance interval training or generic practice drills. Most coaches turn quickness training into circuit training, supersetting one plyometric drill after another. An athlete cannot increase the ability to activate muscles at a high rate by training while fatigued, moving slowly with flawed technique. Quickness practice is quality practice, not quantity practice. The athlete needs to do full-out overspeed efforts for a few seconds followed by generous recovery.

Believe it or not, one professional head coach of athletes training for an anaerobic speed-power start still emphasizes continuous aerobic training as the main (and often only) conditioning and development method! Repetitive continuous aerobic training ultimately practices recruiting muscles for slow movements, which detracts from high-velocity contraction capabilities. Too much aerobic training preferentially activates slow-twitch muscle fibers, detracts from performance, inhibits skill improvement, and blocks development of explosive quickness. Complement and support quickness development with high-velocity anaerobic conditioning.

The athlete must be lean to optimize quickness. Excess fat weight does not contribute to force production and only provides an additional load to overcome. Physical development should prioritize the legs and the speed center, or core of the body (abdominals, lower back, adductors, abductors, hip rotators, hip flexors, hip extensors, and glutes), which initiates and powers all high-speed actions. Muscle hypertrophy in the speed center and leg muscle groups also lowers the body's center of gravity. Excessive upper-body hypertrophy in lieu of lower-body mass raises the center of gravity, weakens dynamic balance and cornering, alters sports technique, and limits first-step quickness and multidirectional control.

Too often, ill-prepared athletes jump right into quick-feet drills. Some coaches and camps are overly concerned about appearing to be on the leading edge by using the "latest" drills with their athletes. Likewise, many personal trainers from a fitness background simply regurgitate memorized high-risk plyometric drills because they lack the knowledge and expertise to implement holistic sport-specific athlete development programs.

For quickness readiness, athletes first need efficiency of movement, which includes coordination, dynamic balance, agility, balanced flexibility, proprioception, and sports technique. They also require great leg and core strength, a low center of gravity, and anaerobic conditioning before progressing to explosive quickness drills. In building the prequickness foundation, balanced flexibility is the most critical. When athletes move past the foundation stage to pure quickness development, my program for them is constructed of 50 percent quick-feet drills and 50 percent micro-Stretching®, two components that in combination hold great potential for performance enhancement. Micro-Stretching (see chapter 3) produces superior flexibility and, even more important, balanced flexibility throughout the speed center. The balanced flexibility contributes not only to the quick-feet drills but also directly to improved quickness. Because the muscles are a linked system and quickness is a skill that relies on perfect biomechanics, explosive technique is impeded by muscle imbalances. Serious muscle imbalances, in strength or flexibility, prevent dynamic balance and equal quickness in all directions.

A hockey player, for example, whose left quadriceps and hip rotators are stronger and more flexible than those on the right will tend to favor the left side. When backing up (gliding) on the ice, this player will have more body weight on the left side. If the defenseman must suddenly cut laterally to the left to angle off an opposing forward, a critical delay will occur before the defenseman can explode to the left because he or she must first shift more weight to the right leg to be able to push off to the left. This brief delay results in losing one-on-one battles. The problem is exacerbated by a tight right side, which limits stride length and power. Less flexible right hip rotators are a weakness that will be exposed when the defenseman opens up to turn to the right from a backward-to-forward skating position. The player will turn at a lower angle, thus limiting defensive coverage options.

More than 99 percent of athletes do not stretch properly. I have been conducting research with Nikos Apostolopoulos on stretching for explosive skill improvement. We have a group of athletes participating in a regular program of micro-Stretching, with no other training whatsoever (no strength training, no speed work, etc.). We measured their power, speed, quickness, and agility before implementing micro-Stretching to improve flexibility in the speed center and to make sure balance exists between flexibility on the left and right sides of the body and between opposing muscle groups. Then we conducted posttests.

The preliminary results are exciting because the tendency is for players to improve their performance with flexibility training only. That includes improved sports technique, more powerful bodychecking, quicker starts, and better mobility. The key is how and when they stretch. Proper micro-Stretching has as much to do with inhibiting muscle-spindle and muscle-tendon receptors as quickness training does stimulating those receptors! A paradigmatic shift to micro-Stretching promises to make a strong contribution to quickness and explosive sports technique. The bottom line is to build the foundation first and then target balanced flexibility along with quickness drills to optimize explosive sports performance.

Stopping and Starting

Skew initial quickness training toward stopping. The majority of injuries occur not in the acceleration phase but during the deceleration and stopping needed to achieve quick direction changes. Such injuries occur because coaches, from teaching technique to training, focus on starting! Stop training includes eccentric strength, stop-and-hold, stop-and-balance, single-leg stop, lateral stop, and stopping on unstable surfaces.

Work also to improve stopping with full stop-and-start quickness drills, such as the lateral crossover stop-and-start drill (see page 108), and emphasize quick and controlled stops. Build from that, first working on minimizing the pause between eccentric and concentric phases and then on accelerating through the full stride.

On the start phase, increase foot quickness by instructing athletes to "pop" the feet off the ground. They should pop off from the toes and minimize ground contact time.

Don't forget about upper-body quickness. During strength training, no matter how much the athlete is thinking "explode," he or she must ultimately decelerate toward the end of each rep to avoid throwing the bar in the air. Medicine balls work well here and help to enhance speed-center quickness such as rotational quickness. Medicine balls help bridge the gap between upper-body power and quickness, allowing the athlete to explode through a full range of motion in a standing, more sport-specific movement pattern. For example, with hockey players I even use medicine balls on the ice, with the players on their skates. Use the principle of the quick-feet drills—rapid countermovement rate and minimal coupling time.

The athlete should always maintain a ready position with knees flexed and hips low. If the athlete has to move into the ready position before becoming set to accelerate, he or she will suffer a critical delay in initiating the required movement.

Athletes should perform at full-out effort until neuromuscular fatigue sets in. Athletes must complete rapid and precise movements to train their neuromuscular systems to organize high-velocity movements. Once athletes become fatigued, explosiveness slows, technique falters, and they finish the drill by practicing the incorrect movement slowly! For pure quickness development, limit initial drills to 5 seconds. After athletes improve, raise the limit to 15 seconds. Allow a generous rest interval to ensure that athletes do not begin the next drill in a prefatigued state.

Regeneration time, the critical part of the quickness equation, must accommodate the individual. A less fit athlete may need supplemental conditioning and physical overload to drive fitness levels up, but during quickness training this athlete, for the time being, needs a shorter work phase and a longer rest period.

In this age of premature sport specialization, young athletes need a variety of quickness drills to develop a base of athleticism and coordinate the body in many dynamic movement patterns. Do not limit youngsters only to sport-specific drills.

Incorporating Quickness Drills in Practice

For progression within a particular drill, increase the number of foot contacts to achieve in a set time, increase lateral distance, increase drill movement-pattern complexity, decrease the time to complete a drill course, use tubing to create an overspeed environment, or use partners to add competition to drills (using shadow drills or quantifying results and keeping score). A further progression is the addition of visual stimuli. For a football player, this could involve catching tennis balls during off-field drills or receiving passes during complex movements on the field. These drills remain constant because the athlete always knows where to go and when to expect the ball.

Next, incorporate visual or auditory stimuli at random times in varied movement patterns. Players may explode into action after a ball is dropped in front of them, attempting to catch it before it hits the ground again. Coaches can also call out directions. These are read-react-and-explode drills.

Although the literature recommends quickness training in the ideal situation, with short bursts and long work-to-rest ratios, competition often calls for quickness in more difficult circumstances. Explosive quickness may be required at the end of a shift, near the end of a match, in overtime, or after drawn-out anaerobic activity. So once the athlete has improved his or her quickness, the final progression is to develop his or her ability to execute coordinated and explosive quickness while fatigued. Top athletes aren't just quicker. To get an edge, they must also be able to mobilize motor units to coordinate explosive complex movements when heavily fatigued. That is game-specific quickness. To develop it, extend a quickness drill past the 15-second limit or extend a regular brief quickness drill performed in a prefatigued state, aiming for quickness-endurance. To accomplish this, lower the rest interval between drills. Whenever you want to drive up quickness again, revert to the ideal quickness environment to stimulate further pure improvements.

Coaches typically place anaerobic conditioning at the end of practice. As the next game approaches, put overspeed quickness drills at the end of practice instead so that the last thing players remember is moving explosively, rather than being exhausted and moving with poor mechanics.

Another tip is to integrate sports skills into dryland, off-court, or off-field quickness drills, and incorporate quickness development into drills done on the ice, the court, or the field to help transfer improvements into game or match performance.

When including additional skill requirements, such as carrying a puck or dribbling a ball, do not sacrifice quickness for puck or ball control. Good athletes can already perform sports skills slowly. To become great athletes, they must learn how to execute sports skills at a high rate of acceleration. Moreover, they must be able to execute skills at top-end acceleration through a variety of movement directions under balanced and off-balance conditions, and in some sports, while withstanding contact.

To help athletes break through to a new level, coaches must sanction failure by motivating players to challenge themselves. Most players will keep their foot speed, technique, and movement patterns within a comfort zone in which they know they can execute well. Athletes must push themselves past the existing limits of their abilities. They will stumble, fall, knock over hurdles, drop balls, and be off balance until eventually they can move effectively and control skill execution at the new level. Short-term failure is a requisite to optimal improvement; the coach should never criticize an athlete's willingness to extend his or her abilities. Part of motivating is assuring athletes that you view their unsuccessful attempts as a positive and courageous effort to improve themselves and, therefore, the team.

Quickness drills are already well received because they are unique, athletic, and dynamic, and because they produce immediate results. Athletes recognize the application to sports performance. Integrate aspects of play and competition into as many drills as possible. Examine children's interactive games to discover what makes them fun to play and add those components into scientifically designed drills. Fostering spirited competition among teammates drives up the work intensity and good-natured jesting. Having fun while competing hard is an incredible combination that produces the best efforts, the best results, and the most enjoyment.

Overspeed Stopping

Purpose
To improve stop quickness, stop control, and balance to achieve an optimal starting readiness position

Procedure
1. The athlete prepares by practicing depth drops, first on two legs, then on one leg, from a box height of no more than 18 inches.
2. The athlete uses tubing and a running entrance to the drill to control horizontal displacement and to create an overspeed condition.
3. The athlete executes lateral stops using a board set at a 45-degree angle. For sideways stops a single leg at a time should be used, but the athlete should practice with both the outside leg and the inside leg.

Key Points
Emphasize "stop fast, balance, and hold." The goal is a rapid and solid stop.

Lateral Crossover Stop-and-Start

Purpose

To improve countermovement rate and reduce coupling time; to practice single-leg stop-and-start moves and crossovers

Procedure

1. The athlete stands sideways to the right of a line on the floor (L_0R_0).
2. He or she transfers weight to the right foot and stands on one leg (R_1).
3. The athlete steps onto the left foot (L_2).
4. He or she crosses the outside (right) foot over the inside (left) foot and plants it across the line (R_3).
5. The athlete plants the left foot to the floor to brake (L_4).
6. He or she touches the right foot to the floor (R_5), then crosses the outside (left) foot over the inside (right) foot and plants it across the line (L_6).
7. The athlete continues executing crossovers back and forth across the line, braking each time with the outside leg.

	$L_0\ R_0$
R_3	$L_2\ R_1$
$L_4\ R_5$	L_6
R_9	$L_8\ R_7$

Key Points

In variation A, the athlete keeps all foot touches close to the line. This focuses on popping the toes off the ground, minimizing ground contact time, and decreasing coupling time. In variation B, the athlete crosses over and lands farther away from the line. This focuses on the braking or stopping action and emphasizes maintaining rapid countermovement. Coaches can mark how wide they want the athlete to move laterally and can control the pace by establishing a target number of line crosses for a set period.

Ankle Tubing Shadow Game

Purpose

To improve stop reaction and stop quickness, stop-and-start moves, lateral quickness, and deceptive tactics

Procedure

1. Athletes partner up, put on ankle tubing (short tubing connecting ankle to ankle), and stand facing each other about two feet apart.
2. One athlete, the offensive player, attempts to evade the other, the defensive player. The offensive player can move only left and right, within established boundaries; he or she cannot move forward or backward or turn and run. Only lateral shuffles are permitted.
3. The defensive player attempts to stay with the offensive player, chest to chest. The defensive player uses lateral shuffles and stop-and-start moves to react to the offensive player's direction changes.

Key Points

Athletes start and remain in a good ready position, with the weight on the toes and the hips dropped. Participants will fatigue quickly, so keep this drill short and allow more rest time than with other drills.

Double-T Stop-and-Start Hurdle Race

Purpose

To develop quick feet; to improve reactions, stop-and-start moves, and cutting

Procedure

1. Mark a course with a starting line, finishing line, and a running line down the middle. Assemble two rows of four microhurdles across the running line, using two hurdles on each side of the line.
2. The athlete sets up at starting line (A_1) in ready position and starts running explosively up the line on the command "go."
3. When the athlete is one stride behind the first row of hurdles (A_2), give a directional verbal command or hand signal indicating that the athlete should turn and run forward over the hurdles to the right (A_3) or left.
4. The athlete quickly steps over the two hurdles indicated, then comes back across the same two hurdles (A_4), lateral shuffles to the next hurdle, and turns to run forward over the two hurdles on the other side of the running line (A_5).
5. The athlete stops, then comes back across the two hurdles to the line and runs up the line to the next group of hurdles (A_6).
6. When the athlete is one stride behind the second row of hurdles, give another directional command or signal.
7. The athlete continues the sequence, completing the drill with a sprint to the finish line.

Key Points

Time each drill repetition so that the athletes can monitor their improvement and compete against teammates. Time from start to finish. Compete for best time.

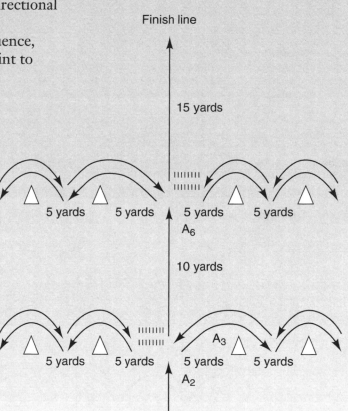

Around, Through, and Over Race

Purpose
To develop quick feet, multidirectional movement, and quick direction changes

Procedure
1. Set up a line of six cones or microhurdles.
2. The athlete begins at one corner of the course and faces squarely in one direction through-out each pass around, through, and over the cones. Each pass should be completed as quickly as possible.
3. At the whistle, the athlete lateral shuffles to the end of the line of cones, runs backward to get behind the line of cones, lateral shuffles back to the first cone, runs forward to the start, and then reverses direction and repeats the series of lateral shuffles and forward and backward running.
4. On the second circuit, the athlete runs backward to the first cone, turns and runs forward between the first and second cones, turns again to run backward between the second and third cones and so on until he or she reaches the end of the line. The athlete then repeats the pattern back to the start.
5. On the third circuit, the athlete does lateral crossovers over each cone, stops outside the last cone, then uses lateral crossovers over the cones to return to the start. Both feet must touch the floor between cones.

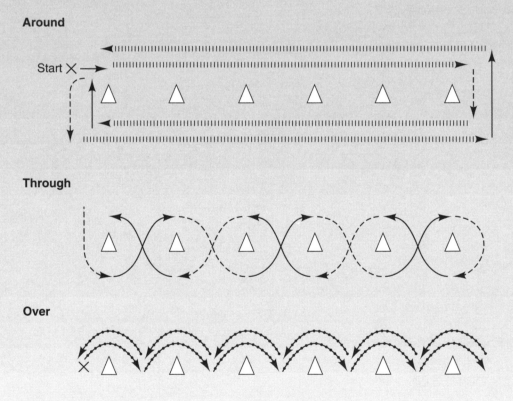

Key Points
The key is to try to make every direction change more quickly. The athlete should not use extra steps to change direction but just plant, cut, and explode!

Backward to Forward Transition

Purpose

To improve quickness and efficiency turning from backward to forward

Procedure

1. Set up a course with seven cones at various positions, leaving enough vertical space between cones for four backward steps plus an angled 5- to 10-yard sprint to the next cone.
2. The athlete backpedals four quick steps straight backward from the cone.
3. In midflight and without reducing speed, he or she turns forward and sprints to the next cone.
4. Without stopping, the athlete turns backward and begins the four-step backpedal again.
5. The athlete continues the sequence until he or she has completed the course.

Key Points

To target a weak turning side, for example, the left, place each subsequent cone farther to the left, so that the athlete turns the same way through the entire course. For equal emphasis, alternate cones to the left and right. For added challenge, mix up the placement so that the athlete, while backpedaling, must look behind to find the next cone to know whether to turn forward, to the left, or to the right.

Zigzag Cutting

Purpose

To develop quick-burst sprinting with lateral cuts and the ability to stop on a dime and explode in the opposite direction

Procedure

1. Set up seven cones in a zigzag pattern, varying the horizontal and vertical distance between cones but placing the cones no more than 10 feet apart.
2. The athlete sprints toward the first cone, plants and brakes just before it, then explodes out toward the next cone.
3. The athlete continues the sequence until he or she has completed the course.

Variations

Modify this drill by having the athlete run around each cone. Depending on placement of the next cone, the athlete will either cut or corner around the cone. This drill can also be done backward and with lateral power shuffles.

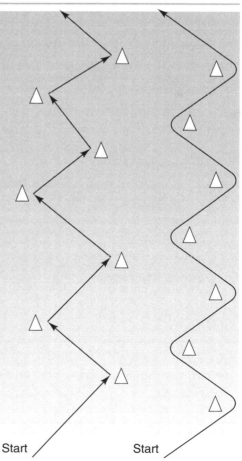

Single-Leg Towel Tag

Purpose

To improve independent leg quickness and balance and reaction skills

Procedure

1. Mark off a small area with clearly identified drill boundaries.
2. One-sixth of the group of athletes are chasers and two-sixths are "it"; half the group rests.
3. Those who are it place a sweat towel out of the top of their shorts, as in flag football.
4. At the whistle, the chasers attempt to capture the towels of the its while the its attempt to prevent the chasers from getting their towels. Players move using only one leg.
5. Once a chaser grabs the towel of an it, the it becomes a chaser and helps chase down towels.
6. The goal of each it player is to be the last one left with a towel.
7. Repeat the game having players use the opposite leg.

Key Points

Define contact or zero contact. For team competition, modify the drill so that the athlete who loses a towel is out but does not become a chaser. Keep going until every towel is grabbed. The coach can time how long it takes the team of chasers to finish the drill, and the six teams can compete for the lowest time. This drill can also be done using two feet.

Follow-the-Leader

Purpose

To improve multidirectional quickness, the ability to read and react, coordination, and mobility

Procedure

1. Split the group into partners or small teams of no more than four athletes.
2. The leader stands ready to explode out at the sound of the whistle.
3. The followers stand six feet behind the leader.
4. At the whistle, the leader tries to evade and lose the followers.
5. The followers try to duplicate the running or skating moves and pattern of the leader, staying as close to him or her as possible.

Key Points

Encourage the leader to be creative and use various types of moves—forward, backward, stop-and-start, cut, spin, roll and so on. Just define whether they have to stay on their feet or not. The followers cannot cut across to catch up to the leader; they must try to duplicate not only each maneuver but also the course of movement itself.

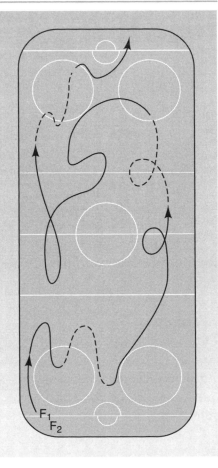

Chaotic End-Zone Tennis Ball Challenge

Purpose

To improve multidirectional quickness; the ability to read, react, and explode; and stop-and-start moves

Procedure

1. Two teams of six players set up in one-half of a basketball court in volleyball format, with two lines of three players for each team.
2. Each team's zone extends from the center-court line to the side and end walls.
3. Each player starts with one tennis ball.
4. At the starting whistle, each player tosses the ball into the opposition's zone. Balls can be placed deep or just over the line, wide or in the center.
5. Players attack each ball thrown into their zone and attempt to throw it back before the ending whistle. They must be heads up, ready to explode into action toward the balls being sent into their zone. The coach times the drill so that there are variations of between 20 seconds and 3 minutes between the starting and ending whistles.
6. The goal for each team is to have fewer balls in their zone at the ending whistle than the opposition has in theirs.

Variation

Start each player with two balls, which they can throw right away on the start whistle. This will really keep them hopping after balls thrown into their zone.

In-Place Lunge Jump

Purpose

To improve leg and hip power, contractile velocity, stride-length speed, and dynamic flexibility

Procedure

1. The athlete stands with the feet shoulder-width apart.
2. He or she steps forward with the left leg into a full lunge position, with the left knee at a 90-degee angle over the left foot (but not past toes), left quadriceps parallel to the floor, and hips low to the ground.
3. The athlete jumps up in place and switches leg positions in midair so that on landing the right leg is in the lunge position described above and the left leg is extended behind the body.
4. The athlete absorbs the landing and quickly jumps back up, switching legs in midair again to land in the original starting position.
5. The sequence is repeated rapidly 5 to 15 times.

Key Points

The athlete keeps hips low to the ground and shuffles legs back and forth. Try a variation in which the athlete jumps as high as possible, achieving maximum hang time.

Lateral Angled Box Shuffle

Purpose

To develop quick feet and improve lateral movement

Procedure

1. The athlete stands with both feet planted in the middle of the board.
2. He or she plants the left foot on the left side of the box.
3. The athlete pushes off the left side of the box with the left foot (L_1) and executes a light foot touch in the middle of the board, first with the right and then with the left , and pops both feet off the board (R_2, L_3).
4. The athlete lands on the right side of the box with the right foot (R_4), brakes, and quickly pushes off in the opposite direction.
5. He or she executes a light foot touch in the middle of the board, first with the left foot and then with the right (L_5, R_6), as rapidly as possible and then pops both feet off the board.
6. The athlete lands on the left side of the box with the left foot (L_7), brakes, and quickly pushes off in the opposite direction.
7. The athlete repeats this sequence for a set period of time.

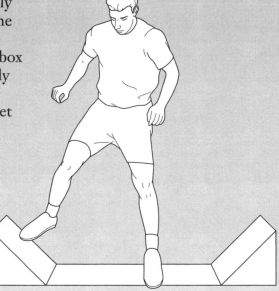

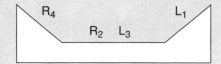
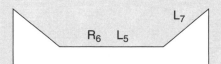

Key Points

Because the athlete completes this drill with lightning quick feet, it is not possible to track the total number of foot contacts. It is more accurate to count how many times he or she touches one side of the box, for example, counting one contact every time a foot is planted on the far right-hand side. The athlete must be up on the toes, with the hips dropped and the knees flexed. When contacting the sides, the athlete should aim for the top half of the angled box to target the hip abductors.

Low-Depth Drop-and-Cut

Purpose

To build lateral first-step explosiveness

Procedure

1. The athlete starts on top of a box 12 to 15 inches high.
2. He or she steps off the box, absorbs the landing, and reacts to the direction signal given by immediately cutting left or right for three or four strides.

Key Points

As the athlete improves, delay the directional signal so that less time is available to read and react. The athlete can also perform this drill by stepping off backward, landing backward, and, in response to the direction command, rotating one leg outward to step forward and sprint for three or four strides. A drill variation with the forward step-off is to have the athlete land and cross over before sprinting.

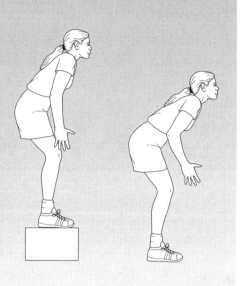

Let Go

Purpose

To improve stride power, velocity change-up, shifting gears, and neuromuscular stimulation

Procedure

1. The athlete begins with a resistance harness, belt, or parachute.
2. At the whistle, the athlete sprints full out (under resistance conditions), using quick, powerful strides.
3. After five or six strides, let go of the resistance device and yell "go."
4. With the removal of the resistance device, the athlete displays a stronger sprint and an accelerated rate of leg turnover.

Key Points

Players begin with full-out, powerful strides, but they must be encouraged to kick in a second effort upon hearing "go" to maximize their acceleration at the let-go phase. This helps teach the nervous system how to command speed change-ups.

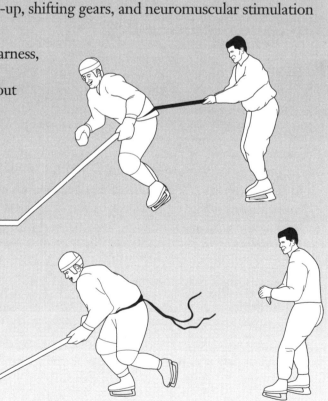

Z-Ball 21

Purpose

To improve read-react-and-explode ability and multidirectional quickness

Procedure

1. Set up boundaries for the game such as half of a basketball court or tennis court.
2. Two players partner up and compete against each other, using a Z-ball, which generates unpredictable bounces.
3. One player drops the ball from the height of the opponent's eyes.
4. Spinning the ball on release is not permitted.
5. The receiving player must keep the hands on the lower quads until the opponent releases the ball.
6. The receiving player attempts to catch the ball in bounds.
7. If the receiving player successfully catches the ball in bounds, he or she gets one point for each bounce. For example, if it bounces three times and the receiver catches it, he or she gets three points. No points are awarded if the ball goes out of bounds, if the ball stops bouncing (and begins to roll), or if the receiver drops the ball.
8. Players alternate dropping and receiving positions until one player scores 21.
9. The first player to drop receives the last drop; if player A drops first and is losing 21 to 18, he or she receives one more drop for a chance to tie. A player must win by two points.

Key Points

The key is staying low and keeping the feet moving to track the ball as it bounces around the floor. This task requires tremendous quickness, agility, and athleticism.

End-Zone Medicine Ball Put

Purpose

To improve upper-body explosiveness (and explosiveness of the legs, speed center, and full body as a linked system)

Procedure

1. Mark off two end zones at equal distance from the center of the room.
2. Two players compete against each other.
3. Holding the ball at arm's length, the first player quickly brings the ball to the chest and then pushes it away for an explosive chest pass toward the opponent's end zone.
4. From wherever the ball lands, the second player executes an explosive chest pass toward the other end zone.
5. Players alternate throws, each trying to work the opponent back until he or she can throw the ball into the opponent's end zone.

Key Points

Players throw with the full body, exploding with the legs. They complete one rep and then rest one rep, allowing for great power. Set a target score, such as a game to five, depending on how difficult it is to reach the end zone.

React-and-Sprint Tennis Ball Drop

Purpose

To improve first-step explosiveness

Procedure

1. Holding a tennis ball in each hand, stand with arms extended at the sides and the tennis balls about six inches higher than the shoulders.
2. Position the player a set distance away from and facing squarely toward you, with slight knee flexion and weight forward on the toes, ready to explode into action.
3. Drop one ball.
4. As it leaves the hand, the player reacts and sprints after the ball, trying to catch it after only one bounce.
5. The player takes an equal number of turns starting from a position facing toward, facing each side, and facing away from you.
6. When the player is not facing you directly, call out "drop" with each drop of the ball; the player must react, turn, and with a quick rotation of the hips, sprint out and cut toward the dropped ball.
7. You can also call out "left" or "right" to mandate the direction in which the player must turn, either toward the dropped ball or in the opposite direction so that the player has to turn and cut back.

Key Points

Coaches who use this drill see immediate improvement in first-step quickness because the player's ability is visually obvious. Players push themselves to the next level using this drill. Individualize the distance or drop height to challenge each player yet offer a chance to break through to new success.

SUMMARY

The ability to initiate skilled movements more quickly than opponents is the foundation for successful offensive and defensive tactics.

The first step in optimizing quickness is building a foundation. Key components include athleticism (balance, coordination, proprioception), anaerobic sprint interval conditioning (not exclusively slow, continuous aerobic training), strength (closed kinetic-chain multijoint and single-leg exercises with squat and lunge variations), and balanced flexibility (through micro-Stretching).

The 100-meter sprint model of acceleration contributes little to developing sports quickness. The mechanical demands of sports quickness are multidirectional with the emphasis on changing direction quickly. Each individual tactic relies on a series of quick biomechanical adjustments and often stop-and-start movements, which are the key to initiating game-breaking plays.

Stopping is the key to starting. Players need a quicker stop to decrease absolute time, to throw off defenders, and to harness the muscle physiology that contributes to a quicker start.

Unless the primary goal is quickness endurance, do not circuit plyometric and quick-feet exercises. Between-drill regeneration time is essential to developing explosive quickness. Don't confuse the most physically exhausting workout with the most effective quickness workout. Quickness drills are designed to stimulate maximal nerve recruitment, to teach the nervous system to command muscles to fire quickly in the correct sequence, and to replicate sports movements and techniques. As with all sports skills that involve neuromuscular adaptation, quickness requires perfect practice.

Multidirectional read-react-and-explode drills that incorporate aspects of play and competition will be well received by your athletes and prove successful for improving quickness. Encourage athletes to push themselves past their comfort zones to extend the boundaries of their abilities. Offer support for venturing and failing, a process that players must go through in order to improve quickness.

The quickest players will always dominate team sports that involve one-on-one confrontations, as well as individual sports whose strategies follow a read-react-and-explode pattern. Lightning quickness is a learned skill. Because successful sports technique, individual tactics, and team systems depend on it, quickness itself is the most important skill for sports performance.

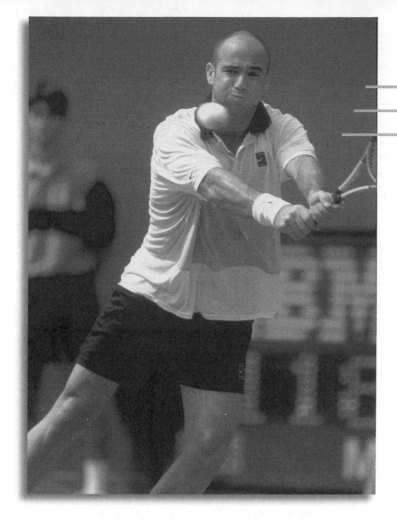

3-D Balance and Core Stability

E. Paul Roetert

A well-balanced athlete has good coordination and control when performing sports actions. When a player absorbs a hit in football or hockey, it is clear that maintaining balance is difficult; air resistance, friction, and gravity also affect how well an athlete can maintain balance. The way in which an athlete resists and handles these outside forces is called stability. The better and more sport specifically athletes train their bodies, the more balanced and stable they will be during sports performance.

119

The exercises described in this chapter relate specifically to three areas of balance and stability: (1) muscular balance, (2) dynamic balance, and (3) core stability. Although listed as separate areas of balance, they are closely related. The section on muscular balance provides a strength basis for athletes in most sports. It highlights single-joint exercises as well as multijoint exercises that are beneficial for general core strength and stability. The section on dynamic balance focuses on exercises that help the athlete control the body's center of gravity while training and competing. The core stability section features core strength exercises, which are designed for sports requiring not just flexion and extension but also rotational movements. The 3-D approach refers to training the top and bottom, left and right, and front and back of the body—in other words, the complete athlete. This type of training ensures muscular balance as well as stability during all sports activities.

MUSCULAR BALANCE

Achieving optimal muscular fitness requires flexibility, strength, muscle endurance, power, and speed. All these components should be included in a well-rounded training program. In some sports or activities such as baseball, tennis, and javelin, the dominant side of the upper body develops more than the nondominant side. Other sports such as running, soccer, and cycling may emphasize the lower body more than the upper body. And if certain patterns or muscular actions are performed repeatedly, muscles develop more in either the front of the body (in football offensive linemen) or the back of the body (in rowers). Competitors in all sports, however, benefit from a well-rounded muscular training program focusing on the front and back, dominant and nondominant, and upper and lower sections of the human body—a program that builds 3-D muscular balance. A well-rounded muscular training program—one that includes single-joint exercises as well as multijoint exercises—will help overall athleticism and coordination, prevent injuries, and, best of all, enhance performance in all sports activities.

Single-Joint Training

As the name suggests, single-joint training exercises focus on the muscle groups surrounding one joint. Single-joint exercises serve an important purpose in preparing the body for more strenuous activities. They promote muscular balance because they recruit or exercise isolated muscles or muscle groups. Although this type of training can be somewhat time consuming, the specific attention paid to each muscle or muscle group can produce significant dividends.

Leg Extension

Purpose

To strengthen the quadriceps

Procedure

The athlete should do the following:

1. Sit on the machine and adjust the backrest (if available) to a location that aligns the center of the knee with the rotating axis of the device. Bend the knee approximately 90 degrees and position the resistance pad just above the ankle.
2. Extend the legs upward against the resistance, straightening the knees fully. It is important not to hyper extend the knees.
3. Slowly lower the weight to the starting position.

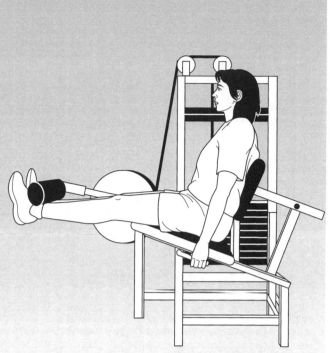

Hamstring Curl

Purpose

To strengthen the hamstrings

Procedure

The athlete should do the following:

1. Lie face down on the machine and adjust the resistance pad so that it hits on the lower third of the calf just above the ankle. The knees should not hyperextend in the starting position.
2. Slowly curl the feet toward the buttocks.
3. Slowly return the weight to the starting position.

Variation

Try bringing the weight up with both legs and then lowering it with one leg, alternating legs on every repetition.

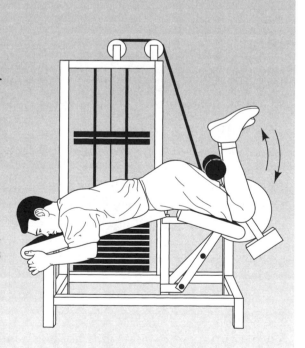

Rubber Tubing Leg Abduction and Adduction

Purpose

To develop the hip abductors, used in lateral shuffling movements, and the hip adductors, used in the split step and recovery phases. Both help stabilize the knee.

Procedure

The athlete should do the following:

1. Attach one end of the surgical tubing to a post or support and the other end to the ankle.
2. Stand approximately an arm's length away from the post.
3. For hip abduction, balance on the uninvolved leg while pulling the working leg away from the midline of the body without swiveling the hips.
4. Hold this position for at least two seconds and return to the starting position.
5. For hip adduction, balance on the uninvolved leg while pulling the working leg slightly past the midline of the body and stop before the hips begin to swivel.
6. Again, hold this position for at least two seconds and return to the starting position.

Multijoint Training

Because most sports require athletes to use a variety of complex movements, training should be performed in a sport-specific manner if possible. For example, to maximize training time and function, multijoint exercises such as squats and lunges are usually more efficient than single-joint exercises. Multijoint exercises do not isolate a single-joint activity; single joint action is uncommon in all sports. Because multijoint exercises are performed in a slow, controlled motion, the likelihood of injury is greatly reduced. This also makes them great lead-up exercises to the dynamic balance exercises described in the next section of this chapter (pages 125 through 127).

Squat

Purpose

To strengthen and balance the gluteals, quadriceps, hamstrings, back extensors, and calves

Procedure

The athlete should do the following (see page 72 for illustration):

1. Stand with the feet shoulder-width apart (the feet should point slightly outward), and hold a barbell behind the neck across the shoulders.
2. Bend the legs in a slow, controlled manner until the thighs are parallel to the ground. While bending, keep looking straight ahead, with the chest out and the back flat. Keep the weight back toward the rear of the feet and the knees over the feet (not forward). If there is a knee problem or a history of knee problems, bend the knees only 45 to 60 degrees, as tolerated.
3. Return to the starting position, keeping the head up and the back flat.

Variation

Try performing the squat while holding dumbbells at each side or a medicine ball stabilized behind the neck with both hands.

Lunge

Purpose

To work muscles in the lower extremities and trunk

Procedure

The athlete should do the following:

1. Stand with the feet six to eight inches apart, holding a barbell behind the neck across the shoulders (a).
2. Take a large step forward and drop the hips until the thighs are parallel with the floor (b).
3. Return the leg to the starting position. It may be necessary to take a few small steps to do so.
4. Keep the trunk erect throughout the exercise by looking straight ahead and keeping the chest out.
5. Alternate legs.

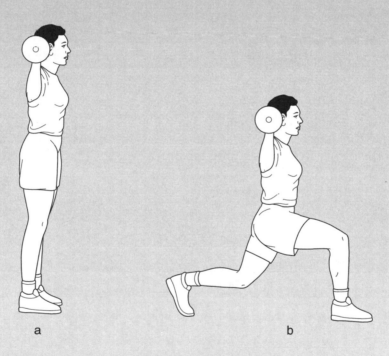

a   b

Variations

1. Crossover lunge. Instead of stepping forward, move the front leg in a 45-degree diagonal lunge (move the left leg in a crossing direction in front of the right leg and foot). Alternate between the right and left legs, using this crossover diagonal pattern.
2. Side lunge. Step directly to the right or left side, sinking into a squat position. Alternate between the left and right sides. If there are knee problems, bend the knee only 30 to 45 degrees to decrease the stress.
3. Dumbbell or medicine ball lunge. Perform the lunge while holding dumbbells at the sides or while stabilizing a medicine ball comfortably behind the neck with both hands.

Step-Up

Purpose
To strengthen and balance the quadriceps, gluteals, and calves

Procedure
The athlete should do the following:
1. Stand with a barbell behind the neck across the shoulders.
2. Using a step 14 to 20 inches high, alternately step up onto the platform and step down.

Variations
Vary the exercise by stepping forward, to the side, and crossing over to step up onto the platform. Try it while stabilizing a medicine ball behind the neck with the hands or holding dumbbells at the sides.

Leg Press

Purpose
To strengthen and balance the gluteals, quadriceps, hamstrings, and calves

Procedure
The athlete should do the following:
1. Lie on the back and adjust the seat or sled to a position where the hips and knees are bent at 90-degree angles (a). The feet should be approximately shoulder-width apart.
2. Straighten the knees and hips by pressing down into the platform until they are almost completely straight (b). Do not lock the knees.
3. Slowly return to the starting position.

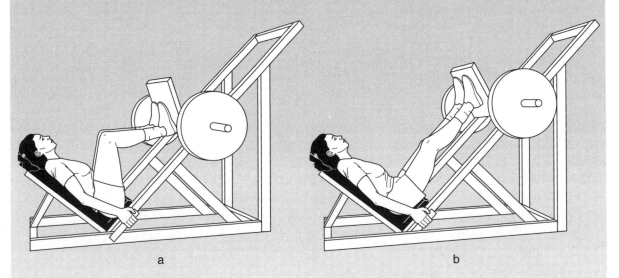

a   b

Variations
Perform this exercise one leg at a time to focus on each leg independently. A second variation is to place a six- to eight-pound medicine ball between the knees and squeeze it as the knees and hips straighten.

Push Press

Purpose

To strengthen and balance the biceps, triceps, deltoids, back extensors, gluteals, quadriceps, hamstrings, and calves

Procedure

The athlete should do the following:

1. Stand with the feet approximately shoulder-width apart with knees and hips slightly flexed.
2. Hold a barbell with the hands in a pronated position (palms facing away) about shoulder high.
3. Perform a knee bend similar to a squat and drive the bar over the head and back down to the starting position.

Variation

Try this exercise using a stretch cord or surgical tubing by standing on the cord with the feet approximately shoulder-width apart with the knees and hips slightly flexed.

DYNAMIC BALANCE

What do the following athletes have in common: a shortstop in softball fielding a ground ball, a basketball player playing man-to-man defense, a soccer player dribbling through several defenders, and a hockey player changing directions at full speed? All these athletes must have tremendous footwork and good balance. Keeping the body under control while moving is called *dynamic balance*.

Having the feet just wider than shoulder-width apart will give an athlete the most stable base of support, as shown in figure 7.1. Of course, this is not always possible during athletic competition. The key is to control the body's center of gravity, the point around which the body balances most perfectly. The center of gravity is usually a little lower in females than it is in males.

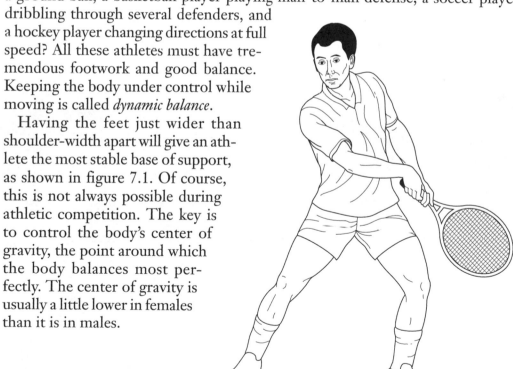

Figure 7.1 A stable base of support allows an athlete to change directions easily.

By keeping the center of gravity between the base of support (the feet), the athlete can more easily change directions. In addition, lowering the center of gravity adds stability. Great athletes in almost every sport have excellent control over their center of gravity and therefore superior dynamic balance.

Some sports depend almost exclusively on an athlete's control of the center of gravity and the ability to balance during the sports activity. As soon as the athlete loses balance, he or she loses the contest. The following sports fall into that category:

- Cycling
- Judo
- Diving
- Skiing
- Fencing
- Speed skating
- Figure skating
- Weightlifting
- Gymnastics
- Wrestling

Other sports require athletes to stay balanced while moving in relation to a moving object (a ball or puck, for example) or teammates. These sports have similar movement patterns and include the following:

- Baseball and softball
- Football
- Basketball
- Soccer
- Ice hockey
- Tennis
- Field hockey
- Volleyball

The following exercises help athletes develop their control over their center of gravity and therefore improve their dynamic balance.

Stork Stand

Purpose
To promote control of the center of gravity

Procedure
The athlete should do the following:
1. Stand on one leg while holding the ankle of the other leg, making sure to point the bent knee straight down.
2. Hold the position for 30 seconds before switching to the other leg.

Cone Jump

Purpose
To increase double-leg strength

Procedure
The athlete should do the following:

1. Line up three cones approximately two feet from each other.
2. Jump forward over all three cones with the feet together. Work to spring off the ground into the next jump immediately after landing each jump.
3. Increase the distance between the cones as improvement occurs.

Variations

A variation is to perform the drill by hopping sideways and by changing directions. An advanced version of this drill is to hop on one leg only. Adequate leg strength and balance are prerequisites for this drill.

Line Hop

Purpose

To increase single-leg strength

Procedure

The athlete should do the following:
1. Place two pieces of tape approximately three feet apart.
2. Hop laterally from line to line, trying to touch down as lightly as possible each time.
3. Continue the pattern for 30 seconds, rest for 15 seconds, and repeat for five sets.

Variations

Perform this movement pattern by moving forward while continuing to hop from side to side. Another variation is to use a deeper knee bend and hold that position for one second on each hop.

Hexagon

Purpose

To measure foot quickness in changing direction backward, forward, and sideways while facing in one direction (which simulates facing an opponent in a match); to test the ability to stabilize the body quickly between direction changes (because stability must be achieved before the next jump can be performed)

Procedure

The athlete should do the following:
1. On the ground, create a hexagon (six sides with angles of 120 degrees; each side 24 inches long) using masking tape or chalk.
2. Stand in the middle of the hexagon and face in the same direction throughout the test.
3. When the person timing the exercise with a stopwatch gives the command "Ready go," jump forward over the tape and immediately back into the hexagon.
4. Continue facing forward, jump over the next side, and jump back to the middle.
5. Repeat for each of the sides.

CORE STABILITY

Most throwing and striking sports require an efficient transfer of force from the ground up to achieve maximum acceleration of the upper limb or implement. This transfer of force is often a function of how well the upper body and lower body are connected. By strengthening the trunk, the athlete creates a solid unit capable of developing and transferring forces from the legs through the trunk to the arms and possibly the implement. The sum of these integrated forces results in optimal acceleration of the ball or implement. This is known as the kinetic-link principle, or kinetic-chain principle. Major sports in which this transfer of forces is critical for good performance include the following:

- Baseball and softball
- Golf
- Basketball
- Javelin
- Discus
- Shot put
- Football
- Tennis

Other sports repeat a certain action or movement on a continuous basis, requiring a strong midsection and trunk to keep the body properly aligned. Balance between left and right sides is crucial for good performance in the following sports:

- Cycling
- Skiing
- Rowing
- Speed skating
- Running
- Swimming

Overtraining of certain muscle groups may become a problem if workouts are not monitored closely. Training programs should be based on proper periodization principles (see chapter 12) such as variation in training and taking appropriate rest periods. In addition, training for muscular balance should not be overlooked.

Most sports require a strong trunk for proper posture or specific patterns of movement within an activity. A strong trunk (rectus abdominis) is the source of many movements and synchronizes the upper body with the lower body. Therefore, all sides of the trunk must be trained—the abdominal muscles for flexion, lower-back muscles for extension, obliques for rotation, and all of them together for stabilization and proper posture. Of course, these muscles never work in isolation. The muscles in the lower body should form a solid foundation and be able to transfer forces from the ground up. The result is optimal core stability.

Crunch

Purpose

To develop core strength in the anterior trunk region needed for most athletic activities.

Procedure

The athlete should do the following:
1. Lie on the back with the knees bent and the feet flat on the floor.
2. Hold the hands behind the head with the elbows to the sides or crossed and resting on top of the chest.
3. Curl the upper body, including the head and shoulders, from the floor until the abdominal muscles contract. Refrain from pulling the head forward with the hands. The upper body should be off the ground by about three inches at the shoulder blades.
4. Then lower the body until the shoulder blades touch the ground and repeat.

Chest Press

Purpose

To strengthen the anterior trunk and develop the pectoralis major and minor, serratus anterior, triceps, and anterior deltoid

Procedure

The athlete should do the following:
1. Lie on the back on a narrow bench with the arms externally rotated at a 90-degree angle to the torso, holding a dumbbell in each hand.
2. While keeping the wrists directly over the elbows and not locking the elbows, extend the hands toward the ceiling.
3. As the hands extend upward, round the shoulders, pushing the hands as far away from the body as possible. This extra motion works the serratus anterior muscle, which supports the shoulder blade.

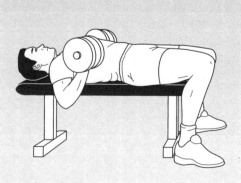
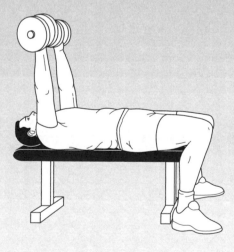

Reverse Sit-Up

Purpose
To work the rectus abdominis through a full range of motion with little use of the iliopsoas (hip flexors)

Procedure
The athlete should do the following:
1. Lie on the back with the knees bent and the feet flat on the floor. Hold hands out to the sides on the floor for stability.
2. Tilt the pelvis by pressing the back against the floor and tightening the abdominal muscles. Hold this flexed abdominal position throughout the rest of the movement.
3. Slowly bring the legs to the chest and then lower them to the ground, keeping the same degree of knee bend throughout the motion.

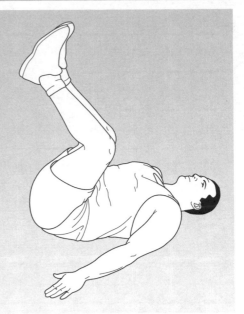

Hip Raise

Purpose
To strengthen the rectus abdominis

Procedure
The athlete should do the following:
1. Lie on the back with the hips elevated, legs straight in the air, and arms and hands out to the sides for stability or under the lower back for support.
2. Raise the hips off the ground and point the toes toward the ceiling while flexing the abdominal wall.
3. With control, lower the hips to the ground and repeat.

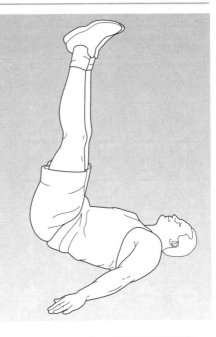

30-Degree Leg Raise

Purpose
To strengthen the lower portion of the rectus abdominis or abdominal wall to improve vertebral stabilization

Procedure
The athlete should do the following:

1. Lie on the back with the hands under the small of the back for support and the legs fully extended with toes pointing upward.
2. Slowly lift both legs together to about 30 degrees.
3. Then slowly lower the legs to just above ground level, but refrain from touching the ground (doing so would allow the muscles to rest during the movement).

Sit-Up With Legs Raised

Purpose

To develop the rectus abdominis and iliopsoas

Procedure

The athlete should do the following:
1. Lie on the back with hips and knees raised at 90 degrees and the hands behind the head with elbows out to the sides.
2. Curl the body up and attempt to touch the chest to the thighs, while refraining from pulling the head forward with the hands.

Seated Row

Purpose

To develop the rhomboids, trapezius, posterior deltoid, and biceps

Procedure

The athelete should do the following:
1. Sit with the knees slightly flexed and the hands holding a cord or band device, cable column, or seated row machine.
2. While keeping the upper body erect and the elbows close to the sides, and without leaning backward, pull the handles toward the chest and upper abdomen area.
3. Slowly return to the start position and repeat.

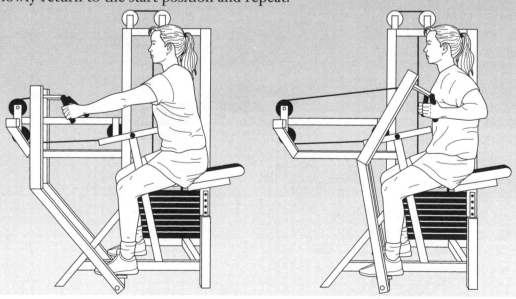

Superman

Purpose

To prevent overuse injuries or chronic lower-back pain by targeting the erector spinae muscles along the spinal column

Procedure

The athlete should do the following:

1. Lie prone on the floor with the arms fully extended overhead.
2. Lift both arms and both legs simultaneously.
3. Hold this position for one to five seconds and return to the start position.

Variation

Lift the right arm and the left leg and then lift the left arm and right leg in an alternating pattern.

Hyperextension

Purpose

To strengthen the erector spinae, which allows the lower back to absorb and exert greater forces during such actions as the service motion in tennis or volleyball and the overhead throw

Procedure

The athlete should do the following:

1. Lie prone on a table with the trunk and upper body hanging off the end.
2. Hold the hands behind the head while a partner holds down the lower body.
3. From a lowered starting position, raise the upper body until it is in line with the rest of the body or until the back is tight.
4. Then lower the upper body to a 30-degree angle or to the point just before the lower back curves.

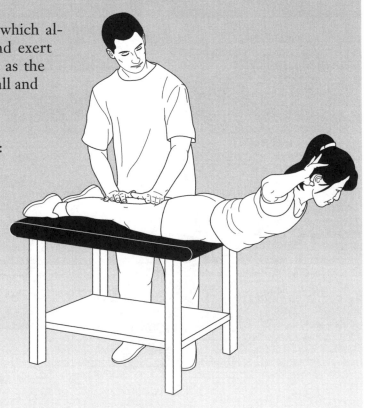

Reverse Hyperextension

Purpose

To strengthen the erector spinae to prevent injury and chronic back pain

Procedure

The athlete should do the following:

1. Lie on the abdomen on a table, letting the legs hang off the end.
2. While keeping the feet together, slowly raise and lower the legs.

Russian Twist

Purpose

To enhance trunk rotation by working the obliques

Procedure

The athlete should do the following:

1. Secure the feet on the floor, with the knees bent and the body leaning back at a 45-degree angle.
2. Hold the arms straight out from the shoulders so that they are parallel with the thighs. Holding a weight increases the resistance of the exercise.
3. Rotate to the side by turning the shoulders until the arms are at a 90-degree angle with the body.
4. Then make a full twist to the opposite side. Over and back constitutes one repetition.

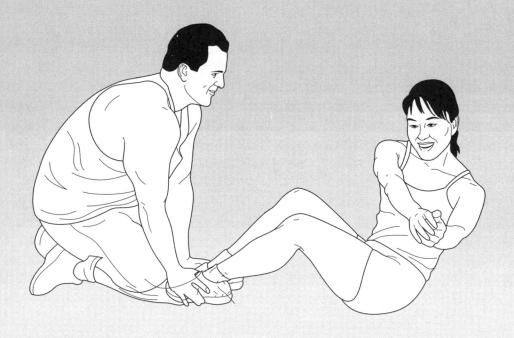

Crossover Crunch

Purpose

To strengthen the internal and external oblique muscles of the trunk, which are responsible for trunk rotation

Procedure

The athlete should do the following:

1. Lie on the back with one knee bent and the same foot flat on the floor. Bend the opposite knee so that the heel rests on the other knee.
2. Hold the hands behind the head with the elbows out to the sides.
3. Curl the upper body so that the elbow opposite the elevated knee moves toward the elevated knee diagonally. Refrain from pulling the head forward with the hands.
4. Repeat this movement on the opposite side.

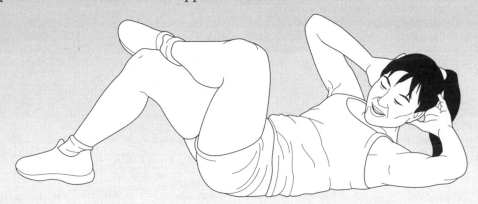

Seated Trunk Circle

Purpose

To strengthen the entire abdomen and trunk more than the basic abdominal exercises

Procedure

The athlete should do the following:

1. Balance on the buttocks with the feet six inches above the floor and the upper body leaning back at a 45-degree angle. The hands are held behind the head with the elbows out to the side.
2. Cycle the legs, alternately bringing each knee to the chest and returning it to the straight position. Do not allow the legs to rest.

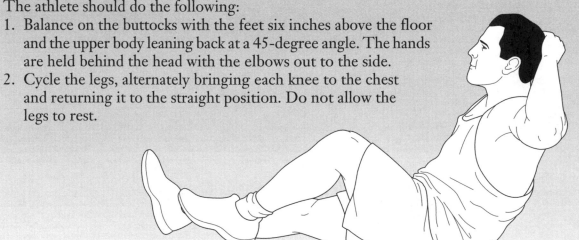

Side Raise

Purpose

To strengthen the trunk and lower-back musculature—rectus abdominis, erector spinae, serratus anterior, transverse abdominis, obliques, and gluteals

Procedure

The athlete should do the following:

1. Lie on the side with the arms at the sides.
2. Have a partner hold the feet down, or if no partner is available, place the soles of the feet firmly against a wall or other support. This makes the exercise easier to perform and better isolates the working muscle groups.
3. Lift the torso off the ground, hold for two seconds, and then lower it back to the ground. During the lift phase, imagine touching the head of the humerus (middle deltoid) toward the ceiling.
4. Repeat the exercise on the opposite side.

Variations

Clasp the hands together above the head and lift the torso and arms toward the ceiling. Increase the time interval during the lift as needed.

Hip Rotation

Purpose

To strengthen the rectus abdominis, obliques, and iliopsoas

Procedure

The athlete should do the following:

1. Lie on the back with the hips flexed and knees flexed, and the arms and hands out to the sides for stability.
2. Rotate the hips and trunk to one side until they touch the ground.
3. Keeping the knees together, rotate them all the way until they touch on the other side. Touching both sides completes one full rotation.

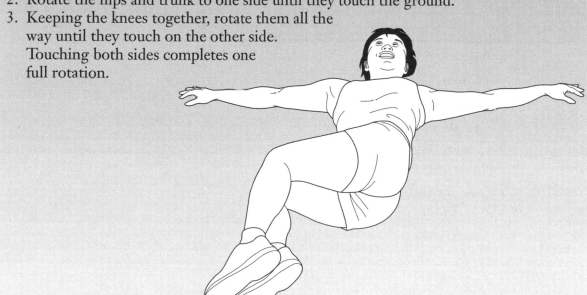

Wood Chop

Purpose

To develop the obliques and rectus abdominis for trunk rotation

Procedure

The athlete should do the following:

1. Stand 8 to 10 feet from a partner, facing sideways, and hold a four- to six-pound medicine ball at shoulder height with both hands.
2. Throw the ball to the partner using a sideways and slightly downward movement pattern; have the partner catch it and release it back to you in the same manner.
3. Catch the ball and release it back to the partner as quickly as possible.
4. Perform the same number of repetitions for each side.

BALANCE AND CORE STABILITY TRAINING PROGRAMS

Because many sports require the athlete to generate force from the ground up, why not train the muscles from the ground up? When designing a training program, think of the muscles of the trunk as a spiral staircase. Start by exercising the legs, followed by hips, midsection (flexion, extension, and rotation), and finally upper body (see sample training programs). Training in this manner follows a logical progression, and different exercises can be plugged into the circuit to add variety. Keep in mind that the goal is to develop balance between muscle groups and to train the muscles from the ground up. Two sample programs illustrate this spiral staircase model:

Spiral Staircase Training Program A

- Squat
- Hamstring curl
- Leg extension
- Leg abduction and adduction
- Crunch
- Superman
- Seated trunk circle
- Chest press
- Seated row

Spiral Staircase Training Program B

- Lunge
- Step-up
- 30-degree leg raise
- Hyperextension
- Hip rotation
- Reverse sit-up
- Reverse hyperextension
- Russian twist
- Wood chop

SUMMARY

Sports and activities can be organized in many different ways. For the purpose of this book, sports are classified in order to understand the training demands and movement patterns. It is possible to look at the muscular activity of each sport and see that certain movement skills are similar and therefore can be trained in a similar fashion. Some sports are quite similar to others in terms of the pattern of movement as well as which muscle groups need to be trained. Of course, some sports fit into more than one category.

Core stability and balance are critical for good performance in almost all sports and activities. Some sports require good balance for movement purposes, some for producing force, some for symmetry. But all athletes, no matter what sport they compete in, benefit from proper preparation. Of course, an athlete cannot perform all the exercises outlined in this chapter every day. Depending on the sport, time of the season, and fitness level of the individual athlete, exercises must be carefully selected for proper performance enhancement and injury prevention. An appropriate training program that includes key exercises will prepare an athlete for successful competition and reduce the risk of injury.

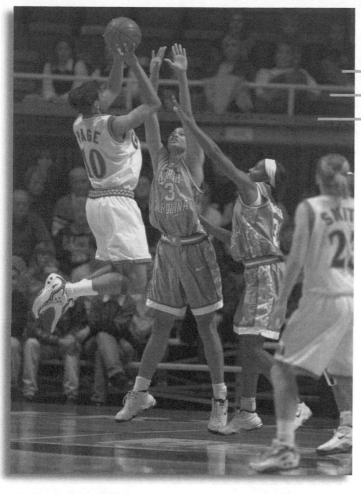

Agility and Coordination

Mark Verstegen and Brandon Marcello

Michael Jordan has the ball with four seconds left in the 1998 NBA finals. It's showtime. MJ holds the ball in his triple-threat position, his eyes processing every aspect of his defender's position. In the blink of an eye, he fakes his body one way and, with incredible efficiency, reacts opposite to the defender's commitment. He explodes past the defender with his first step, gracefully stops on a dime, spins and ascends vertically, and then pauses in midair, creating a stable platform from which to launch the game-winning shot! Another championship goes to MJ and his teammates. This sequence of events is the archetype of coordinated movement, which is the essence of every sport. If we were to break down the sequence, we would be able to fill a whole book.

Agility and coordination are the building blocks that make up sport and the tools that athletes use to express their game, whether it's the smooth yet powerful golf swing of Tiger Woods; the dynamic and graceful synchronization of arms and legs of Mike Powell propelling himself over 29 feet, 4 inches into the long-jump pit; or the wondrous balance and deception of Terrell Davis as he evades three would-be tacklers in a small space. Coaches and spectators often look at coordination and agility as the key components in determining whether someone is an athlete. Try to identify a sport that doesn't require a high degree of coordination or agility. Chances are you won't find one.

The prospect of developing and possessing outstanding coordination and agility is exciting because these movement skills transcend all sports boundaries. Contrary to popular belief, an athlete can do much to improve his or her athletic ability and movement skills. Everyone accepts without question a coach's demand that players practice for hours to improve a particular skill such as free-throw shooting. Coaches use this approach with great success in sports such as baseball, golf, and tennis; they concern themselves with the way the hands and fingers interact while gripping a ball, club, or racket and judge whether making a change might improve performance.

From the way he or she moves the arms all the way down to the way the feet interact with the ground, an athlete needs to develop the most efficient way of moving, stopping, starting, spinning, landing, and so on. Chances are that most athletes have had to figure out these basic movements and develop them on their own. We used to assume that anyone who could walk and run didn't need to take any time to further develop specific movement skills. However, an athlete who trains these skills optimally with the help of the knowledge provided in this chapter can be a significantly better athlete.

Movement is what people refer to as athleticism, the "innate" skills some people have to succeed in many sports, often spectacularly at one. There is no definitive answer as to why some people are able to perform athletic skills better than others. It goes back to the age-old argument of nature versus nurture. Athletes benefit or suffer from the environment to which they were exposed just as they benefit or suffer from the biological parents they "picked" (genetics). Nevertheless, those of us in the performance-enhancement field have yet to meet an athlete, regardless of ability, who has achieved his or her full genetic potential.

The purpose of this chapter is to provide some insight about how athletes learn the most efficient movement systems and to divulge some strategies that facilitate athletes' achieving their maximum potential. We start by briefly defining agility, coordination, and the required physical abilities. Coupling this scientific knowledge with basic movement patterns and sport-specific needs, we then present a model for improving athletic performance.

AGILITY

Agility is not easily defined because it is the culmination of nearly all the physical abilities that an athlete possesses (figure 8.1). When integrated with a coordination system, agility permits an athlete to react to a stimulus, start quickly and efficiently, move in the correct direction, and be ready to change direction or

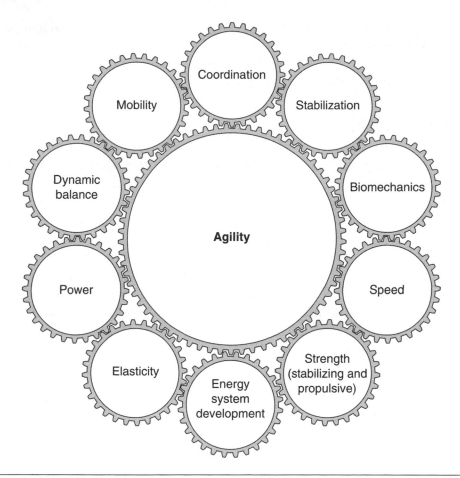

Figure 8.1 The relationship between agility and physical abilities.

stop quickly to make a play in a fast, smooth, efficient, and repeatable manner. People possess several types of agility:

- Whole-body horizontal changes of direction such as faking and avoiding
- Whole-body vertical changes of direction such as jumping and leaping
- Rapid movements of body parts that control movement of implements in sports such as tennis, squash, and hockey

An athlete who possesses high-quality agility can use it to advantage in competition. High-quality agility decreases the potential for injury, improves performance and evasiveness by allowing the athlete to fake or neutralize the competition, and refines the athlete's ability to adjust to an outside object such as a puck or ball.

An athlete can be compared with a computer system; both demonstrate a lot of power and potential. Without agility, however, the athlete is as ineffective as a computer that lacks the appropriate software—great potential but limited performance. There are two critical elements in developing agility, coordination, and skill. The role of coordination is to execute the movements chosen in response to a stimulus. The role of skill is to orchestrate these coordinated abilities into an efficient and effective set of general, special, and sport-specific movements.

These movements should be executed in a manner that uses maximum certainty with minimum time and energy. Specific acts require the use of unique qualities. When athletes struggle to achieve great agility, it is usually due to a deficiency in one or more of the qualities illustrated in figure 8.1.

COORDINATION

Taber's Cyclopedic Medical Dictionary (Thomas 1993) defines coordination as "the working together of various muscles for the production of a certain movement." In the field of exercise science, coordination is recognized as the ability of the body to organize two or more patterns to achieve a specific movement goal. Coordination involves an intricate and complex sequence of activities. Simply stated, these activities encompass reacting to sensory input (stimulus), choosing and processing the proper motor program from learned skills (motor learning), and, finally, executing the action. Information is sent to the brain for prediction, evaluation, and adjustment. The entire process occurs in a matter of milliseconds.

The process of motor learning itself can be broken into four steps:

1. Muscle movements stimulate the sensory receptors.
2. The sensory receptors send information to the central nervous system (CNS), which acts as a processor for the information.
3. The CNS executes, adjusts, or improves this information.
4. The CNS sends the information back to the required muscles via the motor pathways.

Because any external or internal stimulus can affect the outcome at any level of the process, the system is both complex and effective. This is what makes the study of motor learning so challenging.

The process of motor learning is the systematic change of movement behavior leading first to attainment and later to perfection of a certain motor skill. While learning a motor skill is complex and not completely understood, several vital steps can be identified (see figure 8.2).

- *Stimulus identification.* Athletes receive information through an external (exafferent) pathway and an internal (reafferent) pathway. The external pathway comes from external stimuli, whereas the internal pathways receive information relayed to the CNS from ongoing motor behavior. The bottom line is that the information comes in from one, or more likely a combination, of our five basic sensory analyzers: kinesthetic-proprioceptive, tactile, static-dynamic vestibular, optic, or acoustical.

- *Response selection.* The incoming information is processed in this stage. After the information has been processed, the athlete's library of existing motor programs is accessed. A selection is then made to elicit the most suitable response based on the information acquired.

- *Response programming.* Response programming executes the motor program that best fits the situation, simultaneously creating a reference to that choice. This motor program is then executed by passing through the CNS to the

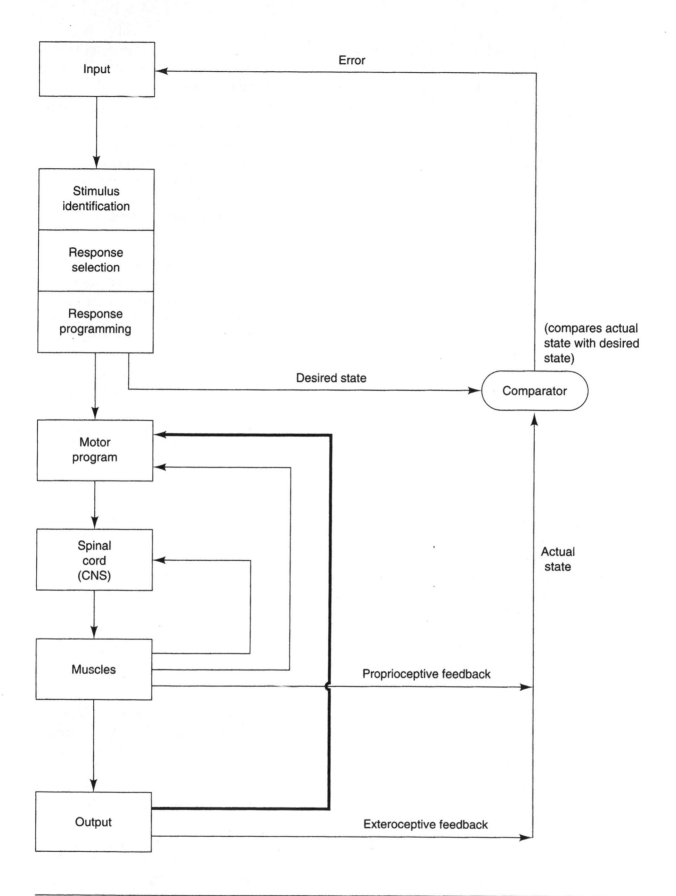

Figure 8.2 The process of motor learning.

appropriate muscles, stimulating the correct motor-unit recruitment and synchronization to produce movement. At every level of this process, feedback is being sent back and compared with the desired outcome.

- *Feedback.* Several types of feedback occur throughout the execution of this process. The muscles relay their force and length, the proprioceptors and kinesthesia report on joint position and body position, and the visual and auditory systems add information about the environment. All this information passes back up the response-produced feedback highway. The information is used to compare the actual program with the desired program and to initiate the *error elimination process* by which the body starts to suppress actions that might hinder the desired performance.

The valuable aspect of this system is that athletes learn from each action—by trial, error, and success. They discover what works and what doesn't. Remembering what was good, discarding the bad, they try again, building on the good. Through this process of adjusting and building on what works (practice), effective motor programs are laid down to be recalled with greater efficiency and effectiveness on the next task.

From the minute a coach starts developing athletes, he or she lays down the motor programs, skills, and habits that will be the basis for all future performance. The athlete's brain learns these habits by creating memorized patterns called *engrams.* These engrams are motor programs that are "burned into" the tissue protoplasm of the brain when practiced a sufficient number of times. These permanent fixtures can be either positive or negative based on the quality of what is put in.

The old saying, "Practice makes perfect" is not entirely true. It is more accurate to say, "Perfect practice makes perfect." Insist that athletes practice perfect techniques in everything they do, from the onset of movement preparation through strength augmentation to energy-system development. Accepting inefficient habits puts athletes at greater risk of injury and compromises their right to athletic success. An athlete who has developed less than optimal motor programs will need substantial time and effort to suppress the existing program and rebuild new, effective motor programs for peak performance. These new programs will be the athlete's tools for future performance, tools that will produce outcomes of better quality with less effort.

There are three main stages in coordination refinement.

- Crude coordination (general)—In this stage the athlete attempts to learn a new task and must consciously comprehend all movements. The athlete must be aware of his or her body in order to control the new task. He or she will rely heavily on visual and auditory input systems because the other senses of the body aren't quite ready to give highly accurate information. This sensory hierarchy will invert itself as the learning process progresses into fine and superfine refinement.

- Fine coordination (special)—In this phase the athlete starts to internalize how movements should feel, relying less on the visual and auditory systems, with the exception of input from the coach, and more on the depth receptors, proprioceptors, and dynamic and static contact receptors. The athlete uses feedback-chain mechanisms that refine the motor skill while inhibiting undesirable actions and enhancing the efficiency of the goal-outcome skill.

- Superfine coordination (specific)—This is the final stage of motor learning, when integration of the automated motor programs that have been cleaned of superfluous activity allows the athlete to execute movement effectively under a variety of conditions.

Within this coordination refinement process, the body learns how to improve the efficiency of desired movements. Efficiency can be increased by improving intramuscular and intermuscular coordination. *Intramuscular coordination* involves the ability to coordinate many neuromuscular units to act simultaneously to perform a muscular contraction. *Intermuscular coordination* is the cooperative interaction of several muscles in order to perform an action. Progressive loading of body weight, resisted movement methods, or assisted movement methods may significantly enhance these abilities.

FOUNDATIONS OF AGILITY AND COORDINATED MOVEMENT

Most sports require athletes to possess general movement skills. In order to excel, athletes should learn and master the building blocks of sport-specific movement.

Balance and Base of Support

Balance—the ability to maintain the center of body mass over a base of support—has long been classified as an important aspect of motor development. It is the underlying component of all movement skills, especially agility (for more on developing balance, see chapter 7).

Defining a few terms will afford a more precise discussion of the contribution of balance to athleticism. *Center of mass* is the hypothetical balance point of the body, which is located at 55 percent of height in women and at 57 percent of height in men (Hay and Reid 1988). The center of mass is a constant and will always lie within the body. Height, gender, and body type affect an athlete's center of mass.

In a static, erect position, the center of mass will be located at the same point as the *center of gravity*. The difference is that the location of the center of gravity shifts with movement; it will fluctuate within the body, and many sport actions will shift it outside the body. This shift of the center of gravity away from the center of mass creates movement.

Balance is traditionally classified into two categories, *static* and *dynamic*. Static balance is inner-zone balance, that is, standing in place while highlighting the intricate systemic feedback system and neuromuscular activity required to stay still. Outer-zone balance is how far outside the inner zone an athlete can go without losing balance. The point where an athlete loses control is the *balance threshold*.

Sport is the essence of *dynamic balance*, of being able to maintain body mass over the base of support while the body is in motion. Consider the critical role of balance within every joint of the body to align and stabilize the entire dynamic kinetic chain to produce or reduce the forces creating movement. Essentially, dynamic balance is efficiently manipulating the balance threshold. Athletes push the edge of this threshold, functionally moving in and out of balance in a way that creates fluid movement. The nature of sport presents further challenges by requiring athletes to compete on various surfaces, against opponents, in variable environmental conditions, and so forth. It should be evident that balance is critical to an athlete's agility and overall performance. Regardless of the location of the center of mass, it is advantageous for an athlete to get back within his or her base of support to keep the center of gravity in check. By gaining control of the center of gravity, the athlete takes the first step toward efficient and successful movement on the court or field.

A solid base of support, or base, creates the foundation on which the athlete can apply *positive angles*. The term positive angles refers to correct placement of the ankles, knees, and hips in relation to the torso (see figure 8.3). These body segments should create proportional angles to allow the athlete to manipulate his or her balance threshold. Positive angles within the base of support enable the athlete to decelerate, accelerate, cut, and jump by creating great leverage between a stable center of mass and the ground. This becomes even more important when outside forces such as other players and obstacles act on the base of support. Great movers in all sports possess awesome positive angles that they exploit in competition. You might have noticed that Michael Jordan would look a little knock-kneed while playing defense or before making a great move to the basket. MJ used great positive angles to be able to stop, start, and redirect his body instantaneously.

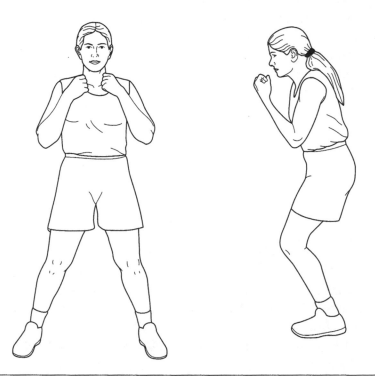

Figure 8.3   Positive angles enable an athlete to manipulate his or her balance threshold to facilitate quick changes in speed and direction.

Posture

Good posture is critical to athletic performance and is seen in an erect trunk. It is the result of good core stability, which in turn is created by a harmony of contractions by the transverse and rectus abdominis, erector spinae, and many other muscles that help stabilize the pelvic and thoracic regions. Stability is gained by drawing in the stomach, as if trying to touch the belly button to the spine while breathing dynamically. This helps create intrathoracic pressure, which acts as a stable platform from which the forces of the legs, hips, torso, and arms can be transferred more efficiently into the ground to create movement and improved balance.

Athletes perform only as effectively as they process information, relying heavily on visual input. Core stability acts as a solid foundation for the head, which should be in line with the trunk. This in turn creates a consistent, stable environment for the eyes to gather reliable information to add to the feedback system. Having dependable information is a critical component in decreasing the potential for injury and achieving a high level of performance in every position, style, and sport.

Once the trunk is stable, the correct stance depends on the sport and situation. For most applications from a static start, the athlete should sit the hips back and lean slightly forward at the waist so that the shoulders and chest are just over the knees. The knees should be aligned slightly inside the toes, and the feet should be nearly flat with the weight forward of the arch and on the inside ball of the foot. (For some sports such as tennis it will make more sense to stagger the feet under the hips.) The torso should be parallel with the forward angle of the shins. The athlete might not feel comfortable in this stance at first but will in time feel well balanced and powerful, and will create positive angles with the ground (see also chapter 7).

Foot Interaction With the Ground

How an athlete's foot interacts with the ground is as important as how a pitcher's hand interacts with a baseball or how a golfer's grip interacts with the golf club. Athletes spend countless hours perfecting technical skills, but how often do they think about how the foot hits the ground? In fact, for most positions in sport, improving foot-ground interaction can offer greater performance rewards than working on specific technical skills.

The calf represents only about 14 percent of the power within the kinetic chain, yet this component either activates or compromises all the bigger muscle groups within the chain such as the legs, hips, torso, and arms. Whether performing agility drills, practicing, or competing, it is imperative to dorsiflex at the ankle, or pull the toe up toward the shin. The toe-up position should become automatic every time the knee lifts up. Assuming this position prepares the leg to reaccelerate back down through the ground by transferring power through the forefoot back up through the kinetic chain. For most activities the foot will actually look as if it is flat, with 75 percent of body weight forward of the instep. It may be possible to slide a pencil under the heel, but the weight is definitely not up on the tips of the toes. If an athlete runs, cuts, or jumps from on tiptoe, the likelihood of injury (cumulative or traumatic) to the ankle, hip flexor, and hamstring increases and performance decreases because he or she is not able to take advantage of the ground reaction forces.

While moving laterally or cutting, the athlete should keep the toes of the lead foot pointed perpendicular to where he or she wants to go. It is common for basketball players and others to shuffle with the lead toe pointed out in the direction they are headed, literally pulling themselves along! This is exactly the opposite of efficient technique; the athlete should push with the back foot. The lead foot should continue to point perpendicularly to the desired direction, enabling the athlete to cut with the weight in the forefoot, specifically on the inside ball of the foot. The athlete lifts the front foot and pushes off the back foot. This applies even when making a transition from a dynamic movement.

Ground Reaction Forces

Ground reaction forces develop from the ability of the body to deliver force into the ground, transfer energy, and produce an equal and opposite reaction that propels the body and limbs in the desired direction. This method of movement takes advantage of innate reflexes such as the phasic spinal cord reflex of crossed extension in which the flexion of one leg elicits extension of all joints of the other leg. The elastic nature of the muscle improves efficiency and performance.

The lifting of the leg should be relatively low for multidirectional movement. The reason the knee and dorsiflexed foot come up at all is to prepare the foot to reaccelerate back through the ground and push the athlete in the desired direction. The sound of the dorsiflexed feet driven powerfully into the ground should be a series of rhythmic, hard, crisp taps. If the tapping is quiet, the athlete probably isn't putting much power into the ground, probably because he or she is trying to run up on the toes. This must be corrected in order to maximize ground reaction forces.

Reaction

Reaction will be improved by using the proper stance and weight distribution as well as taking a positive first step in the desired direction. Improved coordination from evolved motor programs will help. Reaction will be significantly improved with practice in visual, auditory, technical, and tactical anticipation.

Acceleration and Deceleration

Acceleration relies on great posture, a total-body lean, positive shin angles, and aggressive piston-like leg and arm action (see also chapter 9). Deceleration requires great relative strength and technique. Deceleration occurs during cutting and stopping with various levels of abruptness; it is critical to bend or yield to stop.

Starting Quickness

Starting quickness and first-step quickness are related to stance, reaction, and knowing where to go. A balanced stance with great positive angles helps propel the athlete in the desired direction. Make sure the athlete does not false step! The first step should attack the ground with positive shin angles, regardless of the direction the individual is going (forward, sideways, backward). Remember that a first step that strikes out in front of the hip (center of gravity) is too long and will slow the movement. One starting step, the jab step, involves short distance, quick reaction, and a movement backward of the lead foot relative to the center of gravity. (Refer to chapter 6 for more information on quickness.)

Cutting

Cutting, or executing a change of direction, requires rapid deceleration and reacceleration while performing various movements. Cutting can link movement in one direction with the same movement in another direction, or link different types of movement.

Crossover Ability

A crossover is a transition from lateral to backward or forward movement, enabling the athlete to cover a lot of distance in a short time when immediate reaction is not required. The crossover may also occur at speed. The back foot crosses over the front while staying close to the center axis of rotation. The action uses a push off from one or both feet.

Drop Stepping

The drop step is a transitional step that links any forward-facing movement with diagonal crossover runs or that effects the transition from a backpedal to a turn and run. The athlete drops the inside foot while pushing off the outside foot and then aggressively gets the dropping leg back down on the ground with power.

Backpedaling

A backpedal is a preliminary movement, traditionally used while marking or guarding an offensive player or while making a transition into cutting or linear movement.

After athletes master these individual skills, it is time to link them together in a predetermined progression.

DESIGNING AN AGILITY PROGRAM

A drill is an exercise designed to address a specific aspect of a greater skill. Today we see people train by "just doing" a myriad of drills meant to improve speed, agility, or quickness without understanding how the drills will help. Coaches continue to use these drills repeatedly without analyzing them or having a specific goal or outcome in mind.

It is important to classify drills based on how much they contribute (by percentage) to the desired motor ability (mobility, biomechanics, strength, energy-system development, and so forth). Drills should be classified as to whether they are general, special, or sport-specific exercises for a given skill, movement, player, sport, or position.

Evaluate Athletes

To improve and maximize the effectiveness of a training program, it is important to evaluate the needs of the athletes. Every drill prescribed will have some effect on motor programming, the nervous (neuromuscular) system, the energy system, and so on. Thus, to maximize the performance program, it is important to take into account the percentage of contribution and the degree of taxation each drill will have. Compare this with the needs of the athletes.

Evaluate each athlete by answering these questions:

- What is the developmental level of the athlete (age, skill, etc.)?
- What is the current state of his or her movement?
- What is the athlete's limiting factor? Is it coordination? Motor ability (i.e., mobility, strength, etc.)? A combination? See chapter 2 for tests to use in evaluating athletes.

Structure the Workout Plan

This is the fun part—time to attack the limiting factors across all motor abilities. Several methods are available to improve performance, any one of which can help athletes become faster, more agile, and so forth. But only the correct synergy between the relevant variables will maximize athletes' performance *most efficiently*. The workout plan is the culmination of the scientific and artistic aspects of coaching. Remember that no part of the body is totally independent from other parts. Every exercise or drill affects motor programming, the nervous system, the metabolic systems, and so on. Understanding the extent and importance of each variable, as well as which components the drill or exercise focuses on, is critical to proper exercise selection and the success of the program.

Drills and exercises are tools to help athletes accomplish their goals. Drills are powerful tools if they are properly organized, prescribed, progressed, and mastered. To help athletes get the most out of their workouts, coaches should do the following:

- Plan a specific goal for each movement session.
- Strive for perfect technical execution of every rep, every set, every drill, and every skill.
- Remember that quality (proper execution and intensity) is far more important than quantity ("just doing it" or volume).
- Work on simple skills before complex skills; that is, work on preprogrammed (closed) skills before random (open) skills.
- Have athletes master fundamental (general) movement skills before progressing to more advanced (special and specific) skills.
- Attack fundamental limiting factors systematically instead of "shotgunning" everything.
- Provide accurate feedback with visual and auditory cues, and encourage athletes to use sensory input.

- Work on stride frequency (rapid response, quickness, adjustment, deceleration) and stride length (short and long, power).
- Remember: starting is extending and stopping is bending.

Each workout should include the basic components of movement preparation, biomechanics work, neural innervation, and, finally, coordinated movement drills.

Movement Preparation

The goals of movement preparation are to elevate the core body temperature; actively elongate the muscles; activate the nervous system, proprioceptors, and stabilizers; improve kinesthetic awareness; and work on technique by reinforcing critical motor programs daily.

Essentially, movement preparation is warming up in a way that is similar to the way the athlete plays. This segment of the workout is designed to maximize the active ranges of motion required for fluid, high-performance movement. These exercises incorporate and reiterate correct posture, core stabilization, balance, coordination, and range of motion through all planes of movement. Movement preparation is divided into three categories that follow a specific order—from low-level activities that increase core temperature to higher intensity sport-specific dynamic movements that prepare the athlete for training or competition.

1. Warm-up. Start with basic, active movements such as a sprinter's jog, side sweeps, carioca, weaves, spins, or even light games that improve kinesthetic awareness.

2. Joint mobility. This type of work mobilizes and strengthens segments of the body in flexion, extension, and rotation. These drills actively ease the body into motion, gradually elongating and preparing the muscles for more intense dynamic flexibility. Examples include the drop lunge and side lunge (see chapter 7, page 123).
   - Lying supine or prone (hip crossover series, leg-overs, and scorpions)
   - Standing (standing torso rotations and diagonal patterns)
   - Moving (forward, backward, and lateral hand walks; drop lunges; and over-and-under hurdles)

3. Dynamic flexibility. Dynamic flexibility work consists of a progression from walks, marches, and skips through runs, which start at the feet and progress up the body toward the head. These movements start slowly with small amplitude, then progress into large, fast movements that activate the performance systems essential for practice or competition. Two components exist within dynamic flexibility—general and specific. The general component involves movements that target body areas and is not specific to any sport. The specific component matches the types of movements within a particular type of workout session or competition.

Biomechanics Work

This is a fundamental component of every drill or exercise. The material principles—dorsiflexion, positive angles, arms, posture, core, ground reaction—are built in and executed with feedback in every aspect of the athlete's performance. At this point the athletes are thoroughly warmed up and tuned in; this is the time to establish the day's goal or lesson plan. For novice athletes, this training segment may take a significant amount of total workout time.

Neural Innervation and the Stretch-Shortening Continuum

We use neural drills not only to improve the elastic properties of the muscles but also to improve the athletes' motor learning and comprehension of the overall workout. Select these drills by considering first the goal of the training session, then where they fall within the progression from beginning to intermediate to advanced (see table 8.1* on the next page).

1. Rapid response. These drills require high neuromuscular frequency through high velocity and low force. The best analogy is moving your limbs like a sewing machine. Rapid-response exercises improve various types of coordination and lay the foundation for a progression from movement skills to higher level plyometrics. Examples of rapid-response drills would be over-the-line jumps and hops and coordination patterns (see chapter 6, pages 109 to 117) and ladder drills.

2. Short response (minimal yield). Short-response drills require minimal yield (amortization) and possess a low frequency, a higher amplitude, and a higher force. The best analogy is a Super Ball instantaneously rebounding after it hits the ground. In these drills you want your athletes to be "springy," minimizing the time in contact with the ground (switching from eccentric to concentric muscle contraction). Perfecting these drills will help the athletes become more elastic. Examples of short-response exercises are ankle and tuck jumps (see chapter 5, page 88), reactive step-ups (see chapter 7, page 124), and low depth jumps (see chapter 5, page 95).

3. Long response (long yield). These drills require longer yield, lower frequency, moderate amplitude and force, and maximal rate of force development. The action in these drills is analogous to a heavy kid on a pogo stick who compresses the spring along its entire length and then explodes straight up into the air. Long-response exercises develop speed strength by letting the muscles go through a more complete range of motion before executing an explosive, maximal contraction. Examples of long-response plyometrics are squat jumps (see chapter 5, pages 89 to 90) and split jumps.

4. Very long response. These drills require very long yield, moderate to high amplitude and force, and maximal rate of force development. This type of action definitely blends into speed and explosive strength. The movements include some types of resisted movement jumps, certain medicine ball throws, traditional weightlifting movements at various intensities (see chapter 4, pages 69 to 73), eccentric manipulation, and isometric and concentric exercises done with maximal rate of force development.

Movement Drills

This is the actual application of the lesson plan, incorporating into the drills all the elements specifically aimed at attacking the factors that are limiting an athlete's performance. Follow this progression for effective learning:

Table 8.1 Plyometric Continuum

	Rapid	Short	Long	Very long
Upper-body movement				
Pressing	Running or seated fast-arm movements Wall chest pass	Chest pass with partner Punch pass and throw Chest pass with lateral movement	Medicine ball chest pass Explosive push-up	
Throwing	Cuff dribble Walking wall dribble Body blade	Overhead pass	Vertical jump	
Rotating	Rotational twist	Short ball routine	Medicine ball drills: • chopping • swing pass • rotational power throw • rotational overhead throw	
Lower-body movement				
Vertical	Bunny hop Jump rope	Jump rope Pogo stick Tuck jump Jump over obstacle Depth jump One-leg tuck jump	Jump-up to box Vertical jump Power skip Dip-and-drive step-up Squat jump Power step-up Split jump High depth jump	Vertical medicine ball throw Resisted vertical jump Reactive jump
Linear	Jump rope Ladder drill Over-the-line drill Quick skip, jump, hop Run in place Box run Backward or forward jumping jacks	Ankle skip Bounce and go Jump over low obstacle Bounding Tuck jump Depth jump Box bound	Power skip Medicine ball throw and chase Standing long jump Standing triple jump Multiple long jump Medicine ball knee punch Crossover dip-and-drive Crossover power step-up Crossover power skip	
Lateral	Lateral ladder drill Lateral over-the-line drill Lateral bounce	Lateral quick bound Lateral box run Lateral depth jump Lateral box jump (to sprint) Lateral jump over low obstacle Lateral quick hop	Lateral bound Lateral squat jump Lateral dip-and-drive Lateral hop Lateral high depth jump	Resisted lateral bound
Multiplanar	Ladder Over-the-line drill Rotational jumping jack Rotational pogo stick work	Spin jumps Leg external rotational jumps Medicine ball with partner (back to back) Figure 8 throw Medicine ball rotational throw Leg external rotation hop	Medicine ball drills: • chopping • swing pass • rotational power throw • rotational overhead throw Depth jump with spin	

*In each movement category in table 8.1, exercises are listed from those for beginners to those for more advanced athletes. Some drills noted in this table are described in chapters 5 through 7 in detail. For more plyometric exercises, see D.A. Chu, 1998, *Jumping into plyometrics, 2nd ed.* (Champaign, IL: Human Kinetics).

1. Preprogrammed closed skills with variations such as eyes closed, shoes off, resistance or assistance, uneven surfaces
2. Preprogrammed with outside stimulus such as a ball, hand signals, or commands, progressing to random agility (open skills)
3. Random agility progressing from reaction to a single stimulus to reaction to several stimuli or sensory input systems

Closed Skills

In preprogrammed closed-skill movements, athletes know exactly what is expected of them; these drills allow athletes to go through the initial stages of motor learning and to progress within a controlled environment. Closed-skill drills can then be progressed through volume, rest intervals (performing at fatigue), and often resisted movement or assisted movement methods. After the athletes have refined the motor programs within preprogrammed movement, move on to random agility by getting them to react to outside stimuli such as claps, directional signals given by hand, other athletes, kinesthetic awareness, and so on.

Complex Training *Complexing* refers to a protocol that combines some form of training stimulus that activates high levels of neuromuscular excitation with a complementary activity such as jumping or running, with the goal of improving performance. A physiological phenomenon results from the high demand placed on the system by heavy strength exercises; resisted runs, jumps, or throws; or specific plyometrics that improves the summation and synchronization of the desired motor units. These neuromuscular changes last between two and five minutes. There are two main ways to maximize this window. The first way is to extend an already very short set by 7 to 10 seconds, and then take a prescribed rest interval for the set. Second, the athlete can take a two- to five-minute rest if the excitation exercise is more demanding. Empirical evidence indicates that various types and depths of excitation may enhance performance for several hours. As a guideline for trying to match or exceed the previous altered experience, use a ratio of two or three aided reps followed by one or two free applied reps.

Resisted Movement Resistance training provides several benefits:

- Increased coordination through summation and synchronization
- Increased stride length through specific coordination strength
- Kinesthetic learning through nonvisual, nonauditory senses
- Improved biomechanics.

A standard recommendation is to resist specific movements between 5 and 15 percent 1RM. This ensures that the training is enhancing the specific skill, not creating a new motor program. However, using much heavier resistance is effective during specific drills. For example, using an appropriate harness system and attaching a thick or doubled-up bungee cord on the athlete's right hip, then significantly assisting and resisting the athlete during the right-foot cutting action requires the athlete to drop the hips, establish positive angles with the weight on the inside ball of the dorsiflexed foot, and focus on loading and exploding off the outside leg. The same principle holds true in teaching the feel of acceleration by having athletes lunge, march, and run through very heavy sled pulls, push objects, or run up very steep inclines. These exercises teach athletes to have great forward total-body lean, hip separation, back-side extension, and front-side flexion.

When using any type of external resistance or assistance, be sure to follow the product safety guidelines.

Assisted Movement   Assistance training is extremely effective in slightly raising athletes' performance ceiling by exposing the body to higher rates of movement. It is important not to assist athletes beyond 5 to 15 percent of their unaided performance. The goal for the athlete is not to let the assistance do the work but to relax, using efficient biomechanics to "outrun" the device. If assistance negatively alters technique, it is exceeding the athlete's current potential, and the amount of assistance should be lessened. Examples of assisted movement are running downhill at a 3 to 5 percent grade and using assisted pulley and rope systems or bungee cords.

Open Skills

Open skills are required in order to react to an outside stimulus perceived by the sensory input systems. The open skills that comprise random agility—reacting to a ball, an opponent, an obstacle—are essential for success in most sports. To prepare for competition, then, the athlete is enrolled in a chaotic environment to simulate sport through specific movements. Begin training random agility by adding a simple outside stimulus, such as a change of direction given by hand, to mastered preprogrammed work. Another step in the progression is to add assistance or resistance to these now-random drills. The ultimate measure of random agility may be competitive tag games such as mirror tag, shark-in-the-tank tag, freeze tag, and others. This type of game provides an opportunity to evaluate what the athletes have learned and whether they can apply it in a random, chaotic, competitive environment. Use these games to highlight specific instances of success or failure as they relate to the goal of the movement session.

Each of the following drills can be varied to help the athlete progress from closed-skill movements (complex, resisted, and assisted) to open-skill or random linked movements.

Lateral Wave

Purpose

To teach cutting, dynamic balance, positive angles, foot interaction with the ground, and elastic muscle strength

Procedure

The athlete will move laterally between two points three to six yards apart. He or she should do the following:

1. Keep the body erect and stable, and keep shoulders and hips parallel.
2. Rapidly cut to the outside leg, then push back in the other direction
3. Repeat.

Variations

Beginners should work on mastering cutting technique, then progressing volume and speed. More advanced athletes should perform the drill wearing an elastic cord around the waist that is tethered to a fixed object. Add an outside stimulus to make the drill more random, then progress to using resistance and assistance methods while reacting to the outside stimulus.

Crossover

Purpose

To teach the crossover step and develop dynamic balance and elastic strength needed for deceleration

Procedure

The athlete will move between two cones three to six yards apart using a crossover step. He or she will do the following:

1. Keep an erect posture with a solid base of support and keep shoulders and hips parallel.
2. Drive the left leg across to the right by rotating from the core, pushing the left foot through the ground.
3. Square the hips back into a position parallel with the shoulders to help decelerate with positive angles.
4. Repeat, moving to the other side with the opposite leg.

Variations

Progress from walking to doing this drill at all-out speed. Then add assistance and resistance to accentuate the kinesthetic learning and improve deceleration. Progress further to random linked movements by accelerating in all directions in response to an outside stimulus. Apply resistance and assistance from both sides.

Cone Wheel

Purpose

To link various motor skills such as lateral to backward or forward, crossover, drop steps, and so forth

Procedure

1. Set up a circle of cones with a three- to five-yard radius.
2. The athlete starts at one cone and picks a movement pattern to use to move around from cone to cone, linking each movement with other skills.

Variations

Make this drill more advanced by adding assistance and resistance and working on the transitions between linked skills. Have a partner roll balls randomly within the cone area, rolling or throwing the next object the instant the previous one has been caught.

Ball Drop

Purpose

To develop stance, reaction, one-step acceleration, and redirection agility

Procedure

The athlete should do the following:

1. Stand erect with the weight on the balls of the feet and face a partner four or more yards away who holds a ball at the top of his or her reach.
2. Explode toward the ball with a positive first step as the partner releases it. Drive the arms back to enhance acceleration.
3. Try to catch the ball before it hits the ground a second time.
4. Have the partner move back in one-yard increments each time the athlete succeeds.

Variations

Try the drill facing sideways or backward, turning and exploding instantaneously to catch the ball. Have the partner yell the moment the ball is released. Also try incorporating rapid-, short-, or long-response plyometrics or various starting positions. Or use multiple balls so that the object is to get ball two or three.

One-on-One Tag

Purpose

To incorporate acceleration and deceleration from a balanced base and to react to a random situation

Procedure

1. Mark a clear playing area of 10 × 10 yards (for beginners) or 15 × 15 yards (for more advanced athletes) and have athletes form two lines at opposite edges of the box. One line is made up of taggers; the athletes in the other line are "avoiders" (who try to avoid being tagged).
2. Have the first tagger sprint toward the avoiders, decelerate, and gain his or her balance as the first avoider comes out and makes a move to get away from the tagger.
3. Once the avoider is tagged or reaches the opposite edge of the playing area, the next two athletes in each line take a turn.

Variations

Start the line of avoiders facing away from the taggers and call "go" when the tagger is halfway across the playing area. Toss a ball to the avoider before he or she makes a move to avoid the tagger.

Shark-in-the-Tank Tag

Purpose

To incorporate and randomly link together all preprogrammed drills

Procedure

1. Create large playing area with boundaries (approximately 20 × 50 yards).
2. Pick one to five "sharks." Everyone else is a "minnow." The sharks try to catch the minnows.
3. Time how long it takes each shark or team of sharks to tag the minnows.
4. Watch athletes for positive or negative instances of agility and movement. Reward those who are tagged early with some core, balance, stability, strength, and conditioning exercises to do while they are waiting for the game to finish.

Variations

Change the game by increasing the shark-to-minnow ratio up to 1:10, by increasing or decreasing the size of the playing area, or by changing the game to freeze tag (in which the athletes may move to unfreeze tagged teammates). These variations require more strategy, greater energy-system demands, and a higher level of movement skills.

Implement Your Program

To introduce a drill to athletes, clearly define the name, purpose, procedure, key points, and the specific role the drill will play in making the athletes better during competition. The athletes will then have a clear understanding of what they need to do. Offer feedback verbally and visually during the workout through coaching cues, demonstrations, and video. Don't forget that one of the best ways for athletes to learn is by sensory input that is nonverbal and nonvisual (Brisson and Alain 1996). The emphasis of the teaching and the structure of the practice must provide opportunities for the learner to develop skill in all processes involved in the performance of the particular motor tasks. In other words, place athletes in situations in which they will learn by doing and feeling.

Treat drills to improve agility in the same manner as speed work. Have athletes perform these drills while they are fresh, in the prescribed order, and with ample rest for most phases of development. Eventually, athletes will achieve high levels of performance in the required skills. Then use the drills after inducing progressive levels of fatigue; this mimics the conditions athletes experience in the competitive environment.

After athletes master individual skills, it is time to link them together. Start with the same rules used for the progression of preprogrammed (closed) drills, focusing on making efficient transitions from one motor program to the next. Once these various motor programs are seamlessly linked together, progress into random (open) drills. The amount of motor learning that has occurred will be evident in the athletes' execution of the random drills. Only those athletes who have engrained all the specific patterns will express movement skills effortlessly to achieve efficient movement. Inform the others, during and immediately after the session, which aspects of the drill they need to work on.

Follow these guidelines as athletes progress from beginner to advanced stages:

- Beginners—Use the prescribed order at the beginning of the practice. Technique is more important than speed. The goal is to establish the foundation.

- Intermediate—Use the prescribed order, progressing intensity, density, and volume. Have the athletes perform the drills before or during practice.

- Advanced—Vary the order, intensity, density, and volume. Have the athletes perform the drills before, during, or after practice.

During the general preparatory phase of training, the goal is to establish a conditioning foundation. The most effective way of doing this is to spend a lot of time working on movement preparation activities. Teach general and special movement skills. Teach and prepare proper foot interaction with the ground using a variety of rapid-response activities as well as low-level short- and long-response activities. Enhance energy-system work with creative games played barefoot on sand, grass, or turf.

The special preparatory phase builds on the general preparatory phase. Work on mastering special skills in preprogrammed work, mixing altered (resisted and assisted) movements with free movements. Progress all drills gradually after athletes demonstrate mastery so that the athletes are continually challenged. Increase complexity or intensity of rapid-, short-, and long-response drills to improve the athletes' ability to withstand eccentric forces within the ankle, knees, hips, core, and so on.

After athletes have mastered the various special skills and can perform them under altered conditions, start linking them together. Athletes should focus on mastering every combination of preprogrammed drills. Incorporate random exercises. An example of linking using lateral and base movements would be lateral to straight ahead, left, right, and backward accelerations.

Once athletes have mastered special drills and have started linking pre-programmed movements, it is time for them to start applying these actions to sport-specific sequences. This will greatly enhance their speed, and more important, will improve their movement efficiency. When the learned sport-specific linking has been burned into a skill, challenge athletes with a variety of random (open) skills, increasing the complexity and intensity while insisting that they express perfected, engrained motor skills.

SPORT-SPECIFIC DRILLS

This section highlights some major areas of each sport and shows how to combine the special motor programs to create efficient sport-specific movement skills. Linking is the critical element. The ability to link movements together provides the competitive edge in elite-level athletics. The athlete who can link movements can create separation or close ground. He or she has a quicker first step, jump, or cut.

In sport-specific drills, athletes combine special skills and sport-specific links in the most random (open), chaotic environment possible. Clearly, athletes who can execute these links subconsciously in this environment have mastered the movement skills necessary to react during competition.

Football

Football requires diversity of movement skills based on positional requirements. For simplicity, the positions are broken into three main categories, grouping both offense and defense:

1. Line, which includes offensive and defensive lines as well as defensive ends
2. Combo, which includes linebackers, strong safeties, tight ends, and fullbacks
3. Skill positions, which include running backs, wide receivers, defensive backs, and quarterbacks

Line

Defensive ends require great explosion and acceleration skills tailored to running on an arc, quickly regaining balance, and redirecting agility to pursue an agile quarterback or a scampering running back.

Players in the offensive and defensive lines must be able to manipulate balance. They must explode for run blocking, moving past their balance threshold by delivering force to another lineman. At the same time, they must be able to regain their balance immediately when the player they are blocking comes off the block. They must possess the skills to drop the hips within the base immediately, staying on the feet so that they can quickly pick up another player. Athletes who can do this also reduce their chance of injury.

Teaching movement skills to line players is critical. Chances are that they were the big kids who were always sent over to hit the bags and work in the post. Meanwhile, all the smaller kids their age were exposed to countless hours of running, cutting, and agility work. This scenario explains why late-maturing athletes tend to be the best in the end. Offensive and defensive line players will often make the greatest gains and benefit the most from movement skill training.

Combo

Individuals who play combo positions must possess the power and size to deal with the line as well as the movement skills to react and compete with the skill players. Players at these positions will need a lot of integration of movement training throughout their development of hypertrophy and relative strength so that every pound is highly coordinated and innervated. Tight ends and fullbacks must have blocking skills and be able to apply the movement skills that are crucial for skill positions (deceleration, power cuts, spins, and speed cuts in the open field). Linebackers must be proficient in using their lateral and base programs as the foundation for explosive first-step quickness. They must also be able to drop step to open the hips so that they can fall back into coverage using the crossover motor programs. The crossover step will also be useful to them in linking their lateral and base positions.

Skill Positions

Players at skill positions tend to cover more ground and operate in open-field situations more frequently. Wide receivers have the advantage of being able to master preprogrammed (closed) routes and vary them based on their opponents' defense and options within the play. They must be able to cut at speed using the inside leg heavily to cut at angles less than 90 degrees and be proficient in the use of "power cuts," which use the outside foot to redirect at an angle greater than 90 degrees. Players at all skill positions use the same skills, linked with various movements such as backpedaling, drops, crossovers, and so on. These athletes will benefit greatly from kinesthetic awareness drills such as decelerating, drop stepping, and keeping the foot close to the center axis; they can use the skills practiced in these drills to link transitions and transfer to spinning. Players should master general and special skills thoroughly and then spend a majority of their time applying these tools in random movement activities, such as various tag games and competitions. Speed, elasticity, and relative strength will be major long-term developmental goals for athletes at skill positions.

Tennis

Movement skills in tennis are critical to success and often determine both shot selection and the ultimate outcome of each point. Dynamic balance is highlighted in tennis, not just during movement but also in the instant just before ball contact with the racket. Moreover, players must be able to recover their balance to avoid leaving the rest of the court open. Tennis movements are broken into three main areas: close proximity, wide-ball recovery, and baseline to volley.

Close proximity is the area within approximately four meters of the offensive position, usually around the center mark where the players hit the majority of their shots. The critical movement skills are lateral and base, allowing the players to move with perfect balance to offensive or defensive forehands and backhands. In tennis, the base stance allows the athlete to be poised for lateral movement.

Wide-ball recovery occurs out around the doubles alley or beyond. The critical components are squaring up with improved balance and positive angles, linked with a single powerful crossover step, linked with a lateral and base slide. Players must keep the base so that they can make any shot required.

Baseline to volley starts with the multidirectional stance, which enables players to react in a 360-degree arc. They must take a positive first step; link together three to five explosive, accelerative steps; and then link into deceleration and lateral and base (split step), making sure to keep the hips down. This will put them back in perfect position to react to a great volley and recover immediately into a good stance to repeat the action.

Baseball and Softball

Baseball and softball have a variety of positions. On the defensive side of the ball, movement packages are broken into infielders, outfielders, catchers, and pitchers.

Infielders rely heavily on their sensory input reactions to send a message to link their effective stance with a powerful first step, crossover, deceleration, and get-up skills.

Outfielders must use visual stimuli and be able to link that with the correct movement selection (first-step quickness straight ahead, crossover, or a drop step). Outfield movement requires many types of transitions. An outfielder may need to use a drop step, crossover running, acceleration, and absolute speed to fill the gaps. Smooth transitions between these movements will lead to superior performance.

Catchers must work on reacting from the catching position. Starting them in proper position will drive concentric muscle action, because their elastic energy will have dissipated. Catchers must react quickly and possess blocking skills. They must be able to throw to various positions, execute crossover steps, accelerate, and decelerate. Progression of these skills with eyes shut or looking upward can improve agility.

Pitchers require special attention, both on and off the field. They should develop their specific skills from various postpitch positions. They must be able to accelerate or execute a crossover while maintaining balance during total-body deceleration. Practice will decrease the chance of their making an awkward, off-balance throw to which their body is not accustomed and that may result in injury.

Offensively, the roles of assorted baseball and softball players are much more similar. The movements that help players get out of the box quickly and increase on-base percentage are activities that link rotational movements with acceleration skills and transitional backward or forward speed. Softball players can enhance base-stealing skills through drills in which they anticipate the pitcher and then apply acceleration, maximizing the first steps by using the bag. In baseball, players can improve base-stealing performance by assuming the proper stance. Players can do this by sliding back and slightly opening up the right foot to the instep of the left, achieving positive angles with both legs. The back should be flat with a slight lean forward. The player should lean to put 70 percent of the weight on the forefoot, and keep the arms relaxed in front of the body. During the steal, the arm action should be rotating the right elbow back, linking the crossover program to acceleration. The player should aggressively drive the arms and legs "back, back, back." For baserunning, baseball and softball players should practice their stride patterns, using body lean in the turns. Be sure that players run both ways around the bases.

Soccer

A fundamental rule to remember is that movement is king in soccer. Consider that the average player touches the ball less than 2 percent of the time. Of course, a player who develops movement skills can win more balls and increase that percentage! Soccer movement requirements depend on the position. Distance from the goal is a useful way to categorize requirements.

Goalkeepers need to work especially hard on stance, reaction skills from all positions, crossover steps linked to jumping and diving, landing and tumbling, and a modified base stance to give them the best opportunity to react in every direction, including vertical and horizontal jumping.

Fullbacks must work on acceleration and deceleration linked to a modified lateral and base so that they can position themselves to react to the offensive player. To make these linked skills more specific in drills, have athletes take a position against an opponent. As with all positions in soccer, fullbacks will greatly benefit from working on S-style runs.

Front-line players (forwards) should concentrate on being able to link many different skills. They cover significantly greater ground than other players and benefit from being able to link acceleration to transition. Players should train modified absolute speed while being bumped along the way by another player. Many drills require the linking of movements while moving fast. Soccer players should become proficient at all special and specific stride-frequency drills to enhance their ability to dribble at speed.

Basketball

Movement requirements in basketball depend on the position, but the distinctions are becoming blurred as bigger athletes gain more movement skills. The primary movement in basketball is lateral, not vertical. On the defensive side of the ball, every player must have mastery of the lateral and base movements, with the emphasis on both toes facing fairly straight ahead and pushing with the back leg, not pulling with the front leg and the toe opened up. Players must be able to move in this way while keeping a base so that they are always moving within balance and able to react to their opponent. (The stealthy offensive player will exploit the defender who brings his or her feet together!) Players must link movement skills to cutting and crossovers back to the base stance.

On the offensive side of the ball, it is critical to work on a stance that sets up the right positive angles in order to gain the effective first-step quickness that can create separation. Players should then link the stance to acceleration, deceleration, vertical jump, and spinning.

Cycling

Agility and coordination are essential requirements in cycling. Coordination promotes a smooth and efficient pedaling action; cyclists must build specific co-ordination motor programs to pull the toe, heel, and leg up from the six o'clock position to the one o'clock position. Agility comes into play as riders constantly push their balance threshold by leaning and by bumping with competitors. Core stability plays a huge role in efficiently controlling the normal cycling action and in maintaining balance during turns. Serious cyclists should practice and master the special skills of rolling and tumbling to decrease their injury potential in case of a mishap.

Volleyball

Volleyball is a game composed of acts of agility. Defensively, blockers must work on developing the base stance that readies them for lateral movement. They must develop crossover to base components and then link them with vertical jumping. These athletes must learn to link the inertia from lateral movement to a vertical jump by redirecting ground reaction forces. Defensively, backcourt players must master the stance; they must maintain positive angles, keep their weight forward by bending the legs and hips, and maintain good posture in the receiving position.

Offensively, setters need to be proficient at linking every movement skill. This is their world. Outside hitters must be incredibly agile so that they can link several explosive accelerative steps, then decelerate and transfer this energy through positive angles and a stable core to vertical movement. Once airborne, the stable torso acts as a platform that allows athletes to maintain balance, generate spiking forces, and stick the landing without going into the net.

Golf

Golf relies heavily on the coordination system to maximize the kinetic linking required for a flawless swing. Balance and stability play a huge role in the golf swing. Golfers must stay within a stable base of support in order to turn ground reaction forces into rotational movement. They must transfer this energy into a disassociation of the shoulders and hips, creating a coiling effect while maximizing the stretch reflex cycle. Development of club-head speed is a result of the ability to accelerate the body segments while maintaining balance. Golfers also possess a highly evolved sense of kinesthetic awareness and can effectively use sensory feedback.

Gymnastics

Gymnastics is a perfect example of a sport in which athletes master general and special drills and then link them together to produce awe-inspiring physical acts. We believe gymnastics demonstrates the underlying role that balance plays in agility. Kinesthetic awareness is enhanced by a well-developed sensory feedback system. Gymnasts learn to rely on nonvisual, nonauditory cues.

Track and Cross Country

Track and field and cross country are sports in which performance is measurable and finite. They are also sports that require very special motor skills. Agility plays some role within every event, probably reaching its highest expression in some of the throwing events that require spins or rapid deceleration. Agility drills complement all the workouts of runners and jumpers, enhancing coordination patterns and muscle balance in strength and flexibility.

Wrestling

Wrestling relies heavily on agility. This combative sport is built around using balance and leverage to disrupt the balance of the opponent.

SUMMARY

Enhanced movement skills make great athletes. Movement is sport. Athletes are born with an inherent set of gifts that they can maximize with this approach. Success in achieving these goals is up to the athletes. They must realize that these are learnable skills. Every step they take builds the foundation for the future. Ensure success by demanding perfect technique. Perfect practice will lead to peak performance by developing the multisensory feedback system. This system enables athletes to learn rapidly through trial and error. Remember that athletes learn efficiently through nonverbal, nonauditory input. The reward for mastering general and special movement skills is a decreased potential for injury, improved athleticism, and strong, efficient movement programs that link together to produce efficient, high-performance, sport-specific movement.

Manipulating the dynamic nature of balance is the underlying foundation of agility. Athletes need to develop all of the coordination and physical tools, including core stability, mobility, speed, elasticity, power, strength, and energy systems. Doing so enables them to achieve incredible movement skills, sustaining them throughout competition to achieve the ultimate victory—reaching their potential! Enjoy the exciting process of teaching, learning, progressing, and challenging athletes to become great "wired-up" movers.

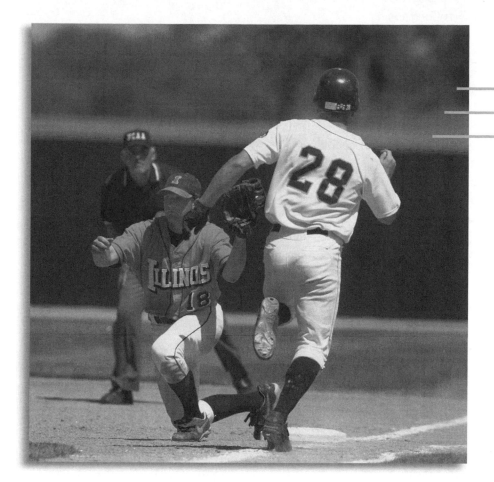

Acceleration and Speed

George Blough Dintiman

*I*n most sports, athletes start from either a stationary or a partially moving posture and attempt to reach maximum speed as quickly as possible. This is referred to as acceleration, or the rate of change of velocity. Speed refers to the point at which athletes can accelerate no more and have reached their maximum rate of movement. At this point, athletes attempt to hold that pace as long as possible and to minimize "slowing" due to fatigue, friction, and air resistance.

Rates of acceleration vary from one athlete to another. In some 100-meter races, Carl Lewis was still accelerating at the 70-meter mark. Although his acceleration rate was less than that of his competitors in the early part of the race, he continued to increase speed longer, allowing him to pass athletes in the final 20 meters. Other athletes also accelerate more slowly only to reach higher speeds later in the race. Speed (maximum miles per hour) can be mathematically determined from world records in sprint events. The current world record of 19.32 seconds in the 200 meters is equivalent to an average speed of 23.5 miles per hour. Splits of world-class sprinters provide a more accurate indicator of just how fast humans can run. Studies indicate that 20-meter segments (from 60 to 80 meters, and from 70 to 90 meters) in a 100-meter race are covered in as little as 1.6 seconds, equivalent to a speed of 27.9 miles per hour.

Sports are played with multiple starts and stops and many changes in direction. It is no surprise that the average speeds players attain during competition are well below their maximums. On only a few occasions will athletes accelerate for 60 meters, the approximate distance it takes a world-class sprinter to reach maximum speed. A triple in baseball, a 100- or 200-meter sprint in track, and a long run in football, rugby, soccer, or lacrosse would approach or exceed 60 meters. What people generally refer to as speed is more accurately termed acceleration to maximum speed.

For decades, acceleration and speed have been recognized as two of the most important qualities an athlete can possess. Skeptics cling to the belief that speed is a God-given genetic quality that one is born with and that no type or amount of training can bring about change. Since 1912, 100-meter world records have improved from 10.6 (Donald Lippincott, USA) to the current record of 9.79 set in 1999 (Maurice Green, USA)—a change of only 0.81 seconds, or 7.64 percent. The 200-meter world record improved from 20.6 in 1951 (Andy Standfield, USA) to 19.32 in 1996 (Michael Johnson, USA)—a difference of 1.28 seconds, or about 7.16 percent. Women's 100-meter and 200-meter times showed larger improvements of 1.3 seconds (9 percent) in the 100 meters and 2.26 (9 percent) in the 200 meters (Lawson 1997).

It is difficult to determine the contribution of new training programs and new equipment (starting blocks, all-weather synthetic tracks, modern shoes) to these improved times. And the change from manual to electronic timing on January 1, 1977, undoubtably eliminated previously inflated times that obscured some of the improvement in the previous analysis.

Although coaches still recruit "fast" athletes, they now realize that every athlete can improve speed. Coaches are also aware that dramatic improvement of acceleration and speed in Olympic-caliber sprinters is difficult to attain; as athletes approach their maximum potential, less room is available for improvement. This is not so, however, for most high school and college athletes, who can improve their 40-yard dash times by as much as 0.7 seconds in only eight weeks.

It is now widely accepted that everyone can improve acceleration and speed, but rarely will any athlete approach his or her genetic speed potential unless the correct training techniques are followed.

Decades ago physiologists uncovered changes to muscle fiber types (fast-twitch white and the intermediate fast-twitch red) following the completion of the training programs discussed in this chapter. Since the early 1970s, researchers have also been aware that stride rate (steps per second), stride length, and speed in short distances improve with proper training. This knowledge has broadened training emphasis from programs that focused mainly on form and anaerobic conditioning to a holistic approach that includes programs that also alter stride rate and length.

If reaction time (RT) or response to a stimuli—the starting gun in track; the center snap or movement of an opposing player in football; the crack of the bat in baseball; the impact of the racket in tennis; the faking action of an opponent in ice hockey, lacrosse, rugby, or soccer—is eliminated, only three areas of change can directly cause improvement of acceleration and speed:

1. Taking faster steps (increasing stride rate) without decreasing the length of each stride

2. Increasing the length of each stride without decreasing stride rate

3. Using sound biomechanics (form)

A fourth area, anaerobic endurance (speed endurance), has an indirect effect on acceleration and speed by reducing slowing at the end of a long sprint and permitting repetitive short sprints to occur at the same rate, relatively unaffected by fatigue.

This chapter focuses on the training programs that affect these four areas and that bring about improvements in acceleration and speed that are specific to various sports.

FACTORS AFFECTING ACCELERATION AND SPEED

No body design is perfect for sprinting. Numerous body types and variations in height, weight, and length of levers have proved effective. Present-day Olympic sprinters are slightly heavier and taller than those of 30 to 50 years ago, but geometrically they are no different. Fast sprinters come in all sizes and shapes, with smaller athletes taking shorter strides but faster steps than their taller counterparts.

Several physiological factors, however, affect both acceleration and speed, including genetic factors such as fast-twitch and slow-twitch fiber percentages, body fat, age, gender, and anaerobic or speed endurance.

Muscle Fiber

Three types of muscle fiber are found in various parts of every athlete's body:

- Slow-twitch red (type I)—This fiber type relies on oxygen to produce energy (aerobic). It develops force slowly, is fatigue resistant (high endurance), and has a long twitch time, low power output, high aerobic capacity for energy supply, and limited potential for rapid force development and anaerobic power.

- Fast-twitch red (type IIa)—This intermediate fiber type can contribute to both anaerobic and aerobic activity. It develops force moderately fast and has moderate fatigability, twitch time, power output, aerobic power, and anaerobic power.

- Fast-twitch white (type IIb)—This fiber type does not rely on oxygen to produce energy (anaerobic). It develops force rapidly, and has fatigability (low endurance), a short twitch time, high power output, low aerobic power, and high anaerobic power.

Muscles with a high percentage of fast-twitch fibers exert quicker, more powerful contractions. Individuals born with a high percentage of fast-twitch fiber in the muscles involved in sprinting have a higher speed potential than those born with a preponderance of slow-twitch fiber, which is more suitable for cross country, marathon running, and other sports requiring high aerobic endurance. Inherited percentages of fiber type are similar in both men and women. Although the theory that slow-twitch fibers can be changed into fast-twitch fibers is controversial, new evidence suggests that prolonged high-intensity training may produce that effect and improve the ratio of fast-twitch to slow-twitch fibers.

Table 9.1   Approximate Percentages of Fast-Twitch Fiber in Speed and Endurance Athletes

Type of activity	Men	Women
Speed-based activities		
Sprinters (100 or 200 meters)	48–80%	72–75%
Ice hockey players	44–62%	——
Shot-putters, discus throwers	50–88%	45–52%
Endurance-based activities		
Cross-country skiers	25–45%	25–50%
Cyclists	25–50%	35–65%
800-meter runners	40–64%	25–55%
Untrained individuals	25–62%	25–72%

Source: Dintiman, George B., 1984. How to Run Faster: Step-by-Step Instructions on How to Increase Foot Speed. Champaign, IL: Leisure Press.

The right kind of high-intensity training (heavy load) will recruit and train the fast-twitch fibers and aid in the improvement of acceleration and speed. Although "training fast to be fast" is a key principle for improving acceleration and speed, it is the intensity (load), not speed, that activates fast-twitch muscle fibers.

Table 9.1 compares the amount of fast- and slow-twitch muscle fiber found in a study of speed and endurance athletes. Postural muscles such as the soleus are composed mostly of slow-twitch fibers whereas large locomotor muscles such as the quadriceps contain a mixture of both fiber types, which permits both jogging, a low-power output activity, and sprinting, a high-power output activity. Numerous studies have found sprinters to possess high amounts of fast-twitch fiber.

Body Fat

Body fat of 6 to 10 percent of body weight for men and 12 to 17 percent for women is desirable for sprinting short distances. It is important to be aware that the lower range for both men and women may be unhealthy even for athletes, depending on the individual. On the other hand, excess fat provides useless weight that negatively affects both acceleration and speed.

Age

Age eventually affects all aspects of athletic performance. The average age of 41 male world record holders in the 100 meters from 1912 to 1999 was 23; for 21 female record holders it was 24.5. Only three male athletes, Barnes Ewell (age 30) of the USA, E. McDonald Bailey (age 31) of Great Britain, and Carl Lewis (age 30) of the USA, set world records after the age of 30. Two record-setting female athletes, Fanny Blankers-Koen of the Netherlands and Shirley Strickland of Australia, were also 30. The late Florence Griffith Joyner of the USA was 29 when she set the current world records in the 100 and 200 meters in Seoul, South Korea, in 1988.

With the onset of hefty endorsement contracts and the resurgence of interest in track throughout the world, sprinters are now motivated to remain active for longer periods. Consequently, Carl Lewis and others have been able to maintain their speed well into their 30s, something unheard of in the past. No physiological reason exists for speed to diminish significantly from age 25 to age 35 unless the athlete ceases training, loses strength and power, or adds body fat.

Gender

Gender is a factor in sprinting. World records by men in the 100 meters are 0.75 seconds faster than those by women. Studies in the 1980s indicated that Olympic male sprinters had a stride rate of about 5.00 steps per second whereas female sprinters had a stride rate of 4.48 steps per second. The faster stride rates and longer strides of males appear to account for the time differences. Although hormonal and anatomical differences exist that have implications for acceleration and speed, now that female athletes are finally receiving proper training, they are increasing in strength and power, and improving at a faster rate than men in both the 100-meter and 200-meter events.

Speed Endurance

Speed endurance (anaerobic energy) will not change stride rate or stride length, at least on the first short sprint. But it will determine the amount of slowing at the end of a long sprint, the pace at which acceleration to maximum speed occurs, and even speed on repetitive short sprints. In other words, athletes with poor speed endurance are unable to accelerate and sprint at the same high level repeatedly during competition because of fatigue. Ideally, athletes run the fourth or fifth sprint as fast as the first. This often does not occur because of inferior speed endurance.

Anaerobic metabolism occurs at the onset of any type of exercise to provide an immediate source of quick energy until circulatory and respiratory adjustments occur. All sprints under six seconds rely almost exclusively on the phosphagen system; those lasting six to nine seconds begin to rely on lactic acid. In short-term, heavy exercise, the only significant energy available is the breakdown of the phosphagens, adenosine triphosphate (ATP) and creatine phosphate (CP), and glycolysis, the breakdown of glucose to pyruvate and lactic acid. Speed-endurance training develops both systems. Sprinting always takes place in the absence of oxygen, a condition under which the skeletal muscles can function for only a short time. When oxygen requirements exceed the ability of the body to uptake oxygen, pyruvic acid forms from glucose and is reduced to lactic acid. This process (anaerobic glycolysis) occurs only in the absence of oxygen, producing energy-rich phosphate bonds to allow muscle contraction to continue. About eight seconds of maximum-effort sprinting nearly depletes these quick-energy stores.

At this point (much sooner for the poorly conditioned athlete) slowing occurs because of lactic-acid buildup. Improved lactic-acid tolerance, increased quick-energy stores, and improvement in the rate that quick energy is available are related to factors such as anaerobic fitness, age, and nutrition.

Mechanics

Although no two athletes run the same way, proper sprinting mechanics are similar for everyone. Removing errors in arm action, body lean, foot contact, overstriding, understriding, and tension can improve acceleration and speed.

TESTING AND EVALUATION

Before personalized programs can be designed to improve acceleration and speed for any sport, the strengths and weaknesses, or limiting factors, of each athlete must be identified. This approach also helps athletes avoid the common tendency to work on strengths and avoid weaknesses. Although chapter 2 covers the subject in detail, the critical test areas for acceleration and speed are briefly discussed in the following sections.

Sprinting Speed

A stationary 120-yard dash with 40- and 80-yard splits, combined with a stride-length test, reveals an athlete's stride rate and acceleration. Unless a high-speed camera is available, stride rate is determined mathematically using the second 40-yard time and length of stride; acceleration is rated acceptable if the difference between the two 40-yard times is less than 0.7 seconds.

Speed Endurance

The drop-off index compares the time taken to cover the last two 40-yard segments in a 120-yard dash—the 40- to 80-yard segment and the 80- to 120-yard segment. A series of 6 to 10 repeated 40-yard dashes using a rest interval similar to the rest period in a specific sport, such as the length of the huddle in football (25 to 30 seconds), also provides an excellent indication of speed endurance. Standards for these two tests devised by the National Association of Speed and Explosion (NASE) are no more than a 0.2-second difference for the drop-off and no more than a 0.4-second deviation from the best time for any of the repetitive 40-yard sprints. This test can be done manually with stopwatches and flags on each finish tape or by electronically timing splits.

Stride Length

Stride length can be easily measured without high-speed cameras by having athletes run naturally through a 20-yard area. It is a simple matter to measure the distance between two footprints.

Athletes can compare their strides to those of top sprinters using the following formulas (which indicate guidelines for ideal stride length):

Male sprinters:	$1.14 \times$ height (+/- 4 inches), or
	$1.24 \times$ height (for athletes under age 16), or
	$1.265 \times$ height
Female sprinters:	$1.15 \times$ height, or
	$2.16 \times$ leg length

Coaches should also watch for understriding and overstriding and make a note of either in order to help each athlete find his or her ideal stride length.

Strength

Use the one-repetition maximum (1RM) for a free-weight squat or the leg press on a Nautilus station to determine a ratio of strength to body weight. A ratio of 1:2.5 or 1:3 or more—a free-weight squat or a leg press score of two and a half to three times body weight—suggests a desirable ratio for optimum development of acceleration and speed.

Explosive Power

The standing triple jump, vertical jump, and double and single 20-yard leg hops provide some indication of an athlete's potential for speed improvement and mild insight into the amount of fast-twitch fiber in the muscles involved in sprinting.

Muscle Balance

The prime movers in sprinting are the knee extensors, hip extensors, and the ankle plantar flexors. Comparing the strength and power of left limbs to right limbs, agonists to antagonists, upper body to lower body, and strength to total body weight provides valuable information. Improving the strength of muscle groups that are already near optimum levels and avoiding areas of weakness is unlikely to produce much improvement in acceleration and speed.

An imbalance usually exists between the knee extensors and the flexors. An even greater imbalance is often found between the posterior leg compartment muscles (plantar flexors) and the anterior compartment muscles (dorsiflexors). A strength imbalance between two opposing muscle groups, such as the quadriceps (agonists) and the hamstrings (antagonists), also produces serious limitations. The strength of the hamstring muscle group is a sprinter's weakest link. It should be improved to 70 to 90 percent of the strength of the quadriceps group. A minimum ratio of 70 percent is recommended for the prevention of injury. Ideally, leg extension (quadriceps muscle group) and leg curl (hamstring muscle group) scores should be the same. In almost every athlete at all ages, however, the quadriceps muscles are much stronger than the hamstring muscles. The average leg curl score in 1,625 middle school and high school football players tested in NASE speed camps was less than 50 percent of the leg extension score.

Flexibility

Because flexibility is joint specific, a single test does not provide an accurate assessment of range of motion (ROM), and it is impractical to measure the ROM of every joint. In addition, the flexibility of some joints is not critical to acceleration and speed. Tests are available that involve little equipment and provide a fair assessment of ankle flexion and extension, shoulder flexibility, and hamstring flexibility.

Body Composition

Unless underwater weighing equipment is available, the most accurate and practical method of determining percent of body fat is the skinfold technique. Measure at least four sites to get the most accurate test. Because people carry weight differently, it is best to measure a site on the upper body (triceps, biceps, subscapula, suprailiac, abdomen), lower body(hip, thigh), front of body, and back if possible.

SPEED-IMPROVEMENT TRAINING PROGRAMS

Although speed-improvement training programs are similar for most sports, each should be sport specific in terms of exercises, repetitions, duration, rest interval, and distance or time. Some forms of training may require more emphasis depending on individual test results.

It is also important to apply the principles of periodization by structuring the training into phases for improving acceleration and speed. Phases of each training area should be organized according to the competition schedule to produce peak performance at the most important times. See chapters 12 and 13 for more on periodizing training.

Functional Strength and Power

The purpose of the functional strength and power program presented in table 9.2 is to develop a strong foundation that optimizes the improvement of acceleration and speed and that develops the required force and tissue capacity for the sport. Periodized weight training in this six- to eight-week phase emphasizes strength, speed, and endurance and involves a program of general exercises for the legs, back, shoulders, chest, arms, trunk, abdomen, and neck starting at 60 percent of a 1RM weight. The Olympic lifts (table 9.3) are added in the second four week microcycle and involve heavy weight, near maximum muscular contractions, low repetitions, and full recovery between sets. Key exercises recommended for improving acceleration and speed follow. Chapter 4 describes the techniques for the execution of many of these exercises.

- Olympic lifts: clean (barbell and dumbbell), jerk (barbell, dumbbell, and machine rack), and snatch (barbell and dumbbell). The suggested program using the Olympic lifts (see table 9.3) includes a wide range of intensity, with loads increased to or near 1RM. Maximize rest between sets to reduce fatigue.
- Legs and back: dead lift, calf raises, front squat, leg extension, and leg curl.
- Shoulders and arms: incline press, bench press, dumbbell arm curls, lat raise, lat pull-down, fly, sprinting arm movements holding dumbbells.
- Hamstring muscle group: Olympic lifts and leg curls. Specific hamstring exercises should be included in each workout because this is a neglected area.

Strength training in the weeks just prior to competition should focus on weight-training exercises that mimic the sprinting action such as sprinting arm movements with dumbbells, kick backs on a leg press station (from a sprinter's starting

Table 9.2 Functional Strength and Power Program for Advanced Athletes

Exercise	Mon.	Tue.	Wed.	Thu.	Fri.
Warm-up: Flexibility	•	•	•	•	•
Power					
Clean, power	M		M		
Snatch, power		M		H	
Jerk, rack	H		M		L
Legs and back					
Pull, clean	M		L		H
Dead lift	H		M		
Squat	L		M		H
Squat, front					M
Shoulders, chest, and arms					
Bench press	H		M		
Incline press		M		H	
Rowing	H		M		L
Flys, supine			L		M
Trunk and abdomen					
Trunk hyperextension			3 × 10 (60%)		3 × 10 (70%)
Sit-ups (bent knee)	3 × 25		3 × 25 (60%)		3 × 25 (70%)
Neck					
Partner four-way neck	3 × 8–12		3 × 8–12		3 × 8–12

Light (L)		Medium (M)		Heavy (H)	
60% 1 × 5		60% 1 × 5		60% 1 × 5	
65% 1 × 5		70% 1 × 5		75% 1 × 5	
70% 1 × 5		68% 1 × 5		85% 1 × 5	
				69% 1 × 5	

position), knee lifts, pull-downs, and other weight machine exercises that simulate exact movements in the start, acceleration, and sprinting phases.

Plyometric Training

Plyometrics revolve around jumping, hopping, and bounding movements for the lower body and swinging, quick-action push-offs, catching and throwing weighted objects (medicine balls, shot puts, sandbags), arm swings, and pulley throws for the upper body. These exercises are critical in developing strength and power in the muscles involved in sprinting. Plyometric training was partially responsible for the unusual progress and success of Russian sprinter Valeri Borzov, a 100-meter gold medalist (10.14) in the 1972 Olympic Games. Borzov progressed from a 100-meter time of 13.0 seconds at age 14 to 10.0 at age 20.

Table 9.3 Olympic Lifts Program for Improving Acceleration and Speed

Monday		Wednesday	
Warm-up		Warm-up	
Cleans		**Jerks**	
Sets	3 to 6	Sets	3 to 6
Repetitions	3 to 5	Repetitions	3 to 5
% RM	66 to 100%	% RM	66 to 100%
Rest	1 1/2 to 5 minutes between sets	Rest	1 1/2 to 5 minutes between sets
Jerks		**Cleans**	
Sets	3 to 6	Sets	3 to 6
Repetitions	3 to 5	Repetitions	3 to 5
% RM	66 to 100%	% RM	66 to 100%
Rest	1 1/2 to 5 minutes between sets	Rest	1 1/2 to 5 minutes between sets

The plyometric exercises in table 9.4 are grouped by level of intensity to allow improved progression from one phase of training to another to reach peak performance. Most of the exercises closely resemble specific sprinting movements and can force similar muscle groups to work at high rates of speed. The proper techniques to perform many of these exercises are described in chapter 5, and many can also be found in *Jumping Into Plyometrics*, Second Edition, by Donald Chu (1998, Human Kinetics).

Sprint Loading

Sprint loading is another key part of a holistic approach to improving acceleration and speed. The program is designed to improve explosive concentric movements such as sprinting. Three basic techniques provide the necessary light resistance that helps improve strength and power in the muscles involved in acceleration and speed.

1. Hill sprints. The degree of incline must allow proper starting and sprinting form. A 10- to 30-yard incline of 8 to 10 degrees should be covered in 2.5 to 3.5 seconds, followed by a near full-speed sprint of 20 to 80 yards at the same incline.

2. Stadium stairs. Stadium stairs or other stairs can be used in the same manner as hill sprinting. Stairs should have the same approximate angles.

3. Weighted sleds. Numerous inexpensive sleds are available. A spare tire with a rope and weighted belt can be made for little cost. Metal and plastic models are available that allow quick and easy weight changes. It is important to use a load that permits proper form and high-speed sprinting. Too much weight decreases both stride length and rate and prevents explosive movements. The objective in all high-speed work is to reduce ground contact time and maintain a stride rate as high as or higher than the stride rate of the sprinting action without resistance.

Table 9.4 Plyometrics to Improve Acceleration and Speed

Intensity	Exercise	Sets × reps	Rest (min.)	Progression
Low (two weeks)	*Squat jump* Double-leg ankle bounce Lateral cone jump Drop and catch push-up	3 × 6–10 3 × 6–10 2 × 6–10 4 × 6–10	2	Add one rep each workout until reaching 10

Low to medium (two weeks)	Lateral cone jump
	Split squat jump
	Tuck jump
	Standing triple jump
	*Backward medicine
	  ball throw*
	Underhand forward
	  medicine ball throw
	Clap push-up
		3 × 8–10
		2 × 8–10
		2 × 8–10
		2 × 8–10
		
		2 × 8–10
		
		2 × 8–10
		2 × 8–10
			2	Add one rep each workout until reaching 10

Medium (two weeks)	*Standing long jump* *Alternate bound* Double leg hop Pike jump *Depth jump* Medicine ball throw with Russian twist Double-arm swings	3 × 8–10 3 × 8–10 3 × 8–10 2 × 8–10 2 × 8–10 3 × 8–10 2 × 8–10	2	Add one rep each workout until reaching 10
Medium to high (two weeks)	*Tuck jump* Single-leg zigzag hop Double-leg vertical power jump Running bound *Box jump* Dumbbell arm swing Medicine ball sit-up	3 × 10–12 3 × 10–12 3 × 10–12 3 × 10–12 2 × 8–10 3 × 12 3 × 12–15	2	Add one rep each workout until reaching 10
High (rest of season)	Single-leg vertical power jump Single-leg speed hop Double-leg speed hop Multiple box jumps Side jump and sprint Decline hops Sprint arm action Medicine ball sit-up	 2 × 8–12 2 × 8–12 2 × 8–12 2 × 8–12 2 × 8–12 2 × 8–12 2 × 8–12 2 × 8–12	1 to 1.5	Stress form and maximum explosion on each rep. Decrease reps from 12 max to 8 max after 2 weeks.

Exercises in italics are described in chapter 5 of this book (pages 88-95). For descriptions of other plyometric drills listed here, see Chu 1998.

Power starts and power sprints are essential aspects of sprint loading. Studies show that the length of acceleration-power starts should be about 60 to 80 yards, or 6 to 8 seconds. Athletes attain peak power at about 0.6 to 0.8 seconds (within 10 yards), and training should involve distances of only 10 to 20 yards. The best way to train high-speed power is to perform sprint loading from a flying start using 6 to 10 repetitions for 10 to 80 yards. The athlete is then near maximum speed when the incline sprint begins.

A sprint loading program for hill sprinting, stadium-stair sprinting, and using weighted sleds is shown in table 9.5.

Table 9.5   Sprint Loading Program

Week	Repetitions	Pulling distance*	Rest (heart rate)	Progression
1	3–5	15 yards	Walk back >120 bpm	Use power starts at 75% speed in hill and stadium sprinting or with no weight on the sled. Complete two sets.
2	3–5	20 yards	Walk back >120 bpm	Repeat power starts at maximum speed.
3	6–8	25 yards	Full recovery	Repeat power starts at maximum speed.
	3–5	30 yards	Walk back >120 bpm	Use power sprints at maximum speed in hill and stadium sprinting with no weight on the sled. Complete two sets.
4	7–9	40 yards	Full recovery	Begin power starts at 90%.
	3–5	40 yards	Walk back >120 bpm	Repeat power starts and power sprints; add weight to sled that allows good form. Complete two sets.
5	7–9	50 yards	Full recovery	Repeat previous workout. Add more weight and complete three sets.
6–9	7–9	60 yards	Full recovery	Repeat previous workout. Add more weight each week. Complete three sets. Include one final run to exhaustion by continuing to sprint as long as possible. Record the distance and try to improve distance pulled each week.

*Actual distance sprinting uphill, sprinting up stadium steps, or pulling sled.

Form Training

Describing ideal sprinting form in a manner that athletes can understand and apply is difficult. Coach Tom Tellez, who trained 100-meter world record holders Carl Lewis and Leroy Burrell and coached the USA Olympic sprint team, provides an excellent summary of this complicated aspect of acceleration and speed (Dintiman, Ward, and Tellez 1997) which is paraphrased here.

Unless athletes are aware of what is natural and what is unnatural, their efforts could slow them down. Often, athletes feel that they have to bear down, stay low, and pull to run fast. The scientific analysis of running suggests just the opposite. Reaching maximum speed depends greatly on how relaxed one can keep the body in a naturally upright position. The human machine is much better at pushing than pulling, partly because the formation of the leg is unsuited to acting as a pulling force. To run faster, remember that sprinting is primarily a pushing action against the ground.

During the running stride, the leg cycles through three different phases: (1) the drive phase, when the foot is in contact with the ground; (2) the recovery phase, when the leg swings from the hip while the foot clears the ground; and (3) the support phase, when the runner's weight is on the entire foot.

Drive Phase

During the drive phase, the power comes from a pushing action off the ball of the foot. Remember that stride length is the result of a pushing action. The goal of the drive phase is to create the maximum push off the ground. The ball of the foot is the only part of the foot capable of creating an efficient and powerful push. Some misinformed sport coaches believe that the pushing action of the drive phase comes from the toes. Pushing from the toes, however, reduces both power and stability and slows the runner. The drive phase contributes to overall speed only when the runner pushes off the ground using the ball of the foot.

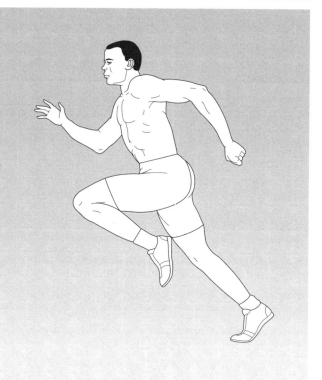

Recovery Phase

During the recovery phase, the knee joint closes and the foot cycles through as it comes close to the body. As the knee joint opens and the leg begins to straighten, the foot comes closer to the ground in preparation for the support phase. An important point to remember about the recovery phase is that the runner does not reach for the ground or perform a stamping action. The leg should remain relaxed and allow the foot to strike the ground naturally.

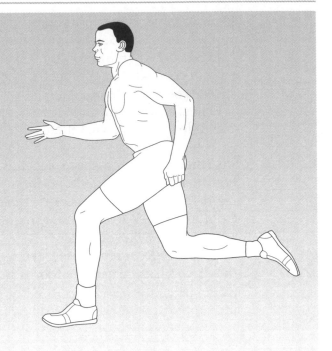

Support Phase

During the support phase, the foot makes initial contact with the ground on the outside edge of the ball of the foot. The weight of the body is then supported at a point that varies according to the speed of the athlete. The faster the speed, the higher the contact point on the ball of the foot. Striking the ground first with this part of the foot maximizes speed but requires great energy. At slower speeds, such as jogging, the contact point moves toward the rear of the foot between the arch and heel. During longer and slower runs, using a flat foot plant saves energy. At all running speeds, the support phase begins with a slight load on the support foot that then rides onto the full sole. Even during sprinting, the heel makes brief but definite contact with the ground. Analysis of the support phase shows that it is impossible to reach maximum speed by running on the toes.

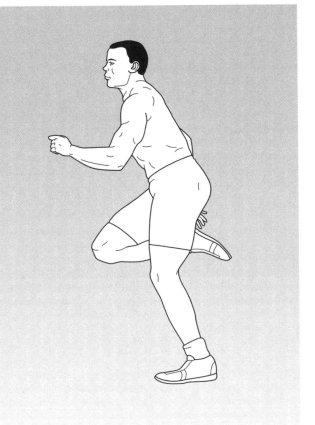

Arm Action

Arm action in sprinting is critical to developing the most efficient stride length. The arms work in opposition to the legs, with the right arm and left leg coming forward as the left arm and right leg go backward (see drive phase) and vice versa. The shoulders should be relaxed, with the swing coming from the shoulder joint. The shoulders should stay perpendicular to the direction of the run. The swing should be strong but relaxed. The hands should also be relaxed. On the upswing, the hand should rise naturally to a point just in front of the chin and just inside the shoulder. During the upswing, the arm angle is about 90 degrees or less, coordinating with the quick recovery of the forward swing of the leg (see recovery phase).

During the downswing, a natural straightening at the elbow corresponds with the longer leverage of the driving leg on the opposite side of the body to allow horizontal drive. As the arm swings down, the elbow will extend slightly. At the bottom of the swing, the hand should be next to the thigh (see support phase). Toward the end of its backward movement, the arm bends and speeds up again to match the final, fast stage of the leg drive. The elbows should stay close to the body; holding the elbows away from the body prevents relaxation of the shoulders and reduces the efficiency of running mechanics. The arm action in sprinting is never forced or tense.

The mechanics of sprinting dictate that athletes who want to run faster must concentrate on pushing off the ground, landing with the proper foot placement, using the correct arm action, and staying relaxed.

Speed Drills

The following bounding, sprinting, and other form workout drills help establish correct neuromuscular movement patterns to improve stride rate and length and to eliminate wasted energy that does not contribute to forward movement. Athletes in practically every sport would benefit by using these drills in each workout for 8 to 10 minutes, following proper warm-up and stretching. Bounding drills are designed to develop the explosive leg power required in starting and acceleration. Sprinting drills are designed to develop the mechanics, strength and power needed to produce maximum sprinting speed.

Straight Bounding

Beginning from a slow jog, bound as high into the air as possible, emphasizing high knee lift. Land on the opposite leg and continue bounding down the field.

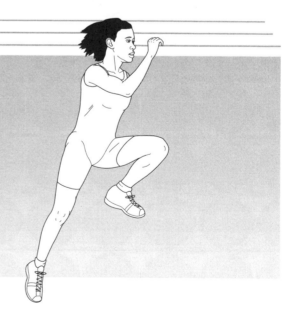

Outside Bounding

This drill is similar to straight bounding except that the foot is placed laterally outside the normal landing position, and the body is projected laterally outward as well as up and forward.

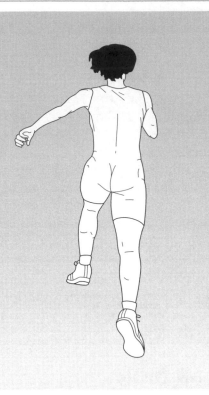

Inside Bounding

This drill is similar to outside bounding except that the foot is placed laterally inside the normal landing position, and the body is projected laterally inward as well as up and forward.

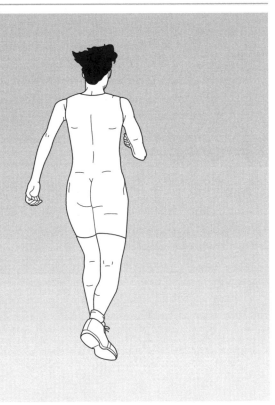

Butt Kicker

From a jog, the lower leg is allowed to swing back and bounce off the buttocks. The upper leg should not move much; focus on allowing (not forcing) the heel to come up to the butt.

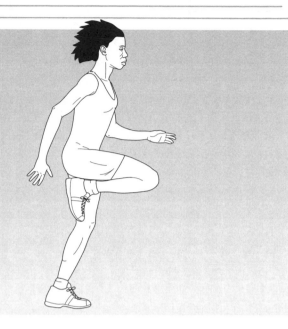

Wall Slide

From a jog, the action is the same as that in the butt kickers except the heel of the recovery leg must not travel behind the body. Imagine a wall of glass running down the back, and do not allow the heel to break the glass. This action will produce knee lift without forcing the action.

Start and Sprint

From a stationary position, start quickly and feel the power being applied behind the body. Ten yards out, quickly shift from running in back of the body to sprinting in front of the body.

Quick Feet

From a jog, increase stride rate and take as many steps as possible in a 10-yard interval. Jog for 10 yards and repeat, emphasizing quick turnover, with the legs moving in front of the body, not behind or under it.

Cycling

Leaning against a wall, bar, or other support, the athlete cycles one leg through in a sprinting manner. Emphasize keeping the leg from extending behind the body, allowing the foot to kick the butt during recovery, and pawing the ground to complete the action. Ten cycles with each leg make up one set.

Down-and-Off

From a high-knee position, the athlete brings the foot down and back up. The emphasis is on decreasing foot-ground contact by hitting the ground with the ball of the foot and getting off as quickly as possible. The effort on the ground should bounce the leg up into a high-knee position. Ten down-and-offs make up one set.

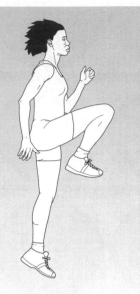

Pull-Through

Extending the leg in front of the body like a hurdler, the athlete brings the leg down and through ground contact in a power motion. Ten pull-throughs with each leg make up one set.

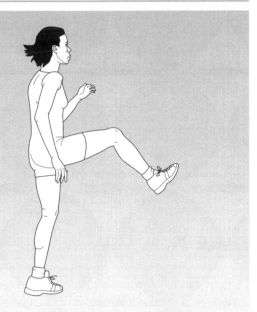

Stick Sprint

Place 20 sticks (18 to 24 inches in length) 18 inches apart on a grass surface. Athletes sprint through the sticks as fast as possible, touching one foot down between each. Emphasize high knee lift and quick ground contact. One run equals one set.

African Dance

While running forward, the athlete raises each leg to the side of the body as in hurdling and taps each heel with the hand. A 10-yard run equals one set.

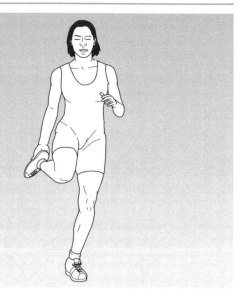

Drum Major

While running forward, the athlete rotates the leg inward to the midline of the body and taps the heel at the midline. A 10-yard run equals one set.

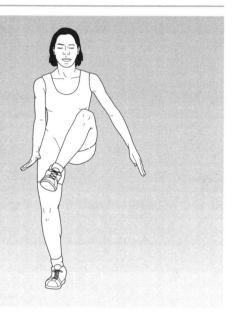

Speed-Endurance Training

As mentioned earlier, speed-endurance training will prevent athletes from slowing down late in the game, at the end of a long sprint, or after sprinting several times with little rest in between. Poor speed endurance becomes evident when a halfback is tackled from behind by a slower player, when a sprinter is passed in the final 10 to 20 meters of a race, when a baseball player runs out of steam and is tagged out at home, or when a basketball player is beaten to the ball by a slower player. High levels of speed endurance provide athletes with a fresh start on each short sprint.

Speed-endurance training programs are designed using the distances of the sprint and the recovery intervals commonly performed in the sport. The number of sets and repetitions simulate the competitive situations that occur in each sport. A typical program for soccer, rugby, and lacrosse would involve gradually increasing the sprint distance from 10 to 50 yards, increasing the number of repetitions from 5 to 15, and decreasing the jogging recovery or rest interval from 20 seconds to 5.

Pickup sprints are an easy, effective program for improving speed endurance in most sports; the sprinting distances and rest intervals are simply adjusted to those that normally occur in the particular sport. In football, for example, short sprints of 10 to 40 yards occur three to seven times at 25- to 30-second (length of huddle) intervals. Speed-endurance training for football players uses these values to develop the foundation of the program. Using pickup sprints, an athlete jogs 25 yards, strides at three-quarter speed for 25 yards, sprints 25 yards, and ends the set with a 25-yard walk. The walking period provides the only rest period between sets. As improvement occurs, lengthen the distance of the segments to 40 and 60 yards. Sprints of longer distances can be used occasionally along with a series of maximum-effort drills (300- and 400-meter sprints, sprinting in place to exhaustion, etc.) at the end of the workout.

Sprint-Assisted Training

The purpose of sprint-assisted training is to increase stride rate and stride length by forcing faster and longer steps than the athlete can take without assistance. Experts feel that such exercises train the nervous system by exposing both the nervous and muscular systems to higher contraction rates. A neurosurgeon, speaking at the national convention of NASE, put it in layman's terms: "After several weeks of sprint-assisted training, the nervous system allows you to continue these higher rates without any assistance." Although this is only theory, research shows that the number of steps taken per second and the length of the stride improve following four to eight weeks of sprint-assisted training.

To achieve maximum results, sprint-assisted training of any kind must be executed according to the following guidelines.

- Begin each workout with a general warm-up routine designed to increase core temperature. Use the large muscle groups first with a slow jog for one-fourth to one-half mile, followed by a faster jog and striding at three-quarter speed for an additional one-fourth mile or more. After perspiring freely, athletes stop and stretch for 8 to 10 minutes. Next are walk-jog-stride-sprint segments (walk 15 steps, jog 15 steps, stride 15 steps at three-quarter speed, and sprint 15 steps), continuing for at least one-fourth mile.

- Expect muscle soreness for one to two days after the first workout. Sprint-assisted training is demanding and will recruit motor units and muscle fibers previously unused.

- Use sprint-assisted training in the beginning of the workout, immediately after completing the warm-up and stretching session. Sprint-assisted training should be avoided if athletes are fatigued from drills, calisthenics, scrimmage, anaerobic training, weight training, or plyometrics. The object is to take faster and longer steps than ever before, not to improve anaerobic conditioning.

- Emphasize quality form in all repetitions. Athletes should avoid sprinting out of control.

The four basic methods of sprint-assisted training are (1) downhill sprinting, (2) high-speed stationary cycling, (3) towing with surgical tubing and pulley devices, and (4) high-speed treadmill sprint training.

Downhill Sprinting

Locate a 50-meter area with a slope no greater than 3 to 7 degrees, which offers only a slight decline. Slopes greater than 7 degrees increase the risk of a fall and produce overstriding, landing on the heels, and ground contact beyond the center of gravity, which produces a braking effect. The braking effect and deviation from natural sprinting form are even noticeable in some athletes when using slopes of no more than 3 or 4 degrees. The ideal area allows a 20-meter sprint on a perfectly flat surface (to accelerate to near maximum speed) followed by a 15-meter sprint on a downhill slope of 3 to 7 degrees (to force higher than normal stride lengths, stride rates, and speed) and ends with a 15-meter sprint on a flat area (to allow athletes to hold the higher speed without the assistance of gravity).

High-Speed Stationary Cycling

During high-speed stationary cycling, the effects of wind resistance, gravity, and body weight are eliminated, allowing more revolutions (similar to steps in sprinting) per second than the sprinting action. This sprint-assisted training technique should be combined with another method, such as towing or downhill sprinting (as shown in table 9.5), to guarantee success.

Towing

Towing, or pulling athletes to sprint faster, is not a new approach. Before the use of surgical tubing and two-person pulley arrangements, motorscooters, motorcycles, and even automobiles were used. Towing produces higher stride rates and increases stride length more effectively than downhill sprinting or high-speed cycling.

Use towing only on a soft, grassy area, after inspecting the surface for broken glass and other objects. Towing requires a 20- to 25-foot piece of elastic or surgical tubing attached to the athlete's waist by a belt. The opposite end can be fastened to another athlete or a stationary object such as a tree or a goalpost to allow individuals to work out alone. Athletes back up to stretch the tubing slightly and run at three-quarter speed with the pull until they make adjustments and master balance. It is possible to stretch the tubing seven times its length (20 feet × 7 = 140 feet) before sprinting at high speed with the pull. Athletes can also make stationary runs from a three-point start. Some athletes have completed stationary 40-yard dashes in 3.7 seconds while being pulled with surgical tubing.

Several towing drills are available:

- Attach one end of the tubing to the front of the waist and the other to the goalpost. The athlete stretches the tubing by walking backward about 20 yards. He or she jogs forward toward the goalpost with the pull. The athlete repeats

Table 9.6 Downhill Sprinting and Cycling Program

Week	Repetitions	Acceleration distance	Sprint-assisted distance*	Progression (repetitions)	Rest (minutes)
1	2–3	10–15 yards (1.5–2 seconds)	20–25 yards (1–1.5 seconds)	Add one to two per workout	2:00
2	4–6	15–20 yards (2–2.5 seconds)	20–25 yards (1.5–2 seconds)	Add one each workout	2:30
3	7–9	20–25 yards (2.5–3 seconds)	20–25 yards (1.5–2 seconds)	Add one each workout	3:00
4	9–10	20–25 yards (2.5–3 seconds)	20–25 yards (1.5–2.5 seconds)	Add one each workout	3:30
5	9–10	20–25 yards (2.5–3 seconds)	20–25 yards (1.5–2.5 seconds)	Add one each wokout	3:30

*Sprint-assisted distance is the actual distance (or time) athletes are sprinting downhill or pedaling at high speeds.

this drill four times, two with a run at three-quarter speed and two with a full-speed sprint. Within the next three sprints, the athlete backs up an extra 5 to 8 yards each time to increase the pull and the speed.

- Repeat the last part of the drill described above using high knee lifts.

- Athletes required to sprint backward or sideways in their sports (defensive backs in football and soccer, rugby and lacrosse players) repeat the drills using those movements.

- Complete the two-person drill by attaching one end of the tubing to the waist and the other to a partner's back. The partner sprints 25 to 30 yards ahead against the resistance, then stops. The other athlete then sprints toward the partner in an overspeed run.

Follow the sprint-assisted training program given in table 9.7 two to three times per week (every other day) during the preseason period and one to two times per week during the competitive season. Keep in mind that using surgical tubing can be dangerous. Provide adequate supervision and a soft grassy area.

Two other pieces of equipment that can be used for sprint-assisted training are the UltraSpeed Pacer and the Sprint Master. The Ultra Speed Pacer is a simple pulley device based on leverage. The pulley can be fastened to a fixed object or held by a partner. Two athletes can also lock on the belts, with one sprinting at a 45-degree angle away from the pulley and the other toward the pulley to receive considerable pull. The device has the potential to provide a strong pull and produce very high stride rates, stride lengths, and sprinting speed.

The Sprint Master machine is precisely engineered to pull athletes at speeds faster than any human can sprint. It attaches to the goalposts of a football or soccer field and provides controlled, variable speed for each athlete. The device increases safety by providing the athlete who loses balance the option of simply releasing his or her grip.

Table 9.7   Sprint-Assisted Training Using Surgical Tubing and the Sprint Master

Week	Repetitions	Distance*	Rest (minutes)	Progression
1	3–5	10–15 yards	2	Three-quarter speed runs only to acclimate
2	3–5	10–15 yards	2	Maximum speed
3	5–7	15–20 yards	3	Maximum speed
4	7–9	20–25 yards	3	Maximum speed
5	7–9	20–25 yards	3	Maximum speed
6–9	7–9	25–30 yards	3–5	Maximum speed with weighted vest, progressing from one to five pounds over three weeks. Used only for the final two repetitions of the workout.

*Represents the total distance an athlete can sprint at maximum speed.

High-Speed Treadmill Sprint Training

In the Virginia Commonwealth University laboratory, the A.R. Young high-speed treadmill (capable of speeds of 0.0 to 26.0 miles per hour) has been used to improve stride length, stride rate, form, acceleration, speed endurance, and speed. Cinematography identifies differences in stride length and rate at various speeds in both treadmill sprinting and unaided, flat-surface sprinting. An expert standing on a stool facing and looking down at the subject corrects form during high-speed sprinting. The treadmill is also an excellent piece of equipment for sprint-assisted training.

Sequence of Training Programs

Although opinions differ among conditioning coaches, there is a logical sequence to using the programs in this chapter, particularly when several training programs are used within the same workout.

Start with a formal warm-up routine involving actions specific to the sport that bring about perspiration. Perform stretching exercises next. Follow immediately with sprint-assisted training, keeping in mind that the purpose is to improve stride rate and length, not speed endurance. Scrimmage and drills are fourth in sequence, completed while the body is still relatively fresh, capable of high speeds under game conditions, and less apt to be injured. Conditioning activities such as calisthenics, speed-endurance training, plyometrics, and weight training are the last items on the workout schedule. It is best to avoid scheduling plyometrics and weight training within the same training session. A final 5- to 10-minute cool-down period may include additional stretching, particularly following a plyometric or weight-training session.

Table 9.8 identifies the role of each training program in altering the four ways of improving acceleration and speed. This information allows coaches and ath-

Table 9.8 Training Programs to Improve Acceleration and Speed	
How sprinting speed is improved	**Specific training programs**
Improved acceleration	Starting-time training specific to the sport Plyometrics Muscle imbalance strength training Functional strength and power training Sprint loading Sprint-assisted training
Increased stride length	Functional strength and power training Muscle imbalance strength training Plyometrics Sprint loading Sprint-assisted training Form training Flexibility training
Increased stride rate	Sprint-assisted training Muscle imbalance strength training
Improved form and speed endurance	Form training Speed-endurance training Sprint loading

Note: The table assumes that athletes already possess an acceptable level of body fat, general conditioning, and strength.

letes to select the major areas of emphasis and to focus on the training programs that are likely to bring about improvement.

SUMMARY

The major areas of emphasis for speed improvement for each athlete depend on the sport and individual testing results. The object is to adjust each training program to simulate the activities of the sport while focusing on the areas of weakness uncovered.

Key points in this chapter include the following:

- In most sports, what is referred to as speed is really acceleration because athletes rarely reach maximum speed during competition.

- Although some athletes are born with more fast-twitch muscle fibers than others and are more genetically suited for sprinting, all athletes, regardless of their genetic makeup, can improve their speed and acceleration with proper training. Sprint loading, strength-power training, speed-endurance training, plyometrics, and sprint-assisted training produce the greatest changes in the exercised fast-twitch muscle fibers.

- Acceleration and speed can be improved by taking faster steps, taking longer steps, and improving sprinting form. Performance deterioration in short sprints as the game progresses can be avoided by improving speed endurance.

- Fast sprinters come in all sizes and shapes; no body type provides a significant edge. Excess body fat can significantly impair acceleration and speed. Although the gap is closing, male sprinters possess better times in the 100 meters and 200 meters, and take faster and longer steps than female sprinters.

- An analysis of correct sprinting form has allowed researchers to identify the significant factors contributing to efficient movement. Research has also revealed a diversity of style and technique among champion sprinters, suggesting that athletes should improve their basic style without trying to mimic the exact technique of others.

- Before a personalized program can be designed to improve acceleration and speed, it is important to evaluate speed, stride length, stride rate, strength, power, flexibility, body composition, and muscle balance. Programs can then be designed to eliminate the areas of weakness that are limiting improvement.

- Apply the concept of working fast to be fast in all training programs.

- All athletes need a solid foundation of functional strength and power before proceeding to training programs designed to improve acceleration and speed. One area that must receive more emphasis in these programs is the hamstring muscle group, the sprinter's weakest link.

- To ensure proper progression and to enable athletes to reach peak performance at the appropriate time for their sport, use periodized training in the speed-improvement program. This approach groups each training program and workout into phases or cycles to help athletes achieve their peak performance at just the right time.

- Plyometric training bridges the gap between strength and speed by using exercises that simulate sprinting movements and use a "down" time (foot-ground contact time) less than that used during the actual sprinting action.

- Sprint loading is a program that involves placing the exact muscles used in acceleration and maximum sprinting under resistance using a sled, a slight incline, or stadium stairs in order to improve power and acceleration while emphasizing correct form.

- Form training can improve acceleration and speed, and should be a part of an athlete's regular workout in all sports. Although the workout drills are difficult to execute correctly at first, once they can be performed with ease neuromuscular patterns become established that ensure proper sprinting mechanics in all activities.

- Speed-endurance training should be tailored to each sport in terms of the typical distance covered, rest interval, and number of repetitions in order to improve training specificity and carryover to a sport.

- Sprint-assisted training forces athletes to take faster and longer steps than they are capable of taking without assistance by using surgical tubing, pulleys, a slope, stationary bicycle, Ultra Speed Pacer, Sprint Master, or treadmill. Full recovery is necessary before performing the next repetition. The purpose of this workout is to train the neuromuscular system so that athletes can eventually take faster and longer steps without assistance. This normally occurs in 6 to 10 weeks.

• If maximum improvement is to occur, the training programs must be sequenced logically. Athletes should begin with a general warm-up, move on to stretching, sprint-assisted training, drills or scrimmage, and end with conditioning activities (calisthenics, plyometrics, or weight training) and a cool-down period that may include brief stretching.

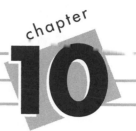

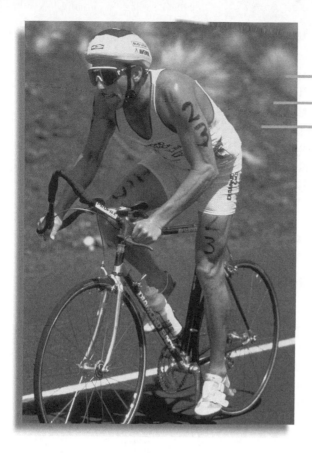

Aerobic Capacity for Endurance

Jack Daniels

Aerobic capacity refers to the greatest amount of oxygen an individual can consume while performing physical exercise. The form of physical exercise that a person might perform can vary greatly, of course, from a simple act involving just a few small muscles to a gross motor movement that demands the use of large muscle groups. With this in mind, an individual's aerobic capacity can range from a limited consumption of oxygen to one that is 20 or more times greater than that associated with rest. For example, running and cross-country skiing are forms of exercise that involve large muscle groups. The amount of oxygen an elite runner or skier can use when exercising at a high intensity can easily be 70 or 80 milliliters per kilogram of body weight per minute, which is clearly over 20 times the resting metabolism of 3.5 milliliters per kilogram per minute. On the other hand, the amount of oxygen that could be consumed while operating an eggbeater may not exceed twice that consumed at rest. Therefore, aerobic capacity is specific to a group of muscles, although we tend to think of it as the most oxygen an individual can consume while engaged in an exercise that brings into play as many muscles as possible.

Aerobic involvement during exercise actually has two major components. The first is the central component, which refers to the oxygen delivery system. The ability of the lungs to oxygenate the blood that is pumped through the pulmonary vessels, the ability of the blood to carry oxygen, and the ability of the heart to pump blood to the exercising muscles are all parts of the oxygen delivery system. The second is the peripheral component, which refers to the ability of the exercising muscles to take in and use the delivered oxygen to convert fuel aerobically to energy for muscular contractions.

Factors of importance here are the degree of vascularization of the exercising muscles and the number, size, and distribution of mitochondria (the intracellular structures in the exercising muscles where oxygen is used to convert fuel—fat and carbohydrate—to energy). In addition, the status of oxidative enzymes (chemicals that aid in the consumption of oxygen at the cellular level) is important in just how much oxygen can be consumed in a given time. In effect, the central component delivers oxygen, and the peripheral component uses some, or possibly all, of the oxygen that it receives.

Clearly, the ideal situation would be to have a central component capable of delivering as much oxygen as the muscles might ever need and for the peripheral component to be able to use as much oxygen as can be delivered. But this is not the case. If it were, we would have no need for the term *aerobic capacity*, which implies that there is a limit to how much oxygen can be consumed by any particular group of muscles.

ENDURANCE AND AEROBIC CAPACITY

Endurance is the relative intensity (to the individual's aerobic capacity) of exercise that an individual can maintain for a period of time. It is better to think of endurance as a *relative* factor rather than an *absolute* one. An improvement in endurance refers to either being able to endure a particular intensity of exercise for a longer period or being able to endure an increased intensity for the same period. Most often endurance is described as the ability to maintain a certain fraction of aerobic capacity for a specific period.

Naturally, an athlete can improve endurance either by increasing aerobic capacity (because even the same fraction of an improved aerobic capacity will lead to performance at greater intensity) or by increasing the fraction of the same aerobic capacity that he or she can maintain for any particular period. For example, early in a season of training a distance runner may be able to sustain a pace that demands 80 percent of his or her aerobic capacity for a period of one hour. Later that season the same runner may be able to endure a pace that demands 84 percent of the same aerobic capacity for the same abount of time. Alternatively, an increase in aerobic capacity may result in an 80 percent intensity being related to a faster pace for one hour.

In a sense, aerobic capacity can be viewed as a somewhat absolute, yet variable, factor and endurance as a relative and variable factor.

Energy Production

To perform any type of physical activity, energy must be provided to the muscles involved. The necessary energy is provided either anaerobically (without oxygen) or aerobically (with oxygen).

Anaerobic Metabolism

The *anaerobic* metabolism of fuel results in the production of pyruvic acid, which later is converted to lactic acid. Both of these by-products of anaerobic metabolism are eventually removed from the body *aerobically*, either during recovery from exercise or, if the intensity is low enough, during continued exercise. Both anaerobic and aerobic processes are going on at the same time, all the time. Anaerobic energy production is more rapidly available than aerobic energy, and athletes rely on it heavily at the beginning of any bout of exercise and during exercise at high intensity. Note that the body also uses lactic acid as fuel that can be burned aerobically.

Aerobic Metabolism

Both carbohydrate and fat are metabolized aerobically in skeletal muscles, with water and carbon dioxide being the waste products of aerobic metabolism. The longer the bout of exercise, the more heavily the body relies on aerobic metabolism for the production of energy. It takes a couple of minutes for the body to adjust to a continuous bout of exercise. While this adjustment is occurring, anaerobic metabolism carries a diminishing share of the load (see figure 10.1). Think of the start of exercise as a rocket taking off. At the start of the process, powerful booster engines produce the bulk of the energy necessary for flight. But the

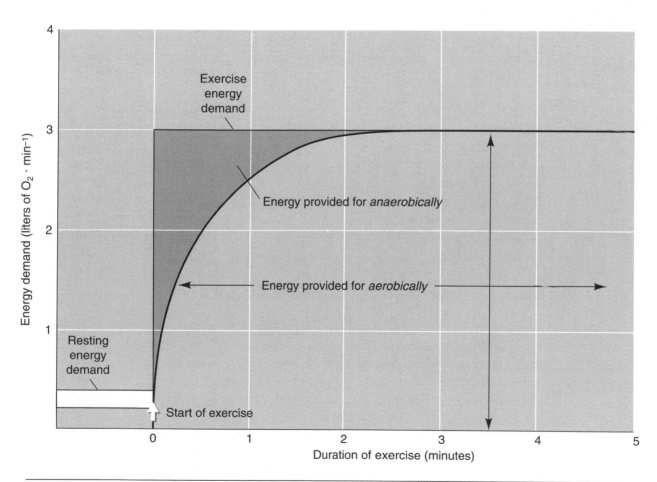

Figure 10.1   It takes a couple of minutes for the body to adjust to a continuous bout of exercise. While this adjustment is occurring, anaerobic metabolism carries a diminishing share of the load.

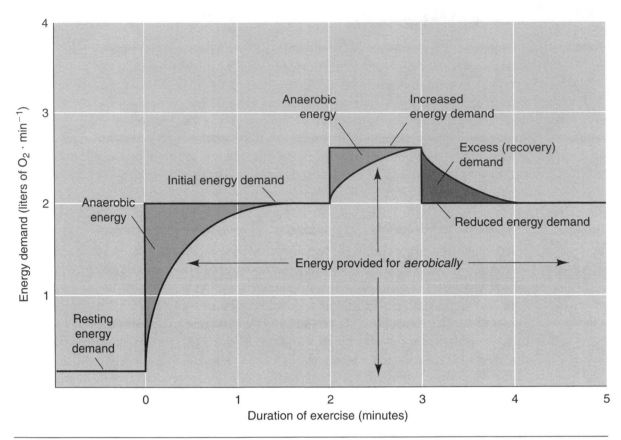

Figure 10.2   If given time to be rejuvenated, the body's "booster engines" can provide considerable power any time it is needed.

boosters can provide power for only so long. Once under way, the main engines take over as the primary energy providers. These engines are capable of functioning more continuously. With adequate fuel and when operating within their capabilities, they can go on for a long time. Still, the booster engines can be called on for sudden bursts of energy at almost any time during the flight. If given time to be rejuvenated, they can produce considerable power whenever it is needed, as depicted in figure 10.2. Furthermore, any time the energy demand exceeds an individual's $\dot{V}O_2$max, anaerobic metabolism must provide all the additional energy.

Aerobic Power for Anaerobic Events

But what about the benefits of high aerobic power in more anaerobic sports or in sports that are intermittent in nature, such as football? Pyruvic acid and lactic acid are removed aerobically, which means that good aerobic capability will have a positive effect on recovery, even from high-intensity exercise. Being able to tolerate repeated bouts of high-intensity exercise is beneficial not only in competition but also in training. An athlete with good aerobic capacity can perform more quality repeats during a specific amount of practice time. So, although a given sport may not be particularly aerobic in nature, additional quality practice time can certainly help produce better performance in a competitive situation.

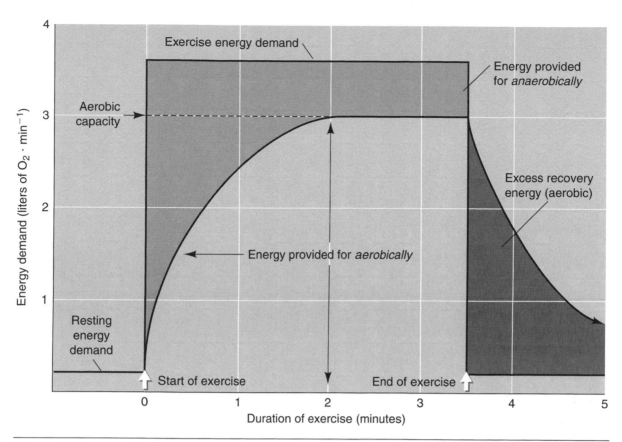

Figure 10.3 Aerobic power plays the dominant energy-production role in competition and serves the competitor well during long practice sessions as well as competitions in which he or she competes in more than one event.

Aerobic Power for Aerobic Events

It should be obvious that a high aerobic capacity is of tremendous importance in sporting events that require prolonged exercise. In aerobic sports the participant relies heavily on his or her aerobic capacity. Aerobic power plays the dominant energy-production role in competition and serves the competitor well during practice sessions in which repeated bouts of exercise are often the goal of training. Furthermore, in track and swimming meets it is common for a competitor to race in more than one event. The enhanced recovery rate associated with a high aerobic capacity plays a significant role in how well the athlete can deal with a second or third event (see figure 10.3).

Relationship of Aerobic Capacity and Economy of Exercise

An athlete with a high aerobic capacity who is not economical when performing his or her sport may not match the performance of an athlete with less aerobic capacity but more economical form. Figure 10.4 shows a typical economy curve generated by the steady-state oxygen consumption ($\dot{V}O_2$submax) of a runner running at 230, 250, 270, and 290 meters per minute (m · min^{-1}). The aerobic capacity of this runner is placed on an extension of the economy curve, and from this,

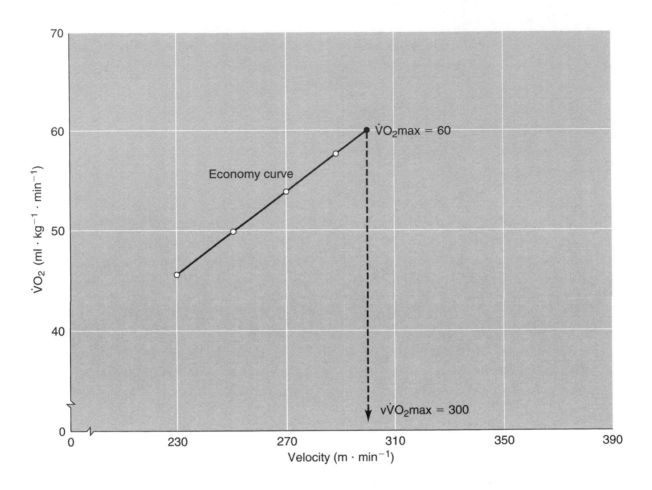

Figure 10.4 The aerobic capacity, economy curve, $\dot{V}O_2$max, and a v$\dot{V}O_2$max of a runner.

a corresponding velocity at $\dot{V}O_2$max (v$\dot{V}O_2$max) can be determined (see figure 10.4). The aerobic capacity for this runner (60 ml · kg^{-1} · min^{-1}) corresponds to a $\dot{V}O_2$max of 300 meters per minute (m · min^{-1}). This v$\dot{V}O_2$max value can be considerably more revealing about this runner's distance-racing capability than the $\dot{V}O_2$max value by itself because it includes the added variable, running economy.

As an example, figure 10.5 shows the economy curve, $\dot{V}O_2$max, and v$\dot{V}O_2$max, for two elite female distance runners. Both these runners raced 3,000 meters in nearly identical times, yet $\dot{V}O_2$max varied by about 20 percent. Notice that v$\dot{V}O_2$max, which adds running economy to the picture, varied only slightly between the runners.

Of course, variations in $\dot{V}O_2$max and economy will occur during different phases of training, and the same athlete may show a marked change in $\dot{V}O_2$max or economy during a single year (or even a single season) of training. The point is that changes in performance may occur in the absence of changes in aerobic power or any other variable chosen as a performance marker.

In keeping with my definition of endurance—being able to endure a particular intensity (running speed, for example) longer, or an increased speed for a specific time—it becomes obvious that a change in economy of exercise also affects

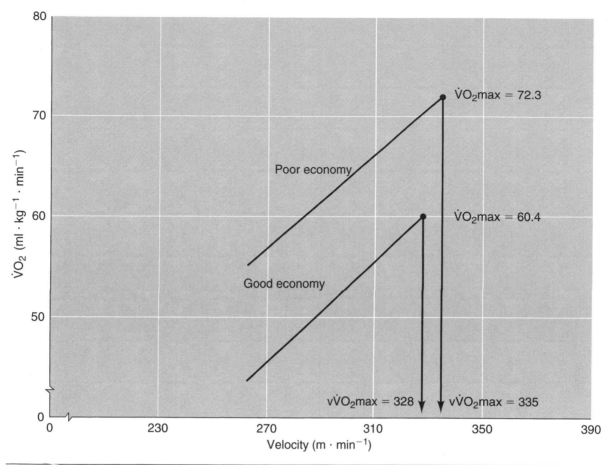

Figure 10.5 The economy curve, $\dot{V}O_2max$, and $v\dot{V}O_2max$ for two elite female distance runners. From Daniels et al. 1984, page 70.

endurance. For example, a distance runner with a $\dot{V}O_2max$ of 60 who races at a 6:00-per-mile pace (268 m · min^{-1}) for 30 minutes at 90 percent of his or her $\dot{V}O_2max$ (54 ml · kg^{-1} · min^{-1}) will increase race speed if improved economy leads to this $\dot{V}O_2max$ (54 ml · kg^{-1} · min^{-1}) being associated with a faster speed (280 m · min^{-1}, for example). Figure 10.6 illustrates this.

So, aerobic capacity, endurance, and economy all play major roles in performance, particularly in sports that demand prolonged, steady exercise at relatively high intensity.

PRINCIPLES OF TRAINING

Before discussing specific training designed to develop or improve aerobic capacity, endurance, or economy, it is useful to understand some of the basic principles of conditioning that affect these components of performance.

Principle 1: Body Reaction to Stress

Actually, two general reactions to stress can be considered. The first is the reaction to an acute bout of exercise, for example, getting up from a bench and running

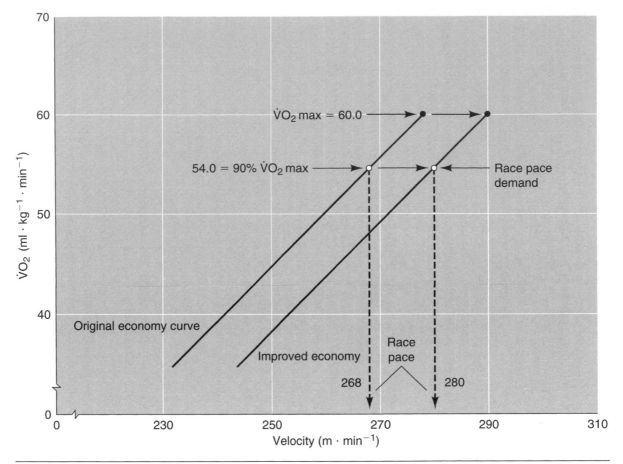

Figure 10.6   A change in economy of exercise also affects endurance.

several hundred meters to the other side of a park. On arriving there, the individual would notice some immediate reactions to this stress: an increase in heart rate, increased breathing, and possibly some leg-muscle fatigue. If some blood were collected, a rise in the lactic-acid level of the blood might be detected. Noticeable sweat might have started to accumulate on parts of the skin. All these reactions would take place any time the individual attempted such a bout of exercise, regardless of his or her level of fitness.

The second type of reaction to physical stress is in the form of changes that take place in the body as a result of chronic stress—undergoing a particular stress repeatedly, maybe in a single session of exercise but perhaps with regular frequency on different days. For example, one might get up from the same park bench and run to the other side of the park five times each week for several weeks. When chronic stress of this type (which we would usually refer to as *training*) is imposed on the body, the body makes changes that will allow the individual to perform the same bout of exercise with greater ease. The heart muscle will get stronger, as will the running muscles and the ventilatory muscles. Changes will take place in the muscle cells that will result in lower accumulations of lactic acid in the blood. The soreness associated with earlier bouts of exercise will disappear as the body strengthens itself against this particular activity. A desirable training effect will take place; the individual will attain a new fitness level.

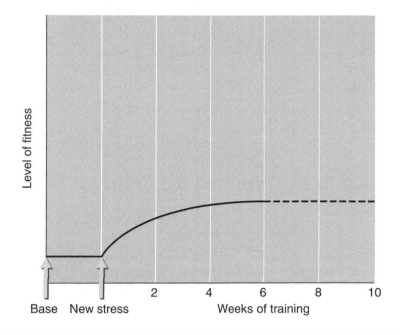

Figure 10.7 Exercising at a greater degree of stress produces an increase in fitness that levels off after a period of time.
From Daniels 1998, page 19.

Principle 2: Predictable Rate of Improvement

A person at a stable level of fitness who begins to exercise at a greater degree of stress will reach a higher level of fitness. The rate at which the individual will achieve this new fitness, however, is not linear. Rather, as weeks of performing the same routine go by, the benefits become less until the person reaches the new fitness level. Further training at this particular stress will not produce further improvements in fitness. Figure 10.7 depicts how a person might achieve a new level of fitness by regularly performing a consistent schedule of training.

A beginning runner might train three days each week, running two one-mile runs in 12 minutes each, with a 5-minute recovery between the two runs (written as 2 × 1 mile at 12:00 with 5:00 rest, 3 × week). Each training session involves a *workload* (two miles in this case), an *intensity* of training (12:00 pace for the miles being run), and an amount of *recovery* time between individual work bouts (5 minutes). *Frequency* of performing this training (three times each week) is also indicated. All training can be described in this manner: workload, intensity, recovery (sometimes there is a single work bout so recovery between bouts is not a consideration), and frequency. Furthermore, increasing the stress of any of these factors will lead to achieving a new level of fitness.

Principle 3: Limits to Improvement

Principle 2 suggests that as long as a person keeps increasing the stress of training, fitness will continue to improve. Everyone, however, has limits. These limits are often seasonal. A young beginning runner may have an immature body that can take only so much stress before it starts to break down. A college student may try to add additional training time to an already crowded schedule, resulting in insufficient rest and illness. For numerous reasons, an individual might not be able to go beyond a particular state of fitness one season and then move to much greater heights in the next season of training.

We must also accept that each individual has absolute limits to how much he or she can achieve in any sport. Certainly, differences exist in body structure, degree of motivation, level of opportunity, and quality of direction (coaching) available. All these factors play a part in the degree of success that an individual can reach.

Principle 4: Diminishing Returns

This principle of training implies that as the stress of training continuously increases, the benefits of the training become less. A beginning runner who increases training from 20 to 40 miles each week will not realize as great an improvement with the additional 20 miles as he or she did when training went from no running to running 20 miles each week. The greater the stress, the less the increase in benefit.

At some point of increased stress, a decrease in fitness may occur if accompanying rest and recovery time are inadequate, a condition typically referred to as *overtraining*. A good approach to avoiding overtraining is to be aware of how training feels to the athlete, not just how fast the training sessions are going. Also, if an increase in training stress is not associated with better performance, the athlete should reevaluate what he or she is doing; it may be time to back off for a while.

Principle 5: Accelerating Setbacks

This principle goes hand in hand with principle 4. It states that relatively minimal training stress is associated with few problems (injuries, illnesses, overtraining, loss of interest, etc.), but, at some point of increased stress, even a small amount of additional stress can result in a much greater chance of something going wrong. Figure 10.8 depicts how principle 4 (upper curve) and principle 5 (lower curve) appear if fitness potential and chance of a setback are both plotted against increased training stress.

Principle 6: Specificity of Training

This principle refers to the fact that the part of the body that is stressed is the part that stands to benefit from that stress. The running muscles must be stressed to become more efficient during the act of running, the heart must be stressed for it to become stronger, and so forth. This principle does not deny the benefits of cross-training, but it does suggest that an athlete carefully consider the consequences to avoid producing undesirable results (for example, too much gain in muscle mass that is nonproductive in the sport of primary interest).

Principle 7: Ease of Maintenance

The ease of maintenance principle states that once an individual achieves a certain level of fitness, the degree of stress necessary to maintain it is not as great as was necessary to reach that level of fitness in the first place. Part of this effect

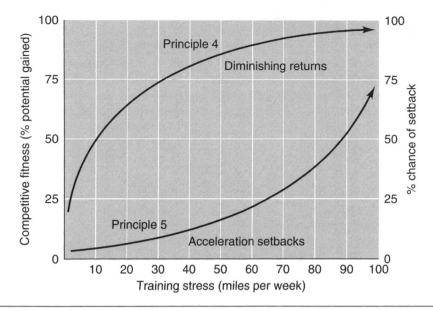

Figure 10.8 Increasing training stress beyond a certain point can lead to diminishing returns and a greater chance of injuries and overtraining.
From Daniels 1998, pages 26 and 28.

comes from an elevated level of confidence achieved through specific performances, but part of it is strictly physiological. Various systems of the body will continue to perform at an achieved level with only occasional stress, allowing the individual to attend to another, possibly weaker, system with greater enthusiasm.

INGREDIENTS OF SUCCESS

In addition to an understanding of the basic principles of conditioning there are several other attributes that are necessary for athletic success.

Ability

Every individual is born with specific physical characteristics that largely determine potential success in a given sport. It is easy to see that a very tall person may have good potential for a sport like basketball but not necessarily for gymnastics. On the other hand, small individuals are designed more for gymnastics than for throwing the discus. In many sports like boxing, wrestling, and weightlifting differences in body size are so important to competitive success that weight classes have been established to level the playing field.

Although not as obvious as differences in anatomical design—height and weight—physiological makeup varies greatly among individuals. Some people have systems ideally designed to perform endurance activities. Others seem to be put together to excel at sprinting. Add to these variations that an immature body is different from a fully developed one, that males differ from females, that physical characteristics vary across a wide range of ages, and it is apparent that addressing the issue of training for sport is not always straightforward. It is difficult to say that a set amount of stress will produce the optimum training effect for anyone.

Motivation

Even among individuals with equal or nearly equal ability to perform a particular physical activity, vast differences exist in the desire shown toward the same activity. Being tall and coordinated doesn't guarantee success on the basketball court if the person's motivation is in another area, such as music or art. With thoughtful and enthusiastic direction, an outside influence can sometimes instill motivation, but intrinsic motivation is normally essential to achieving real success in any sport or physical endeavor. The athlete involved must be the one with the motivation, not a parent or coach.

Opportunity

Further muddying the waters of developing an ideal approach to training is the extent of opportunity available to the individuals involved. In many sports, climate, facilities, and equipment are major concerns. Skiers need snow, swimmers need water, rowers and paddlers need water and boats. Money can be an obstacle, as in sports like yachting and equestrian events. Naturally, just having the opportunity to compete against others is a factor in how far an individual can develop in any sport.

Direction

Another ingredient that should be addressed is the matter of having a coach or teacher, or at least a training plan to follow. Possessing this ingredient may be a detriment if the plan or person directing the training of an individual or team is not in tune with proper training principles or is not patient enough to let the athletes progress at a reasonable rate. The most serious fault that someone in charge of the conditioning of others can make is not being sensitive to individual differences and needs.

Age and Body Composition

Before reaching physical maturity (in the late teens for most individuals), age can be a major factor in the success that an endurance athlete might achieve. When one realizes the important role that muscle mass plays in oxygen consumption—the greater the mass of exercising muscle, the greater the need for oxygen to feed that mass and the greater the weight the runner must carry—it is easy to accept the various degrees of success that youngsters reach as distance runners. Some late-maturing individuals have light bodies to carry around and often have great success when they start out as distance runners. When they mature, many have a rapid growth spurt, adding not only additional muscle mass but also fat deposits and larger bones. An immediate effect is a drop in endurance as the body struggles with its new dimensions.

On the other hand, some individuals grow steadily, and the adjustment is gradual enough for them that performance may never take a backward slide, even temporarily. In either case, once the body has had a chance to adjust to its new dimensions, performance will usually continue to progress as long as training continues.

Actually, over time, from very young ages to about 18, the major physiological change that accompanies an improvement in performance is better economy. $\dot{V}O_2$max (ml · kg^{-1} · min^{-1}) often remains nearly constant as increases in total oxygen consumption are matched by increases in body mass. The improvement in running economy appears to be partly associated with normal growth and partly with training that may take place during the growth years. Even in the absence of an increase in relative $\dot{V}O_2$max, the improvement in economy results in v$\dot{V}O_2$max becoming significantly better. This change is directly associated with a change in performance, as described earlier. Figure 10.9 shows the changes that took place in relative $\dot{V}O_2$max and running economy among a group of young runners who were followed over a period of five years.

A word of caution is appropriate regarding body mass as it relates to the performance of a distance runner. First, oxygen consumption ($\dot{V}O_2$) can be expressed in either *absolute* or *relative* terms. Absolute oxygen consumption refers to the actual amount of oxygen that an individual consumes each minute, usually expressed in liters or milliliters per minute. For example, a runner might be consuming 3,000 milliliters of oxygen per minute while running at a maximum aerobic effort. If this runner weighs 60 kilograms (132 pounds), then he or she will have a relative $\dot{V}O_2$ of 50 milliliters per kilogram per minute (3,000 ml ÷ 60 kg = 50 ml per kg). If this represents the individual's $\dot{V}O_2$max, it can be improved in either of two ways—by increasing the absolute 3,000-milliliter maximum or by reducing the body mass, which is divided into the absolute $\dot{V}O_2$ to arrive at a relative $\dot{V}O_2$max. Remember that relative $\dot{V}O_2$max is the one more closely associated with running performance.

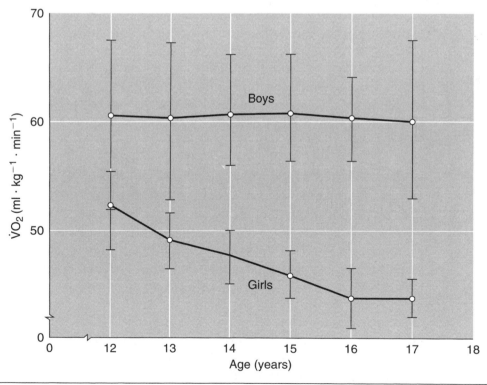

Figure 10.9 The changes in muscle mass, fat deposits, and bone size that occur as athletes reach physical maturity affect their relative $\dot{V}O_2$max.
From Daniels et al. 1978, page 202.

The danger comes in getting overzealous in an attempt to reduce body mass (in hopes of increasing relative $\dot{V}O_2$max). If the body is carrying unnecessary body fat, some drop in body mass will improve performance. But if one curtails nutrition to the extent that muscle mass or energy stores are reduced, the result will be a reduction in *absolute* $\dot{V}O_2$max. Continued loss of weight will not improve performance and, in fact, can degrade performance. Growing youngsters sometimes try to avoid growing up "too much" by reducing their food intake so much that muscle growth is held back and nutrients are not adequate to sustain nutritional needs.

COMMON PROBLEMS IN GAINING ENDURANCE AND AEROBIC POWER

Given the many factors that influence success in sport, it is not difficult to appreciate that some individuals have much greater success than others do in particular sports. Unlike sports in which skill plays a dominant role, some sports that rely on high aerobic capacity or superior endurance actually have rather limited skill components. Of all competitive sports, distance running probably demands the least from its participants in skill development. Conditioning is the most important element in the success of runners. Even in endurance sports with a high technique component, such as cross-country skiing and distance swimming, at some point conditioning the aerobic system becomes of primary importance.

Rushing to a Goal

Nothing can become a greater problem for an endurance athlete than shortcutting a sound, consistent training plan. Not adhering to the simple training principles presented earlier in this chapter can lead to a setback that curtails training for an undetermined time. Training setbacks are a particular problem because they not only stop steady progress toward a goal but often motivate the participant, once he or she regains health, to try to make up for lost time by training even harder. This increase in training stress usually leads to further setbacks.

Copying the Champion

The careers of many potentially outstanding endurance athletes have undoubtedly been cut short by trying to duplicate the training habits of a current champion or record holder. This is particularly true among young, inexperienced athletes, who idolize the outstanding individuals in their sport and will attempt to do exactly what their hero does in training. A key word here is *does* because beginners in a sport often don't realize the many hours and years of training that the current stars went through as youngsters. They just read about what the champion does now and figure that is what they need to do.

Not Listening to the Body

Not even the best thought-out training plan in the world will always be right for everyone. It seems so simple to lay out a training program and conscientiously follow it to the letter. How can a person go wrong? How can a person overtrain if the program is a proven, successful approach to greatness? The answer is that no matter how perfect the plan, things go wrong now and then. People become injured, people become ill, people have other things to do in their lives that sometimes limit the rest or nutrition they get. Some days don't go so well, and this is when it pays for an athlete to listen to his or her body. A variety of methods are available to examine the effects of training, such as monitoring heart rate, timing segments of a training session, taking blood samples to check on blood-lactate levels, and so forth. But the simplest and most often overlooked method is learning to read the body. Most great athletes excel at this (which is probably why they became so great), but enthusiastic beginners often overlook this important aspect of training. Endurance athletes need to learn to *feel* how things are going. They need to know when to end a workout and when to change a workout to something that may be just as stressful but of a different nature. Learning to read the body takes some time but is well worth the effort.

Assuming Everyone Is the Same

Not recognizing individual differences is often the weakest part of a training program for youngsters and older individuals. Youngsters mature at far different rates, and some oldsters age rapidly. But this problem is not limited to the young and old. Besides normal physiological changes that take place among individuals, a variety of psychological factors come into play. Because people react differently to the same training stresses, it is not uncommon to see two distance runners, for example, attain quite different race times even though they have followed the same program and are equally motivated. Recognizing individual differences goes hand in hand with learning to listen to the body.

Not Caring for Illness and Injury

In the heat of training for an important competition, it is tempting to try to train through an injury or illness. Some injuries will clear up just as fast during normal training as they will by taking time off; other injuries need true rest, at least from specific stresses. Learning which injuries fall into which categories is not easy, but experience and a good coach can go a long way in making the determination.

Lacking Flexibility

Just as trying to train through an injury or illness is not always desirable, not being willing to alter training or competition schedules can be counterproductive. Situations sometimes dictate a change in plans. A typical example is when an important planned training session with a specific time goal coincides with adverse environmental conditions that negate any chance of meeting the hoped-for time. Two ways to deal with this situation are to change the workout completely or to move the same workout to another day in the same week when conditions may be more conducive to success. A third possibility would be to go on with the planned workout but to go by feel rather than time for the various stages of the session.

Lacking Confidence in the Training Plan

An athlete will usually achieve better results by following a less-than-ideal training scheme presented by a person in whom the athlete has complete confidence than he or she would by adhering to a sound plan set up by a coach in which the athlete has less confidence. Clearly, the ideal situation is having confidence in someone who is presenting a good program. It is always beneficial to commit to a program, but if results are not reasonable for the effort put forth, the athlete may want to try a different approach.

Underestimating Aerobic Fitness and Endurance

It is not uncommon for an endurance athlete who has lost a couple of races during the final "sprint" to the tape to feel that he or she must do more speed training. Spending more time on speed (anaerobic) training may actually detract from aerobic fitness, which can cause the athlete to be so far behind the leaders that he or she receives no benefit from a kick to the finish. Often, a better explanation for losing races in the final minute is not being aerobically fit enough to run away from an opponent during the middle part of a race. A strong finishing kick is accomplished by athletes who arrive at that part of a race with high energy reserves, not necessarily superior all-out speed.

MEASURING AEROBIC CAPACITY

An athlete's aerobic capacity, or $\dot{V}O_2$max, can be measured by a "max" test. During a max test the subject should be constantly monitored to evaluate the stress being imposed so that the test can be terminated if necessary. Tests of less-fit individuals should include monitoring of the subject's heart rate, blood pressure, and ventilatory responses. The electrical activity of the heart may also be monitored with an electrocardiograph. The tester should ask the subject periodically how he or she is feeling and whether it is possible to go on another minute or half minute before the test ends. With fit individuals (those involved in regular, strenuous training and competitions), it is good to monitor these variables, but in field tests it may be possible only to ask the subject to express his or her feelings. An important consideration is that with most trained endurance athletes the individual will reach $\dot{V}O_2$max before he or she feels that the test must be terminated. Thus it is best to be able to monitor the rate of carbon dioxide produced ($\dot{V}CO_2$) as well as the rate of oxygen uptake ($\dot{V}O_2$) throughout the test. The ratio of these two respiratory values provides a good measure of how hard the subject is working and when it is appropriate to stop the test.

Regardless of the extent to which a max test is being monitored, the subject should first perform a normal warm-up (as if getting ready to compete in a race) and then be fitted with any equipment necessary for the test itself. If the test is being conducted on a treadmill and the person is unfamiliar with treadmill running, let the subject perform at least some of the warm-up on the treadmill.

If resting values are to be recorded before the test gets under way, it is best to take them while the subject is sitting and has recovered from any warm-up routine. The tester should make sure the subject understands how the test will be conducted and when it will be terminated. Then the actual test can begin. With runners, I prefer the following protocol.

1. Start the treadmill at the speed of the individual's 10,000-meter race pace (if only a 5,000 time is known, use a pace just a little slower than 5,000-meter race pace, which is 30 to 40 seconds per mile slower than current one-mile race pace).

2. The individual runs at this speed throughout the entire test but on a level (0 percent) grade for only the first two minutes.

3. Each minute after the second minute has been completed, the treadmill will be elevated 1 percent. The speed stays the same.

4. Any physiological variables that are being monitored should be recorded during the final 15 seconds of each minute.

5. About 10 seconds before the end of *each* minute, the tester asks the subject if he or she can go on for another minute. If the answer is yes (indicated by a thumbs-up sign), then the current treadmill grade is increased by 1 percent and the test continues. If the answer is no (indicated by a back-and-forth horizontal waving of the hand), then the tester may ask the subject if a half minute more is possible. Based on the response, the test is either terminated or continued for a final half minute.

6. If recovery data are to be collected, the subject should be seated (on a chair on the treadmill), with the feet elevated or the legs moving somewhat to stimulate circulation. Final blood collection for determination of maximum lactate accumulation should be made about two to three minutes after the test ends.

If a running max test is being conducted *over ground* on a running track or road (to simulate race conditions more closely), then the following protocol is used.

1. For the first 400 meters of the test, the subject runs at about 10,000-meter race pace or a little slower.

2. After completing 400 meters of running, the subject increases the pace to one that is equal to his or her most current 5,000-meter race pace.

3. The subject holds the 5K race pace for three more 400-meter laps of a track (or equivalent distance on a road) with 30-second expired-air collections beginning with the third of these three laps.

4. Upon completion of lap four (1,600 meters of running), the subject increases the pace to one that is as hard as he or she can go for a final 400 meters of running. Expired-air collections (lasting about 30 seconds each) are continually collected during this final all-out run.

5. Heart rates can be monitored and recorded during the final 400 meters of running (or immediately upon termination of the final 400 meters if a heart-rate monitor is not available).

6. If recovery data are to be collected, the subject should sit quietly with the feet elevated or with the legs moving around somewhat to stimulate circulation. Blood samples for maximum lactate determination should be taken about two to three minutes after the test ends.

In over-ground running tests, the test administrators must be driven alongside the subject throughout the test to make the expired-air collections. Figure 10.10 shows an over-ground running test being administered.

MEASURING ENDURANCE AND ECONOMY

A good test for endurance is one that measures blood-lactate accumulation upon termination of a series of increasingly faster submaximal runs. Economy is often measured during a similar series of submax runs, but it can also be evaluated using just one or two submaximal efforts.

Blood samples and expired-air samples can both be collected during the same series of runs. Following a normal warm-up, use the following protocol, which is practical for either a treadmill test or an over-ground test. Hook up the subject for collecting expired air samples and for monitoring heart rates.

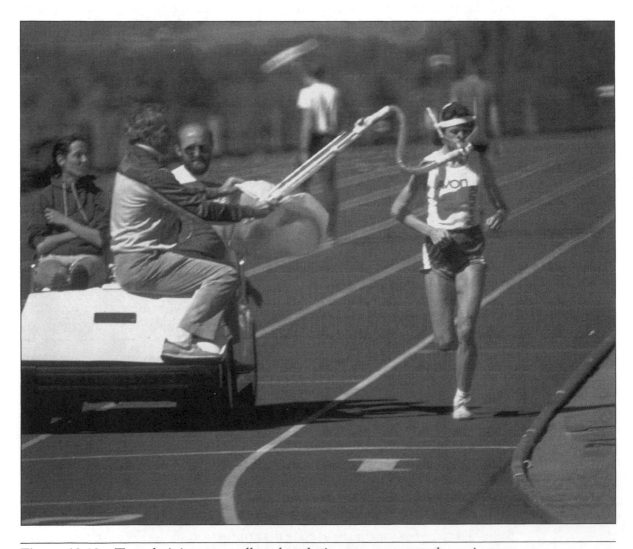

Figure 10.10 Test administrators collect data during an over-ground running test.

1. From the following chart of running velocities (in meters per minute) and corresponding mile paces, pick the *fastest* velocity that is *slower* than the current 5,000-meter race pace.

190	210	230	250	270	290	310	330	350	370
8:28	7:40	7:00	6:26	5:58	5:33	5:11	4:53	4:36	4:21

2. Count back three or four paces, depending on whether a four- or five-stage test is used, to determine the first (slowest) test speed.

3. The subject runs for five minutes at the first test speed, and an expired-air sample is collected for the final 60 seconds of the five-minute run. Heart rate is also monitored during the final 15 seconds of the run.

4. After the five-minute run, a blood sample is collected during a 60-second break that the subject receives after each run.

5. Heart rate is recorded, expired air is analyzed for determination of $\dot{V}O_2$ and $\dot{V}CO_2$, and the blood sample is used to determine blood-lactate accumulation.

6. A similar five-minute run is performed at each progressively faster test speed (selected from the preceding chart), until the fastest speed identified in step 1 has been completed.

7. $\dot{V}O_2$, blood lactate, and heart rate are determined and recorded for each of the four or five submaximal tests that are completed.

Plotting these data will generate a heart-rate response curve, a blood-lactate profile, and an economy curve.

Using Economy Data

The resulting economy curve can be used to compare running economies among athletes or for the same athlete at different stages or seasons of training. This is accomplished by comparing the $\dot{V}O_2$ values at identical test speeds. In addition, by extending the economy curve out to the individual's $\dot{V}O_2$max, a value for $v\dot{V}O_2$max can be determined. Figure 10.11, on page 212, illustrates.

A single value for running economy can be calculated by converting the $\dot{V}O_2$ at any measured velocity to a standard value that represents the "cost" of running one kilometer. For example, a $\dot{V}O_2$ of 50 milliliters per kilogram when running at a velocity of 250 meters per minute would result in one kilometer of running costing 200 milliliters per kilogram per kilometer ($1,000 \div 250 \times 50 = 200$). Similarly, running at 300 meters per minute with a $\dot{V}O_2$ of 60 milliliters per kilogram would also cost 200 milliliters per kilogram per kilometer ($1,000 \div 300 \times 60 = 200$). This method of expressing running economy has the advantage of comparing an individual's economy over a variety of velocities.

Using Blood-Lactate Data

The blood-lactate profile can be used as a measure of endurance. A simple way to accomplish this is to connect the lactate data points and determine the $\dot{V}O_2$ and running velocity that correspond to a standard lactate value. This is done in figure 10.11, using a blood-lactate value of 4.0 millimoles per liter ($mmol \cdot L^{-1}$) of blood. The corresponding $\dot{V}O_2$ and running velocities can then be expressed as a percentage of $\dot{V}O_2$ and $v\dot{V}O_2$max, respectively. The values for percentage of

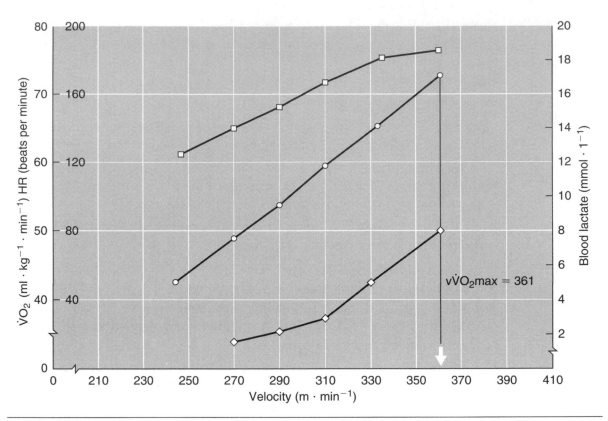

Figure 10.11   A comparison of the oxygen consumption ($\dot{V}O_2$—circles), heart rate (HR—squares), and blood-lactate level (Bla—triangles) of an elite runner.
From Daniels 1998, page 50.

$\dot{V}O_2$max and v$\dot{V}O_2$max are 85 and 89 in figure 10.11, which are typical values for a trained distance runner.

Heart-Rate Data

The heart-rate data collected during the submaximal and maximal tests can be compared with data from subsequent test sessions. In addition, a percentage of max heart rate can be determined that corresponds to the blood-lactate value of 4.0 millimoles per liter (about 90 percent in figure 10.11).

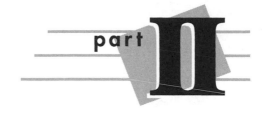

part **II**

Developing a Sports Performance Training Program

With the information provided in part II, you will be able to apply the scientific principles from part I to meet your sport-specific conditioning needs. Chapter 11, "Incorporating Sport-Specific Skills into Conditioning," features a number of sport-specific drills from coaching experts for the following nine sports:

Baseball—Fernando Montes
Basketball—Bill Foran
Distance Running—Jack Daniels
Football—Kent Johnston
Golf—Pete Draovitch
Hockey Peter—Twist
Soccer—Vern Gambetta
Tennis—Barrett Bugg and E. Paul Roetert
Volleyball—Courtney Carter

Eric Lawson, of the United State Olympic Training Center provides an overview for the chapter.

Tudor Bompa's chapter 12, "Periodizing Training for Peak Performance," takes a close look at what is involved in setting up an annual periodization plan for athletes of different sports and specifically discusses factoring in training phases for strength, endurance, and speed. Chapter 13, "Designing Periodized Training Programs" combines the information from chapter 12 with a way of setting up a specific periodized training program for each of the nine sports covered in chapter 11. Todd Ellenbecker's chapter 14, "Restoring Performance After Injury," covers applying fitness components to effectively rehabilitate injured athletes while keeping them as fit as possible for their specific sports.

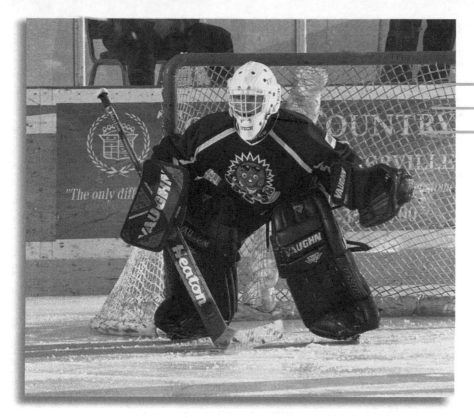

Incorporating Sport-Specific Skills Into Conditioning

OVERVIEW
Eric Lawson

*T*he days of the generalized "one program fits all" strength and conditioning model are quickly coming to an end. It is clear now that incorporating sport-specific skills into strength and conditioning programs helps athletes target specific performance requirements and helps coaches account for individual athletic idiosyncrasies.

Today's strength and conditioning expert should work in conjunction with the head coach, athletic trainer, positional coach, sport psychologist, sport nutritionist, and the athlete to meet the specific performance needs of the sport and the athlete. Working together, this sport-performance enhancement team ensures that the athlete can improve performance and also mitigates the likelihood of injury.

In attempting to formulate a comprehensive strength and conditioning program for a particular athlete, the sport-performance team begins by determining the athlete's requirements, that is, assessing the athlete's strengths and weaknesses. See chapter 2 for specific tests and a functional assessment form (page 42).

Assessing the Athlete

The specific performance concerns of an athlete fall into the following categories: sport-specific movements, planes of motion, muscular action, metabolic demands, strengths (offensive and defensive), and weaknesses (offensive and defensive). A strength and conditioning coach can arrive at the specific performance concerns by using the entire body of knowledge available, starting with the head coach's input followed by input from the positional or assistant coach. Then he or she can gather information from the physiologists, trainers, psychologists, and, if available, biomechanists. The strength and conditioning coach should spend many hours in practice and film sessions to become familiar with the metabolic and kinematic demands of the sport.

Generally, the higher the level of the athlete, the more specific the training protocol. Younger and inexperienced athletes should spend more time with foundational strength building (see chapters 4 and 7).

Tailoring Drills to a Particular Sport

When determining specific skills to train athletes for their sport, think about the types of training the sport requires: foundational strength, neuromuscular power, kinesthetic proprioception core stability and functional strength, dynamic flexibility and range of motion (ROM), speed, agility, quickness, and metabolic conditioning.

The next step is to determine the power-to-strength requirements and the specific metabolic requirements of the sport and to emphasize the most important components within the drills you choose. One way to accomplish this is to review kinematic and repetitive-motion analyses and then to design appropriate speed and agility drills for the sport.

Take volleyball, for example, as a typical interval sport with short exercise periods (6 to 7 seconds) of high intensity alternating with 12- to 14-second rest periods; these metabolic requirements are primarily supported by the ATP-CP (alactic anaerobic) and the O2 (aerobic) systems. Thus, the conditioning drills are formulated to tax the ATP-CP and O2 systems and to simulate the movements and metabolic requirements of competition. To tax the ATP-CP and O2 energy systems effectively for a sport like volleyball, the scheme of sets and repetitions should allow for 5 to 10 seconds of intense activity interspersed with 9- to 12-second rest intervals; the goal is to elevate and keep the heart-rate reserve (HRR) between 75 and 85 percent and to maintain a steady pace for a minimum of 20 minutes. The entire conditioning volume depends on the intensity and duration of the practice and the athlete's current juncture in the periodized cycle (see chapters 12 and 13).

Elite-level volleyball play also requires repetitive, explosive movements; therefore, many coaches use drills that stress repetitive arm swing, dig position, defensive position, transition steps, and print block positions. The conditioning program menu should contain a variety of drills to help thwart mental and physical staleness.

When devising the overall plan for increasing an athlete's jumping and game-day quickness, keep three major determinants in mind: muscle mass, proportion of fast-twitch muscle units, and the effectiveness of the voluntary neuromuscular activation, that is, the ability to activate many motor units quickly during a voluntary contraction (Schmidtbleicher 1992). The speed of a movement is always the result of the produced acceleration impulse. Therefore, speed-strength performances are characterized by the steepness of the rise in force and the height of the force maximum.

The weight-training and core-stability portion of a program blends general closed kinetic chain total-body exercises with sport-specific exercises. The core-stability routines incorporate medicine balls, physio balls, and bands and are designed to develop core strength and kinesthetic proprioception (see chapter 7). The routines are usually performed immediately following a light warm-up.

The model for successfully incorporating sport-specific skills into training integrates many areas of expertise and knowledge. Today's strength and conditioning coaches must understand the specific physical requirements of the sport they are coaching. Interactions with positional coaches and athletes and access to the scientific body of knowledge for a particular sport are critical for proper development of a comprehensive strength and conditioning program. The age of specialization and individualization has arrived.

BASEBALL   Fernando Montes

Baseball has long been known as America's pastime. The game is rich in tradition and, when it comes to sport-specific strength and conditioning, rife with myth.

The challenge for the strength and conditioning professional is to understand the traditions of the game and the myths that surround strength and conditioning. The first major obstacle is the player. The baseball player of today lacks the overall fitness and conditioning of competitors in other sports. The source of this problem is not the game of baseball but the lack of early physical development and exposure to basic movements in early childhood. The basic issue cannot be overlooked; it must be addressed as a fundamental training issue throughout the overall training program.

First, you should establish the needs and current physical limitations of each player. It is important to have a starting point from which to work when designing movement agility drills. This framework is helpful in keeping you focused on quality preparation and good program design.

Consider the following steps before planning a sport-specific movement program for baseball players.

1. Determine and understand the following areas:
   - The athlete's current physical development—what type of strength does this athlete have? Can he or she negotiate these drills with his or her current level of strength?

- The athlete's training history—what exposure has this athlete had to this type of training?
- The athlete's fitness level—what kind of shape is the athlete in? Is the energy system that he or she will use ready?
- The position the athlete plays—which movements match the player's needs and the position he or she plays?
- The basics of a drill continuum—understand the levels of drill adaptation from basic to advanced drills.
- The training parameters—consider the number of athletes you need to train, the location and equipment available, and the feasibility of performing the drills both indoors and outdoors. Evaluate when in the training program to conduct the drills, how much time to assign to them, and what total volume to use.

2. Understand the factors for drill selection.
   - Body control—how much does this come into play in the position the athlete plays?
   - Balance—establish the specific kind of balance needed by the individual for the position he or she plays (pitching, hitting, fielding, and baserunning).
   - Timing—determine the time it takes to execute these movements by position (pitching, baserunning, fielding, hitting).
   - Chaotic movements—what reactive situations take place in baseball?

3. Identify the skills and movements unique to each position.
   - Basic athletic position—what type of stance is needed in hitting, fielding, pitching, and baserunning?
   - First-step movement—what type of start is needed for hitting, fielding, pitching, and baserunning?

4. Identify the movements and specific injury information of the individuals and any potential hazards by position.
   - Identify what potential injury zones are common to baseball (e.g., pitcher fielding a bunt, base runner sliding into a shortstop, etc.).
   - Identify the injury history of individual athletes.

5. Evaluate the drill using the SMART test:
   - **S**pecific—does the drill meet the needs of the player and the position he or she plays?
   - **M**easurable—is this drill measurable in testing or progression?
   - **A**ttainable—will this drill achieve the desired expectations and training goals?
   - **R**ealistic—is the drill realistic in its implementation?
   - **T**ime manageable—can the desired training goals be accomplished in a timely manner?

Before designing any sport-specific movement drill, ensure that all aspects of the program design meet the needs of the sport and the individuals being trained. Only then can expectations and training goals be reached. The following drills may meet the needs of your athletes.

Single-Hoop Agility

Purpose

To identify specific movement limitations in body control and foot movement for players of all positions in order to work on baserunning and fielding skills

Procedure

1. Use a hoop or mark a circle that has a 12-foot diameter.

2. The player starts at any point around the hoop but must end at the same location.

3. The player sprints around the hoop as fast as possible without allowing the body to pull away from the hoop. He or she should stay as close as possible to the hoop throughout the drill.

4. The athlete should lower the inside shoulder as he or she rounds the hoop while keeping outside foot placement away from his or her center of gravity. This action prevents falling and facilitates body control as the athlete negotiates future obstacles or hoops.

Limitations

- Poor body control as the athlete rounds the hoop (player moving away from the hoop)
- Foot placement too close together as the athlete rounds the hoop (the feet become tangled up)

Variations

- Double-hoop figure-8 agility—Follow the instructions used in the single-hoop drill, however there are two 12-foot hoops forming a figure-8. The athlete must continue to adjust both body control and foot placement as he or she moves through the second hoop.

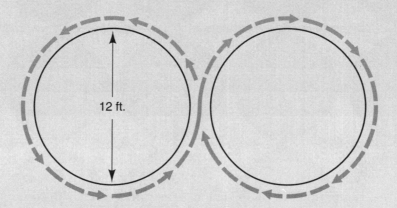

- Figure-8 rabbit run—The player negotiates around the two hoops in the figure-8 pattern while being chased by another player. The lead player should stay as close to the hoops as possible throughout the drill and prevent the chasing player from tagging him or her.

- Four-hoop rabbit run—This drill includes four 12-foot diameter hoops. The player should sprint as fast as he or she can around the hoops in a figure-8 pattern, staying as close to the hoops as possible throughout the drill, and prevent the chasing player from tagging him or her. After the lead player has completed one figure-8 pattern, he or she can go in any direction using any combination of hoops.

Three-Cone Movement

Purpose
To teach body control and change of direction in preparation for future agility drills and to identify specific movement limitations

Procedure
1. The coach assigns the starting position and the type of athletic (baseball-specific) stance the athlete should use for the drill. The coach then assigns the specific movement (i.e., speed carioca, carioca step, shuffle, sprint, backpedal, and so forth).
2. Using the assigned movement, the player negotiates the cones as quickly as possible, moving in a straight line from cone #1 to cone #2, back to cone #1, and on to cone #3.
3. The athlete should repeat as assigned.

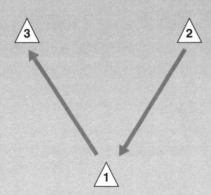

Limitations
Poor body control and weight shift during reactive change of direction

Variation
Three-cone T—Same as the previous drill, but the player moves from cone #1 up the line until parallel to cones #2 and #3. The athlete changes direction and moves toward cone #2, then changes direction again and moves to cone #3. Once at cone #3, the player returns by changing direction again until he or she reaches the middle between cones #2 and #3. The player then returns to cone #1 (starting position).

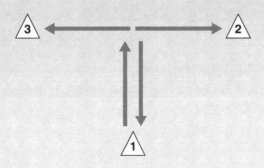

Agility Bag Lateral In-Out Shuffle Step

Purpose

To develop the lateral shuffle-step movement

Procedure

1. Set up 6 to 10 agility bags in a straight line about five feet apart from one another.
2. The player starts in good athletic position, with weight over the balls of the feet.
3. The athlete negotiates the agility bags using a lateral shuffle step as quickly as possible.

Limitations

Poor lateral movement patterns, poor hip flexibility, inadequate foot quickness, and improper foot placement

Variations

The coach can add other movements at the end of the agility drill, such as agility hoops and quick-foot ladders.

Agility Bag Ball Pickup

Purpose

To teach basic sprint and backpedal movements to prepare for reactive and chaotic movements

Procedure

1. Set up 6 to 10 agility bags, cones, and baseballs as shown in the diagram.
2. The player starts in a good athletic position, with weight over the balls of the feet.
3. He or she moves quickly around each agility bag to field each baseball.
4. The athlete backpedals and straddles the bag while placing the ball on the assigned cone.
5. The player repeats the pattern until he or she has picked up all the baseballs.

Limitations

Poor concentration, lack of foot quickness, and poor foot placement

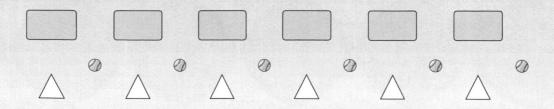

BASKETBALL   Bill Foran

Basketball is a game of high-intensity work followed by a quick recovery period. This sequence continues throughout a game. Conditioning is paramount. If basketball players are not in top physical shape, their skill level drops considerably during the game as fatigue sets in. The worst way to lose a game is because of fatigue.

Basketball players must be able to run the court efficiently, have a quick first step, read and react to game situations, move in any direction at any time, and jump high and quickly in rapid succession. To accomplish this, basketball players need a strength base and a conditioning base. The player who is well conditioned will obtain the best results from sport-specific functional training.

A conditioning base is developed through a 6- to 10-week progressive program of 400s (meters), 200s, and 100s on a track, football field, or soccer field.

A strength base is developed through a total-body weight-training program with emphasis on the power center of the body (hips and legs) and the core (midsection). The upper body needs to be strong, balanced, and flexible, but it is third priority behind the legs and midsection.

The sport-specific conditioning drills for basketball include on-court conditioning drills with and without a basketball, jumping and quick-feet plyometrics, agility drills, and medicine ball drills.

On-Court Conditioning Drills

After athletes have developed a conditioning base, they are ready to build on that base with on-court conditioning drills that involve sprinting, dribbling, and shooting skills. There are many different on-court conditioning drills. Five are listed here, but be creative and come up with others.

Five and One-Half

Purpose
To develop basic on-court conditioning

Procedure

1. The athlete runs five and one-half lengths of the court as fast as possible (baseline to baseline five times and then a finish at half-court).

2. After each run, the athlete should rest two to two and one-half times his or her running time. For example, if an athlete runs the drill in 32 seconds, he or she should rest between 64 and 80 seconds before the next run.

Variation
Add dribbling a basketball to the drill for variety.

Suicide Shuttle

Purpose

To develop basic on-court conditioning

Procedure

1. Players start at one baseline, run to the closest free-throw line and back to the baseline, run to half-court and back, run to the opposite free-throw line and back, and then run fullcourt and back.

2. The rest is two to two and one-half times the running time.

Variation

Add dribbling a basketball to the drill for variety.

Sideline Touch and Elbow Jump Shot

Purpose

To develop basic conditioning as well as shooting skills

Procedure

1. The player shoots a jumper at the right elbow of the free-throw line.

2. He or she then sprints to the opposite sideline, and sprints back to the left elbow for another jumper.

3. The player then sprints to the other sideline and back to the right elbow for a jumper.

4. This continues for a set time or until a certain number of baskets are made. Have another player serve as a rebounder or passer during this drill.

Variation

Have the athlete lateral slide to the sideline and sprint back.

Endline Touch and Top-of-the-Key Jump Shot

Purpose

To develop basic conditioning as well as shooting skills

Procedure

1. The athlete shoots a top-of-the-key jumper within a comfortable range, then sprints to the opposite baseline and back for another jumper.

2. The player repeats this for a set time or until a certain number of baskets are made. Have another player serve as a rebounder or passer during this drill.

Corner Touch and Perimeter Jump Shot

Purpose
To develop basic conditioning as well as shooting skills

Procedure
1. The athlete shoots a perimeter jumper, then sprints to one of the court's four corners and back for another perimeter jumper.
2. The player then sprints to a different corner and back for a jumper.
3. This continues for a set time or until a certain number of shots are made. Have another player serve as a rebounder or passer during this drill.

Plyometric Drills

After developing a strength base in the hips and legs with squats, lunges, step-ups, and so on (see chapters 4 and 7), jumping plyometrics are the best way to improve the vertical jump. A good jump-training program involves box jumps, weighted box jumps, double jumps, and single-leg hops.

Be aware that box jumps can be dangerous if done incorrectly. Make sure the height of the box is appropriate for the athlete's jumping ability. Soccer shin guards may protect an athlete from a badly bruised shin if he or she loses concentration and misses a jump. Do not allow an athlete to hyperflex the knees on landing. If this occurs, the box is too high.

The quick-feet plyometric drill (page 225) helps athletes practice moving their feet as fast as possible.

Box Jump

Purpose
To improve vertical jumping ability

Procedure
1. The athlete stands in front of the box (the starting height is usually between 20 and 30 inches), jumps as high as possible, and lands softly on the box.
2. He or she then steps down. The athlete repeats these steps for 10 jumps.

Variation
After the athlete can do three sets of 10 jumps, he or she is ready for weighted box jumps. The athlete executes weighted box jumps by holding dumbbells in each hand (5 to 10 pounds for starters) while performing the box jump. The athlete *must not* jump down. The player performs 10 jumps. During weighted box jumps the athlete should not use the arms. The arms should stay in a fixed position, either straight or slightly bent.

Double Jump

Purpose

To improve vertical jumping ability and jumping quickness

Procedure

1. The athlete starts on a small box (12 inches high) and jumps off the box to the floor.
2. As soon as his or her feet touch the floor, the athlete jumps onto a higher box (20 to 30 inches) as quickly as possible.
3. The athlete steps down, returns to the starting position, and repeats the jump up to 10 times.

Single-Leg Hop

Purpose

To improve vertical jumping ability, balance, stability, and one-legged power

Procedure

1. The athlete stands in front of a small box (8 to 16 inches high) on one foot.
2. He or she hops with one leg up on the box and holds the position for one to two seconds.
3. The athlete then hops down on the same leg and holds the position for one to two seconds.
4. The player hops back onto the box for up to 10 repetitions, using one leg throughout the entire exercise before repeating the sequence using the other leg.

Quick-Feet Plyo

Purpose

To develop quick foot movements

Procedure

1. Mark four spots 12 to 18 inches apart on a good surface (not concrete).
2. Number the spots 1 through 4 in this pattern:

3   **2**

4   **1**

3. The athlete follows the number pattern with the feet, moving as quickly as possible.
4. Count the number of times the athlete lands on the starting spot during the allotted time.
5. Allow enough rest time for a good recovery between drills (20 to 90 seconds, depending on the fitness level of the athlete). Do four to six two-feet drills and four to six one-foot drills per workout.

Variations

Several different movement patterns can be set up using the same four spots. Players can do the drills with two feet for 10 to 20 seconds or with one foot for 10 seconds.
- Two-number patterns—1-2, 1-4, 1-3, 4-2
- Three-number patterns—1-2-3, 1-3-2, 1-4-3, 1-3-4
- Four-number patterns—1-2-3-4, 1-4-3-2, 1-3-2-4, 4-2-3-1

Agility Drills

Of all the movement skills basketball players need, being able to read and react, to move in any direction quickly and under control, may be the most important. Agility drills performed all out with proper technique will help develop these movement skills. Be creative and design your own agility drills using cones and quick-feet ladders (see chapter 8 for several ideas). They should last 10 to 20 seconds with all-out effort and can involve quick starts and stops, changes of direction, and movements in all directions.

Lane Shuffle

Purpose
To learn to move in any direction quickly and with control

Procedure
1. Players start on one side of the lane and move laterally as quickly as possible to the other side of the lane and back.
2. They continue the back-and-forth movement for 20 seconds.
3. Count the number of times players cross the lane.

Around the Lane

Purpose
To learn to move in any direction quickly and with control

Procedure
1. Players start at the baseline where the lane sideline intersects it. They sprint up the lane line to the free-throw line and then move laterally across the free-throw line to the opposite lane line.
2. They backpedal to the baseline and move laterally back to the starting position.
3. Players immediately repeat the movements, moving in the opposite direction.

Lateral Resistance Quick Step

Purpose
To learn to move in any direction quickly and with control

Procedure
1. Attach resistance-training rubber tubing or bands to each athlete.
2. Athletes move laterally against the resistance for three quick steps and come back to the starting position under control.
3. They immediately repeat the explosive quick steps, performing the drill for reps (5 to 10) or time (15 to 30 seconds).
4. Players then execute the movement to the opposite side.

MEDICINE BALL DRILLS

Medicine ball drills are functional and versatile; they are effective for developing strength (especially core strength), power, and quickness. The following two drills develop core strength, and the third teaches athletes to sit deep and stay low on defense. Feel free to be creative and design your own drills.

Side Toss

Purpose
To develop core strength, power, and quickness

Procedure
1. Two athletes face each other about 10 to 12 feet apart.
2. One athlete holds the medicine ball with both hands next to the right hip.
3. He or she fully rotates the midsection to the right and tosses the ball while rotating back to a neutral position.
4. The athlete tosses the ball to the right side of the partner, who rotates to the right as well and then tosses it back.
5. After each partner does 10 tosses, the athletes repeat the drill on the left side.

Over Under and Under Over

Purpose
To develop core strength, power, and quickness

Procedure
1. Two athletes stand back to back about a foot apart.
2. The partner holding the medicine ball lifts it over his or her head and hands it to the other partner, who passes it between the legs and back to the other partner.
3. After 10 reps, they reverse the direction for 10 more reps.

Deep Squat Overhead Pass

Purpose
To develop core strength, power, and quickness

Procedure
1. Two athletes stand facing each other about 10 to 12 feet apart.
2. They both assume a deep squat position with heels on the floor, knees over the feet, head up, shoulders back, and hips as low as the knees.
3. In this position, the partners play catch using overhead bounce passes for 20 passes.

DISTANCE RUNNING   Jack Daniels

Although it is useful to understand the principles of training and the needs of the body in preparing for athletic performance, what most coaches and athletes want to know is what types of workouts they should do and why. The following types of sport-specific training do not so much highlight specific "drills" that a distance runner—track or cross country—would do as provide guidelines as to the most important sport-specific conditioning workouts for endurance athletes.

Cellular Adaptations

A variety of changes take place in and around the exercising muscle cells as a function of exercise. These include improved blood supply to the muscle cells; increased number, size, and distribution of the mitochondria (sites of aerobic metabolism); and increased enzyme activity (chemicals that aid in the process of metabolism). Fortunately, most of these desirable adaptations do not require exercise at more than moderate intensity. For runners, this means easy running of the type used on warm-up runs, cool-down runs, and long, easy runs. Running at an intensity of about 70 percent of the runner's $\dot{V}O_2$max (about 75 percent of maximum heart rate) is adequate. This intensity could be referred to as "conversational." Keep in mind that running at greater intensities will produce more fatigue but not necessarily a more rapid, or better, training adaptation.

Easy Runs

Purpose
To encourage cellular adaptation

Procedure
The easy runs can vary widely in duration. Runners do easy running as a warm-up for a more intense session, during recovery between harder runs, and as a cool-down following a demanding session. The amount of running performed for these various reasons is a function of personal preference, with the runner doing as much as necessary to accomplish an adequate warm-up or recovery. If an easy run is all that the runner is performing in a particular training session, the duration of the run will typically vary from about one-half hour to as much as two and one-half hours. The shorter easy runs are just that—easy runs used to recover from harder training days that still produce some beneficial effects. The longer easy runs are performed specifically to train the body to exercise for prolonged periods as well as to stimulate even greater cellular adaptations.

To determine the length of a long run, place a relative limit on the amount of time spent running. For example, identify a long run as one that is not more than 25 percent of the total mileage for the week, or two and one-half hours, whichever is the lesser amount. Obviously, the 25 percent value is appropriate only for those training more than four days each week.

During long runs the runner should be aware of good mechanics, use a comfortable, rhythmical breathing pattern, and consider taking in some fluids while running. A true long run would normally be performed not more than once each week and in some programs only a couple times over a three-week period.

Lactate Threshold

As discussed in chapter 10, each runner has an intensity, or speed of running (lactate threshold), beyond which lactic-acid clearance cannot keep up with lactic-acid production. At this point blood lactate accumulates at a rapidly increasing rate. A runner's lactate threshold is a good indicator of how long the runner can endure a particular intensity. Marathon runners, for example, race the majority of a marathon just below "threshold" intensity, and a blood-lactate measurement at the end of a marathon would usually show lactate levels that are no different from normal resting values (about 1 mmol per liter). The higher the intensity (the farther above lactate threshold) at which a race is run, the faster blood lactate accumulates, with 800- and 1,500-meter races showing very high levels even though they last only a few minutes. The longer the race, the slower blood lactate accumulates until the intensity associated with lactate threshold is reached, after which lactate clearance can keep up with or exceed production. Blood lactate then may actually decrease as the race progresses.

To improve a particular function in most types of running, that function must be stressed but not overstressed. For training performed with a goal of increasing lactate threshold (endurance), choosing the proper intensity of training is particularly important.

If a trained runner were to run a race that takes about one hour to perform, the pace that he or she would average for the race would closely mimic threshold pace. Threshold pace is the preferred intensity for any threshold training used in a running program. "Comfortably hard" is a good, subjective way to describe threshold pace. A heart rate of a little over 90 percent of maximum would also give a good estimate of threshold intensity.

The best measure of whether a runner is performing at threshold intensity is to perform a series of runs that last about 5 to 12 minutes, each at what is felt to be threshold intensity, and measure blood lactate following each run. If the resulting value stays the same after each run, that indicates that the pace properly reflected threshold intensity. On the other hand, if blood lactates climb with each subsequent run, the pace was too fast. If lactates steadily decrease, the pace was too easy. Naturally, weather and terrain will cause the running pace to vary somewhat even with the same intensity of effort.

Another way to estimate whether a pace is too fast is to become aware of breathing patterns. Having to breathe more rapidly than a two-two rhythm (taking two steps while breathing in and two steps while breathing out) is usually a sign that threshold intensity has been surpassed.

Two basic types of training fall into the category of threshold training: tempo runs and cruise intervals. The intensity (speed of running) is the same for each—threshold intensity.

It is typical to include one session of threshold training in each week's schedule, but some phases of training may include no threshold runs while others may have two sessions per week.

Distance Running

Tempo Runs

Purpose

To stress the lactate-threshold system and thereby increase the lactate threshold (endurance)

Procedure

A tempo run is typically a steady run that is about 20 minutes in duration. The runner performs a tempo run following a good warm-up and follows it with a good cool-down. The tempo run itself is run at a steady pace throughout, with the emphasis on going neither too fast nor too slow. The runner should relax and concentrate on the task rather than what is going on around him or her. The runner should usually perform a tempo run on a calm day over flat terrain so that he or she can maintain a consistent intensity of effort throughout.

Cruise Intervals

Purpose

To stress the lactate-threshold system and thereby increase the lactate threshold (endurance)

Procedure

Cruise intervals are minitempo runs separated by brief recovery periods. A session of cruise intervals might involve five or six repeated one-mile runs with a one-minute recovery after each one. It is usually best to repeat runs that are 4 to 15 minutes in duration, with a recovery time that is about one-fifth as long as the preceding run time. A rule to keep in mind regarding sessions of cruise intervals is that the total amount of "quality" running (total time or distance at threshold pace) should not be greater than 10 percent of the total mileage accumulated for that particular week. Minimum and maximum durations of quality running can also be set at 25 minutes and 40 minutes, respectively.

Aerobic Capacity ($\dot{V}O_2$max)

To stress the capacity of the running muscles to produce energy through aerobic metabolism, running intensity needs to be about equal to the pace at which a runner could race for 10 to 15 minutes (one to three miles, depending on the runner's ability). It is common for coaches and runners to consider 5,000-meter pace as most closely reflecting $\dot{V}O_2$max intensity. This rule, however, produces a rather conservative estimate for runners who take 20 minutes or longer to race a 5,000.

Subjectively, the intensity of running appropriate for aerobic capacity training can be referred to as "hard," and this type of training is indeed the hardest that runners will encounter. If heart rate is used to monitor a training session designed to stress aerobic capacity, the slowest pace that elicits maximum heart rate is the pace to shoot for. Of course, any pace faster than that will also elicit maximum heart rate, but the goal is to work as hard, aerobically, as possible, and to minimize anaerobic involvement. Going too fast in this type of training session may produce the desired results, but it puts much greater stress on the body and requires a longer recovery period without producing any greater benefit.

Interval Training

Purpose

To stress the capacity of the running muscles to produce energy through aerobic metabolism

Procedure

This is hard training that typically involves repeated runs of three to five minutes in duration at a speed the runner could maintain for only 10 to 15 minutes. The recovery time (which should be active in nature) between individual work bouts is usually about equal to the time spent in the previous quality run.

Interval training can involve a series of shorter runs (even as short as 30 seconds each), but the accompanying recovery periods must then be kept even shorter. Furthermore, when performing shorter work bouts, it is important not to run too fast, which is tempting because the runs are so short. It is better to shorten the recoveries than to speed up the runs. In other words, each runner will have an appropriate interval training pace, which he or she should adhere to regardless of the duration of the individual runs within the session.

An upper limit to place on the quality portion of an interval session is 8 percent of the total mileage for the week or 10,000 meters, whichever is less.

Interval training is demanding. Even during a phase of training when intervals have top priority, it is not common to include more than one (sometimes two if no races are scheduled for that week) interval sessions in a single week. Furthermore, interval training is best scheduled for a period of several weeks during a single season, then set aside in favor of other types of training.

Speed and Economy

Improvements in speed and economy tend to reflect as much attention to biomechanical changes as to physiological changes. In fact, much of the training associated with speed and economy is more anaerobic than aerobic in nature.

What the runner is trying to do in this aspect of training is to minimize unnecessary movement and perform the most work with the least effort. The runner is trying to learn to run faster while staying relaxed, which demands shorter bouts of exercise separated by relatively long periods of active recovery.

For the distance runner, the speed of running used to improve speed and economy need not be nearly as fast as what would be appropriate for a sprinter. Training at an individual's current mile pace is adequate in almost all cases. Still, the training can be referred to as "fast," whereas training designed for lactate threshold and aerobic capacity improvement was referred to as "comfortably hard" and "hard." Bear in mind that fast is usually not as demanding as hard, primarily because the faster training sessions are made up of shorter work bouts and longer recovery periods.

Distance Running

Repetition Training

Purpose
To minimize unnecessary movement and to perform the most work with the least effort

Procedure
Repetition training is similar to interval training in that it involves repeated work bouts separated by periods of recovery, but the reps are typically shorter, faster, and separated by periods of "full" recovery. The shortness of the work bouts caters to the faster speed of the runs, which in turn demands longer recoveries. The speed of repetitions is usually at current one-mile race pace. If the individual is training for races shorter than one mile, rep pace is more often adjusted to coincide with race pace.

Running relatively fast not only develops better speed but also improves running economy. The prolonged recovery periods ensure good recovery and allow the runner to feel good enough to perform each subsequent run in a relaxed way with good technique. The key is to learn to run fast and relaxed and to feel in control of desirable running mechanics.

Most repetition sessions involve individual runs (work bouts) that last up to about two minutes each (distances of 200, 400, and 600 meters are common). The runner performs enough quality runs in the session to reach about 5 percent of the week's total mileage or a maximum of four miles.

Usually one repetition session per week is adequate. During a phase of training that emphasizes reps, however, the runner often performs two sets of reps in the same week. Although interval training may be eliminated from the latter weeks of a training program, it is common to include at least some reduced repetition sessions throughout a season of training.

Various types of training and the corresponding levels of intensity are shown below. E/L is easy/long; T is threshold; I is interval; R is repetition.

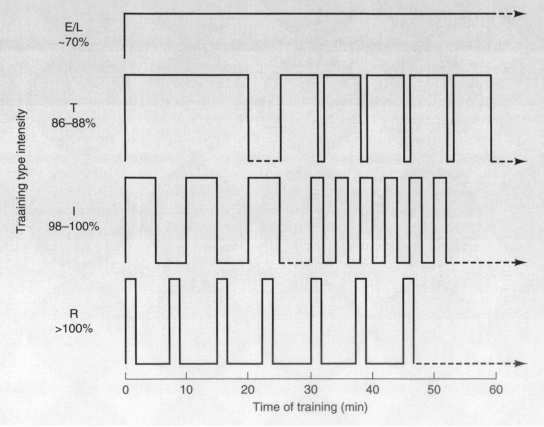

Table 11.1 presents lists of performances that can be converted to "VDOT" values. In short, VDOT values are based on performance-based VO_2max values to provide an estimate of an individual's aerobic capacity based on actual race time. To use table 11.1, a runner first finds his or her best VDOT based on a recent race performance (the performance that generates the highest VDOT is used when more than one performance is considered). The identified VDOT is then used with table 11.2 to establish the paces for each type of training.

Table 11.1	**VDOT Values for Popular Race Distances**								
VDOT	**1500**	**Mile**	**3000**	**2-mile**	**5000**	**10,000**	**15,000**	**Half-Marathon**	**Marathon**
30	8:30	9:11	17:56	19:19	30:40	63:46	98:14	2:21:04	4:49:17
31	8:15	8:55	17:27	18:48	29:15	62:03	95:36	2:17:21	4:41:57
32	8:02	8:41	16:59	18:18	29:05	60:26	93:07	2:13:49	4:34:59
33	7:49	8:27	16:33	17:50	28:21	58:54	90:45	2:10:27	4:28:22
34	7:37	8:14	16:09	17:24	27:39	57:26	88:30	2:07:16	4:22:03
35	7:25	8:01	15:45	16:58	27:00	56:03	86:22	2:04:13	4:16:03
36	7:14	7:49	15:23	16:34	26:22	54:44	84:20	2:01:19	4:10:19
37	7:04	7:38	15:01	16:11	25:26	53:29	82:24	1:58:34	4:04:50
38	6:54	7:27	14:41	15:49	25:12	52:17	80:33	1:55:55	3:59:35
39	6:44	7:17	14:21	15:29	24:39	51:09	78:47	1:53:24	3:54:34
40	6:35	7:07	14:03	15:08	24:08	50:03	77:06	1:50:59	3:49:45
41	6:27	6:58	13:45	14:49	23:38	49:01	75:29	1:48:40	3:45:09
42	6:19	6:49	13:28	14:31	23:09	48:01	73:56	1:46:27	3:40:43
43	6:11	6:41	13:11	14:13	22:41	47:04	72:27	1:44:20	3:36:28
44	6:03	6:32	12:55	13:56	22:15	46:09	71:02	1:42:17	3:32:23
45	5:56	6:25	12:40	13:40	21:50	45:16	69:40	1:40:20	3:28:26
46	5:49	6:17	12:26	13:25	21:25	44:25	68:22	1:38:27	3:24:39
47	5:42	6:10	12:12	13:10	21:02	43:36	67:06	1:36:38	3:21:00
48	5:36	6:03	11:58	12:55	20:39	42:50	65:53	1:34:53	3:17:29
49	5:30	5:56	11:45	12:41	20:18	42:04	64:44	1:33:12	3:14:06
50	5:24	5:50	11:33	12:28	19:57	41:21	63:36	1:31:35	3:10:49
51	5:18	5:44	11:21	12:15	19:36	40:39	62:31	1:30:02	3:07:39
52	5:13	5:38	11:09	12:02	19:17	39:59	61:29	1:28:31	3:04:36

(continued)

Table 11.1 *(continued)*

VDOT	1500	Mile	3000	2-mile	5000	10,000	15,000	Half-Marathon	Marathon
53	5:07	5:32	10:58	11:50	18:58	39:20	60:28	1:27:04	3:01:39
54	5:02	5:27	10:47	11:39	18:40	38:42	59:30	1:25:40	2:58:47
55	4:57	5:21	10:37	11:28	18:22	38:06	58:33	1:24:18	2:56:01
56	4:53	5:16	10:27	11:17	18:05	37:31	57:39	1:23:00	2:53:20
57	4:48	5:11	10:17	11:06	17:49	36:57	56:46	1:21:43	2:50:45
58	4:44	5:06	10:08	10:56	17:33	36:24	55:55	1:20:30	2:48:14
59	4:39	5:02	9:58	10:46	17:17	35:52	55:06	1:19:18	2:47:47
60	4:35	4:57	9:50	10:37	17:03	35:22	54:18	1:18:09	2:43:25
61	4:31	4:53	9:41	10:27	16:48	34:52	53:32	1:17:02	2:41:08
62	4:27	4:49	9:33	10:18	16:34	34:23	52:47	1:15:57	2:38:54
63	4:24	4:45	9:25	10:10	16:20	33:55	52:03	1:14:54	2:36:44
64	4:20	4:41	9:17	10:01	16:07	33:28	51:21	1:13:53	2:34:38
65	4:16	4:37	9:09	9:53	15:54	33:01	50:40	1:12:53	2:32:35
66	4:13	4:33	9:02	9:45	15:42	32:35	50:00	1:11:56	2:30:36
67	4:10	4:30	8:55	9:37	15:29	32:11	49:22	1:11:00	2:28:40
68	4:06	4:26	8:48	9:30	15:18	31:46	38:44	1:10:05	2:26:47
69	4:03	4:23	8:41	9:23	15:06	31:23	48:08	1:09:12	2:24:57
70	4:00	4:19	8:34	9:16	14:55	31:00	47:32	1:08:21	2:23:10
71	3:57	4:16	8:28	9:09	14:44	30:38	46:58	1:07:31	2:21:26
72	3:54	4:13	8:22	9:02	14:33	30:16	46:24	1:06:42	2:19:44
73	3:52	4:10	8:16	8:55	14:23	29:55	45:51	1:05:54	2:18:05
74	3:49	4:07	8:10	8:49	14:13	29:34	45:19	1:05:08	2:16:29
75	3:46	4:04	8:04	8:43	14:03	29:14	44:48	1:04:23	2:14:55
76	3:44	4:02	7:58	8:37	13:54	28:55	44:18	1:03:39	2:13:23
77	3:41+	3:58+	7:53	8:31	13:44	28:36	43:49	1:02:56	2:11:54
78	3:38.8	3:56.2	7:48	8:25	13:35	28:17	43:20	1:02:15	2:10:27
79	3:36.5	3:53.7	7:43	8:20	13:26	27:59	42:52	1:01:34	2:09:02
80	3:34.2	3:51.2	7:37.5	8:14	13:18	27:41	42:25	1:00:54	2:07:38

Table 11.2 Training Intensities Based on Current VDOT

VDOT	E/L Pace		M Pace	T Pace			I Pace			R Pace			
	km	mile	mile	400	1000	mile	400	1000	1200	mile	200	400	800
30	7:37	12:16	11:02	2:33	6:24	10:18	2:22	–	–	–	67	2:16	–
32	7:16	11:41	10:29	2:26	6:05	9:47	2:14	–	–	–	63	2:08	–
34	6:56	11:09	10:00	2:19	5:48	9:20	2:08	–	–	–	60	2:02	–
36	6:38	10:40	9:33	2:13	5:33	8:55	2:02	5:07	5:07	5:07	57	1:55	5:07
38	6:22	10:14	9:08	2:07	5:19	8:33	1:56	4:54	–	–	54	1:50	–
40	6:07	9:50	8:46	2:02	5:06	8:12	1:52	4:42	–	–	52	1:46	–
42	5:53	9:28	8:25	1:57	4:54	7:52	1:48	4:31	–	–	50	1:42	–
44	5:40	9:07	8:06	1:53	4:43	7:33	1:44	4:21	–	–	48	98	–
45	5:34	8:58	7:57	1:51	4:38	7:25	1:42	4:16	–	–	47	96	–
46	5:28	8:48	7:48	1:49	4:33	7:17	1:40	4:12	5:00	–	46	94	–
47	5:23	8:39	7:40	1:47	4:29	7:10	98	4:07	4:54	–	45	92	–
48	5:17	8:31	7:32	1:45	4:24	7:02	96	4:03	4:49	–	44	90	–
49	5:12	8:22	7:24	1:43	4:20	6:55	95	3:59	4:45	–	44	89	–
50	5:07	8:14	7:17	1:42	4:15	6:51	93	3:55	4:41	–	43	87	–
51	5:02	8:07	7:09	1:40	4:11	6:44	92	3:51	4:36	–	42	86	–
52	4:58	7:59	7:02	98	4:07	6:38	91	3:48	4:33	–	42	85	–
53	4:53	7:52	6:56	97	4:04	6:32	90	3:44	4:29	–	41	84	–
54	4:49	7:45	6:49	95	4:00	6:26	.88	3:41	4:25	–	40	82	–
55	4:45	7:38	6:43	94	3:56	6:20	87	3:37	4:21	–	40	81	–
56	4:40	7:31	6:37	93	3:53	6:15	86	3:34	4:18	–	39	80	–
57	4:36	7:25	6:31	91	3:50	6:09	85	3:31	4:15	–	39	79	–
58	4:33	7:19	6:25	90	3:45	6:04	83	3:28	4:10	–	38	77	–
59	4:29	7:13	6:19	89	3:43	5:59	82	3:25	4:07	–	37	76	–
60	4:25	7:07	6:14	88	3:40	5:54	81	3:23	4:03	–	37	75	2:30
61	4:22	7:01	6:09	86	3:37	5:50	80	3:20	4:00	–	36	74	2:28
62	4:18	6:56	6:04	85	3:34	5:45	79	3:17	3:57	–	36	73	2:26
63	4:15	6:50	5:59	84	3:32	5:41	78	3:15	3:54	–	35	72	2:24
64	4:12	6:45	5:54	83	3:29	5:36	77	3:12	3:51	–	35	71	2:22

E/L is easy/long; M is marathon; T is threshold; I is interval; R is repetition.

Distance Running

(continued)

Table 11.2 *(continued)*

VDOT	E/L Pace		M Pace	T Pace			I Pace			R Pace			
	km	mile	mile	400	1000	mile	400	1000	1200	mile	200	400	800
65	4:09	6:40	5:49	82	3:26	5:32	76	3:10	3:48	–	34	70	2:20
66	4:05	6:53	5:45	81	3:24	5:28	75	3:08	3:45	5:00	34	69	2:18
67	4:02	6:30	5:40	80	3:21	5:24	74	3:05	3:42	4:57	33	68	2:16
68	4:00	6:26	5:36	79	3:19	5:20	73	3:03	3:39	4:53	33	67	2:14
69	3:57	6:21	5:32	78	3:16	5:16	72	3:01	3:36	4:50	32	66	2:12
70	3:54	6:17	5:28	77	3:14	5:13	71	2:59	3:34	4:46	32	65	2:10
71	3:51	6:12	5:24	76	3:12	5:09	70	2:57	3:31	4:43	31	64	2:08
72	3:49	6:08	5:20	76	3:10	5:05	69	2:55	3:29	4:40	31	63	2:06
73	3:46	6:04	5:16	75	3:08	5:02	69	2:53	3:27	4:37	31	62	2:05
74	3:44	6:00	5:12	74	3:06	4:59	68	2:51	3:25	4:34	30	62	2:04
75	3:41	5:56	5:09	74	3:04	4:56	67	2:49	3:22	4:31	30	61	2:03
76	3:39	5:52	5:05	73	3:02	4:52	66	2:48	3:20	4:28	29	60	2:02
77	3:36	5:48	5:01	72	3:00	4:49	65	2:46	3:18	4:25	29	59	2:00
78	3:24	5:45	4:58	71	2:58	4:46	65	2:44	3:16	4:23	29	59	1:59
79	3:32	5:41	4:55	70	2:56	4:43	64	2:42	3:14	4:20	28	58	1:58
80	3:30	5:38	4:52	70	2:54	4:41	64	2:41	3:12	4:17	28	58	1:56
81	3:28	5:34	4:49	69	2:53	4:38	63	2:39	3:10	4:15	28	57	1:55
82	3:26	5:31	4:46	68	2:51	4:35	62	2:38	3:08	4:12	27	56	1:54
83	3:24	5:28	4:43	68	2:49	4:32	62	2:36	3:07	4:10	27	56	1:53
84	3:22	5:25	4:40	67	2:48	4:30	61	2:35	3:05	4:08	27	55	1:52
85	3:20	5:21	4:37	66	2:46	4:27	61	2:33	3:03	4:05	27	55	1:51

E/L is easy/long; M is marathon; T is threshold; I is interval; R is repetition.

Distance Running

FOOTBALL

Kent Johnston

Speed pays enormous dividends for almost every athlete in almost every sport. The faster an athlete can perform, the better. For this reason, I find specific speed and agility drills to be most important for football players of all positions. Once a football player has acquired the necessary basic strength and aerobic fitness, he is ready to develop his speed and quickness through drills that develop reaction time (the motor reaction to a signal), movement time (the ability to move a limb quickly), and general running speed (the frequency and synchronization of the arms and legs).

Some of the most important components of a football player's speed development include the following:

- Starting strength—the power required to begin a movement, such as the initial push required by an offensive lineman off the snap. Starting strength involves reaction time, thus the neurological center is important. It also is one of the first abilities we lose to age, so older athletes have to emphasize it more in training. You can improve starting strength in the weight room by using techniques such as pausing partway through a repetition. You can also improve starting strength by using visual or audio cues to trigger the explosive movement.

- Acceleration—the ability to gain speed, beginning with the initial movement (starting strength) and continuing until reaching full speed. Acceleration in the weight room is defined as bar speed.

- Maximum velocity—top speed that can be held for only a few seconds. Most football players seldom attain maximum velocity during a game; starting speed and acceleration are much more important for football. Still, there are drills and sprinting form fundamentals that can help any athlete run faster.

- Lateral speed and agility—the ability to change direction as quickly as possible while maintaining body control and mechanics. Outside of the weight room, if I were asked to choose only one method of training for football, I would choose lateral speed and agility drills (see chapters 8 and 9 for more agility drills).

- Power endurance—the ability to perform a maximal explosive effort over and over again. An offensive lineman not only has to explode off the snap, he has to do it 60 to 80 times a game. Power endurance is built by doing a high number of repetitions in an exercise.

- Speed endurance—the ability to run or accelerate at full speed over and over again. A wide receiver has to run pass pattern after pass pattern at nearly full speed. Speed-endurance drills help increase speed and are good general conditioners.

The following four drills help football players develop all six of these components of football-specific speed.

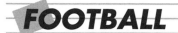

Lying-Start Sprint

Purpose

To develop starting speed, acceleration, maximal velocity, and power and speed endurance

Skills Used

Explosive starts, acceleration, and good sprinting form

Procedure

1. Set a distance of between 10 and 30 yards, and have the athlete start from a lying position at the start line.
2. At the starting sound from the coach, the athlete quickly gets up and sprints at 100 percent of maximum speed to the finish line.
3. The athlete walks back to the starting line and repeats the exercise for a total of 10 repetitions.

Variations

Try longer sprints from a three-point starting stance (track start) or from a flying start (standing start from 10 yards behind the "starting line"). The number of repetitions the athlete does of these variations depends on the intensity of the sprint. For example, if the athlete is to sprint at 60 percent of maximum speed, he should do more repetitions than if he is sprinting at 80 percent to 90 percent of maximum speed. The amount of rest between each sprint will also depend on the intensity and volume. For 80 percent to 100 percent maximal sprints, athletes should rest 90 seconds (or full recovery) between sprints. Try mixing in sets of different intensities of sprints.

Build Up Acceleration

Purpose

To develop starting speed, acceleration, maximal velocity, and speed endurance

Skills Used

Changing speed, acceleration, and good sprinting form

Procedure

1. Mark off a 40- to 60-yard course.
2. The athlete starts from a three-point stance (track start) and accelerates up to 75 percent of maximal speed by the halfway point of the distance.
3. At the halfway point, the athlete holds the speed at 75 percent through the end of the sprint.
4. The athlete walks back to the starting line to recover and repeats the exercise for a total of 6 to 10 repetitions.

Football

Four-Corner Agility

Purpose
To develop starting speed, acceleration, lateral agility, and endurance

Skills Used
Explosive starts, lateral movements, and quick changes of direction

Procedure
1. Mark off a 20- by 20-yard to 40- by 40-yard square using cones to mark the corners.
2. The athlete starts from a three-point stance at one cone.
3. Using quick movements, he performs a lateral shuffle to the second cone, turns and backpedals to the third cone, cariocas to the fourth cone, and sprints back to the start.
4. The athlete performs three repetitions with one minute of rest between them.

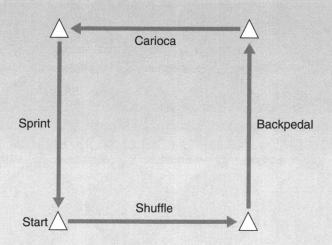

Variations
Choose other lateral movements, shuffles, or sprints for each leg of the drill and try changing directions.

Ladder Backpedal Sprint

Purpose

To develop agility, general conditioning, and acceleration with changes of direction

Skills Used

Explosive starts, acceleration, deceleration, backpedalling, and quickness in changing direction

Procedure

1. The athlete starts from a two-point stance with the back to the starting line.

2. He backpedals 10 yards, pivots to the right 180 degrees, sprints 10 more yards, and touches the line with either foot.

3. The athlete then backpedals 10 yards, pivots to the left 180 degrees, and sprints 10 yards back to the starting line.

4. He rests 60 seconds before repeating the drill.

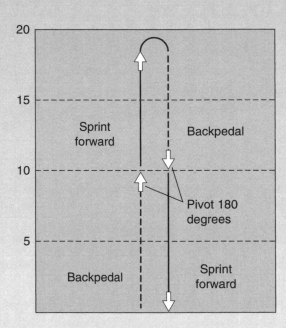

Key Points

• Shoulders and body weight should be kept slightly forward during backpedaling.

• The athlete accelerates after the turn.

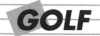

GOLF

Pete Draovitch

History has shown that golfers are typically not willing to spend long hours working out to improve their game. But just as in sports such as football, basketball, and baseball, the role of fitness in golf has evolved and increased in importance. With younger, more athletic players taking up the game, fitness may be not just an advantage but a necessity for competition at an elite level.

The power demands of golf are unique. A player must launch a ball 300 yards during a drive and follow that blast with a 65-yard wedge shot to the green. Golf requires physical development similar to that of other athletic activities. The amount of force the hips generate can equal that developed by the hips of an elite discus thrower. Like a gymnast or diver, the golfer needs a powerful trunk to create the stability that protects the spine. The arms must possess the same combination of firmness and softness that an NFL receiver needs to make a catch. A sense of mobility, stability, and coordination is necessary to execute every golf shot.

The four fitness components of the golf swing are sport-specific muscular strength, functional flexibility, dynamic postural balance, and segmental coordination. Perhaps the most important element, however, is motor learning. Research has shown that motor output is guided by sensory input except in the case of ballistic movements such as jumping, punching, throwing, and swinging a golf club. These brief, all-or-nothing, high-speed movements cannot rely on the sensory system for feedback during the short period of their execution. Training the body to move with the forces required by a discus thrower, elite-level gymnast, or NFL receiver is difficult. Golfers ask the lower part of the body to create an explosion like that produced by an NFL running back trying to break tackles, and at the same time, ask the middle of the body to become a rigid lever for transferring forces. To add to the complexity, golfers should also let the arms hang like pieces of spaghetti (to borrow a line from Jack Nicklaus). Lee Trevino noted that the arms should hang from the body such that if you allowed golf balls to roll out of your mouth, they would land directly in your cupped hands. Given factors such as structural and functional imbalances, swinging outside the limitations of the body, and not knowing what it feels like to make a great swing, golfers are often faced with trying to improve a skill by trial and error.

According to research, sensory analyzers fall into five basic categories:

- Proprioceptive, or body movement and awareness
- Tactile, or sense of touch
- Vestibular, or balance and equilibrium
- Optic, or visual
- Acoustic, or auditory

Any time we attempt to teach a new skill, we must first make the person aware of his or her limitations. After the player becomes consciously aware of a limitation, we attempt to correct it consciously. Following the conscious correction, we try to ingrain the correct motor program into the brain so the player can

Golf

subconsciously recall it. The task of hitting a ball correctly and consistently is extremely difficult, as any of us who have tried the game know. The problem is that a player cannot know how to hit a good shot if he or she has not felt what it's like to hit a ball correctly. Using the following functional screen movement, however, can help teach a player how an efficient golf swing *should* feel.

Golf Functional Screening

Before beginning a program, the player should undergo baseline fitness testing (see chapter 2) in combination with some specific golf activities. The functional screening movement that follows provides invaluable information about imbalances within the body by exposing structural and functional limitations. Other golf-specific drills reveal coordination and balance shortcomings.

Starting Position

Attach tubing to a door at about shin level. The player wraps the waistband around the left shoulder and turns in a clockwise direction until the tubing is wrapped once around the body. The player assumes a golf stance. A jump-rope handle may be adjusted to rest along the rib cage so that the tubing does not rest directly on the body. Once the player has assumed the golf stance, he or she is ready to do the drill.

Movement

The player stands away from the anchored location to develop a workable tension in the tubing. He or she then assumes the address position and crosses the arms so that they rest on the chest. The tubing should be resting so that it comes off the left hip between the seven and eight o'clock positions. (In the address position, straight ahead is twelve o'clock.) The player assumes the golf stance and takes a backswing. The tubing will create resistance to help build the muscles during the backswing. The tension created in the tubing will help pull the player forward as he or she attempts the downswing. This helps with weight transfer from the back leg to the front leg. If the player does not develop stability in the front leg, the tubing will pull him or her forward, simulating the sliding motion common among recreational golfers. Sliding results in loss of power and reduced club-head speed at impact.

End Position

The player returns to the starting position. To alter the degree of difficulty or work on individual components, adjust the tension in the tubing by having the player move farther away from or closer to the anchor point. I sometimes use this drill with rehabilitation patients directly on the driving range. Because no door is available for an anchor point, I drive a tent peg into the ground and secure the tubing to it. If you are going to do this, however, you should work in groups of two. After every golf shot the person monitoring the routine should be certain that the tent peg is still firmly in the ground.

By working with a partner, the golfer can use all five of the sensory analyzers. The partner helps by providing auditory feedback. The eyes will automatically work. The vestibular and balance systems get to experience the feeling of a good, effortless golf shot. The tactile analyzer is being satisfied because the golfer feels the tubing creasing in the correct areas if he or she is properly making the shoulder turn. Finally, the body now knows, proprioceptively, what it feels like to hit a good golf shot.

Golf Drills

It is difficult to relieve a golfer's limitations without developing a custom program for the individual. Nevertheless, we can identify some common shortcomings that contribute to inconsistent golf. These include poor coordination, a faulty swing, weak hip-girdle musculature that causes sliding in both directions, and poor balance. Finally, the right side of the right-handed golfer will often be shortened and tight, and the left side will be elongated and weak. The opposite effect will occur in left-handed golfers. The primary focus of a custom program should be to correct neuromuscular imbalances created by the nature of the sport.

Although it is not possible to choose four drills that relate specifically to *every* golfer's swing, the following drills address the most common limitations. Perform two to three sets of 8 to 10 repetitions of each drill.

Hip-Trunk Separation

Purpose
To disassociate the hips from the trunk during the golf swing

Skills Used
Strength and flexibility in the trunk and coordination between the upper- and lower-body segments

Procedure
1. The player assumes a golf stance in front of a mirror and places the hands across the chest.
2. Hinging at the hips, not bending at the back, the player rotates loading on the back leg while the upper body assumes the backswing position. By using this action, the player disassociates the lower body from the upper body, which is what creates separation in the golf swing. The motion should not be painful. To decrease the stress, the player should remain in an upright position.
3. The player returns to the starting position.

Key Points
- The player should go only as far as the point where he or she feels a light stretch.
- It is best to do the drill in front of a mirror because this provides immediate feedback.

Variation
To feel loading on the back leg, the player may want to stagger the stance a bit, with the right leg back for the right-handed golfer. Doing this will allow the player to feel more loading on the right side.

Golf

Hip-Trunk Separation and Connection

Purpose

To disassociate the hips from the trunk and to feel the transfer of weight to the front side

Skills Used

Weight shift and rotation

Procedure

1. The player assumes a golf stance in front of a mirror and places the hands across the chest.

2. The player performs the motion described in the Hip-Trunk Separation drill but finishes the motion by transferring the weight from the back foot to the front foot, centering the hips toward the target. The player hinges at the hips, not the back. This action creates movement recall, which the player needs to consistently reproduce the golf swing.

3. The front of the body faces the target, with weight rolled onto the left foot and the toes of the right foot providing the main support on the ground.

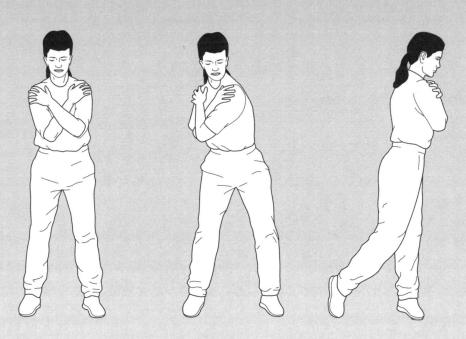

Key Points

The player should swing within the limitations of the body so that the body is not over-stretched. Purposeful movement within a limited range of motion will provide better feedback than movement through a much larger range, which provides feedback that may become harder to decipher as body strength and flexibility improve.

Variations

The variations are the same as those for the Hip-Trunk Separation.

Tubing Abductor and Adductor

Purpose

To improve single-leg balance and develop strength of both the hip abductors and adductors

Skills Used

Strength, flexibility, balance, and posture

Procedure

1. Attach tubing to the door and place a waist belt around the waist.

2. The player walks outward from the wall, creating tension in the tubing.

3. He or she lifts the outer leg off the ground and attempts to balance on the inner leg. This stretches the inside part of the leg.

4. The player raises the inner leg off the ground and attempts to support his or her weight with the outside leg. This works the outer muscles of the buttocks and leg.

5. The player returns to the starting position so that the tubing offers minimal tension and he or she is able to balance with both feet on the ground.

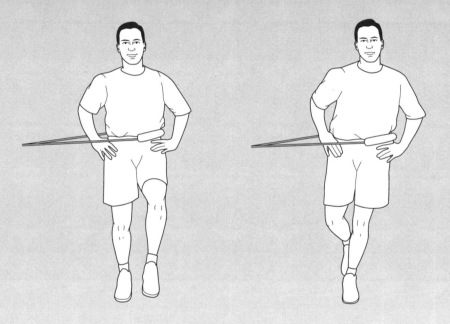

Key Point

When the leg farthest from the tubing attachment is being worked on, good balance is difficult to achieve, especially when the leg is loaded. The player may have to move in a bit at first. Balance will improve within a few weeks.

Variation

If loading with tubing is too difficult, the player may begin doing something as simple as standing in a doorway with the eyes open and progressing to eyes closed. When the player is able to accomplish this for approximately 10 seconds, he or she can move outside the doorway and initiate the progression again.

Golf

Double-Leg Rotation Stretch

Purpose

To improve flexibility of the right side of the body and the hip girdle for the right-handed golfer. (For left-handed golfers, substitute the opposite side throughout these instructions.)

Skills Used

Flexibility of tight side created during repetitive golf swing

Procedure

1. The player lies on the floor on the left side with the knees pulled toward the chest.
2. He or she rolls the right shoulder back to the floor while keeping the knees still. The right elbow stays close to the body.
3. The left arm is placed on the right knee so that the knees are held close to the ground as the player rolls the right shoulder toward the floor.

Key Points

- The player should roll only as far as the point where he or she feels a light stretch.
- The player must keep breathing and must not overstretch.
- Keeping the hip girdles flexible and the trunk and abdominal muscles strong helps to ensure pain-free golf.

Variation

The player may attempt to do this in a seated position if he or she is unable to get on the floor.

Golf

HOCKEY

Peter Twist

A sport scientist's exploration of the biomechanical, anatomical, physiological, bioenergetic, and neuromuscular demands of ice hockey produces an extensive "to do" list for the coach, and this is without even addressing the sport skills, individual tactics, and team systems that will ultimately be needed for competition.

The foundation of the game relies on an unnatural mode of locomotion—moving on thin blades across a slippery surface, that is, skating. The complexity of skating is exacerbated by the read-react-and-explode requirements of hockey, which call for repetitive stop-and-start movements, tight turns, backward skating, crossovers, and lateral movement, often while receiving contact. Add to the mix carrying a long stick, controlling a tiny puck, passing, shooting, physically warding off opponents, and delivering bodychecks, and it becomes obvious that designing and prescribing a conditioning program specific to this unique sport is an intriguing coaching challenge.

Performance enhancement and game preparation must draw on a multidimensional conditioning paradigm. Hockey is a high-velocity anaerobic sprint sport, including acceleration, deceleration, abrupt stops, and explosive starts. Although the anaerobic system fuels full-out 45-second shift activity, the aerobic energy system can play an important role in between-shift recovery. The aerobic system also makes an on-ice metabolic contribution if training is intense enough to elevate the lactate threshold. As a full-collision sport, hockey requires large muscle mass and exceptional strength, but it also demands high relative strength for efficient movement. Extraordinary visual skills and the ability to execute fine motor skills under fatigue and duress are critical components. Furthermore, hand-eye coordination, reaction abilities, core power, balanced flexibility, proprioception, unilateral balance, coordination, and agility all contribute to success. Speed is important but quickness and speed endurance are even more crucial.

The are numerous factors to take into account in developing a conditioning program for hockey: the individual player's position, role on team (pure scorer versus fourth-line physical checker), physical maturation, past training experience, injury history, coach evaluations, scouting reports, physiological assessment data, on-ice testing, schedule density, and travel schedule.

Coaches attempt to develop a better athlete and an improved hockey player, not just a stronger, more fit person. Fitness training has little to do with developing better hockey players. General strength and fitness simply produce the foundation on which sport-specific conditioning is built. Individual player-developmental programs must consider hockey movement patterns, range of motion, joint angles, contraction types, sequential activation of muscle firing, velocity, sprint duration, force, time-motion analysis, work-to-rest ratios, fatigue indexes, and positional demands.

Some of these considerations, such as movement pattern and mechanics, drive exercise construction and drill design. Others, such as lifting tempo and sprint duration, affect the variables that coaches manipulate to generate specific adaptations. A meticulous study of the characteristics of the sport should drive exercise prescription. Without developing the exact physical tools that players draw

Hockey

on for successful execution of skills, repetitive technical practice produces few results.

Sport-specific conditioning must also incorporate skill rehearsal, individual tactics, and segments of team systems. In a game, hockey players must cooperate with their teammates, quickly moving into position for passes. They must be able to read the play and position themselves to block opponents or draw them away from the play. Sport conditioning programs to improve hockey players must address game demands and incorporate technique and offensive and defensive tactics. Offensive players select from a repertoire of maneuvers and deceptive tactics to beat a defender. Likewise, defensive players and backchecking forwards draw on select techniques and tactics to defend successfully in a one-on-one confrontation.

For example, a dryland drill designed to improve the anaerobic system and lateral movements under fatigue can also demand shifty moves and fakes common during one-on-ones. A "forward" may try to move quickly to evade the "defensive player" (a training drill partner), who in turn works hard to shadow and contain his or her training partner. On the ice, a drill designed for quickness and reaction skills may require the player to retrieve a puck quickly from the corner and execute a breakout pass. These are two-layered drills. The basic goal in the second example—to improve foot quickness and reaction skills—is masked within a drill that practices a segment of a team system (a breakout).

Two-on-Two, Nets Back to Back

Purpose
To condition stopping quickness, agility, explosive quickness, mobility, puckhandling, anaerobic conditioning, one-on-one tactics, and visual awareness

Skills Used
Multidirectional skating, passing, shooting, containment, angling, offensive and defensive tactics, communication, and mental skills such as rethinking their positioning, remembering which net they are attacking, and deciding how they will defend

Procedure
1. The game takes place inside the neutral zone. Game boundaries are boards to boards and blue line to blue line.
2. Two skaters (SA, SA, SB, and SB on diagram) and one goalie are active on each team. Skaters attack and defend. They can pass to their goalie or to their stationary passer. Goaltenders are encouraged to quarterback plays, move to support the play (i.e., turn it into a three on two), and be prepared for quick counterattacks.
3. Each team also has one stationary passer (PA and PB) who is locked into position at the center red line against the boards. Passers can receive passes and send passes but cannot move from their exact position.
4. Resting players remain outside the neutral zone. Depending on the number of players, they can be resting or participating in other drills. But the next four players (two per team) must be ready to jump into the play on the whistle, which signals a "shift" change.

Hockey

5. Two coaches, one near each blue line, have a pile of pucks that they are ready to inject onto the ice.

6. Nets are right at the center red line, back to back. The game begins when a coach sends a puck into the neutral zone.

7. Any time a goal is scored or the puck travels over the blue line, a coach *immediately* fires a puck back into the game, reminding wandering players by yelling "puck." Coaches should dump most pucks toward the net to maintain non-stop attacking and defending, but sometimes they can send the puck over to a stationary passer.

8. Skaters are credited with 1 point per goal. A goalie who scores earns his or her team three points.

9. At each shift change, the coach dumps a puck in on the whistle. Finishing players must clear the neutral zone without touching the puck or interfering with new skaters. Two new skaters jump in, one for each team. Two new stationary passers also jump in.

Key Points

- Play continues with no stops, and players change shifts without hesitation, immediately jumping into play.

- Skaters must keep their heads up, cycle to the net, support the play, and move relative to their passer at the boards.

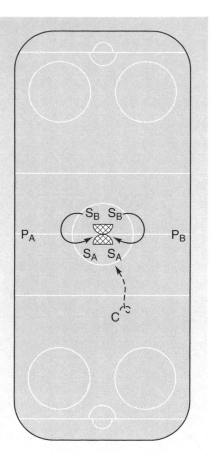

Partner Medicine Ball Full-Body Put With Lateral Shuffle

Purpose

To condition anaerobic endurance, generating explosive power under fatigue, lateral movement, and linking full-body power application into multijoint full-body put

Skills Used

Lateral movement, transfer of power from low to high, and mental toughness

Procedure

1. To establish game boundaries, test each athlete for his or her best-effort, full-body throw using the heaviest medicine ball and add 12 feet to that length. For example, a 20-foot full-body put sets the length from end zone to end zone at 32 feet. The width is 12 feet. Mark the boundaries with cones.

2. Two players position themselves in diagonally opposite corners, 6 feet out from their end-zone line, standing upright, each with a medicine ball at the feet.

3. The drill begins on the whistle. Each player squats down, picks up the ball, and throws from the legs up, aiming down the sideline.

4. As soon as they release, they must use quick lateral shuffles to get to the ball the partner threw.

5. Again they squat down, pick up the ball, and throw it down the sideline. They immediately shuffle across to pick up the ball the partner is throwing.

(continued)

Hockey

6. The goal is to prevent the partner from sending a ball into the player's own end zone within a set time and, likewise, to throw as many balls as possible into the partner's end zone. If a ball crosses an end-zone line, the defending player still continues the drill, gets to the ball, and throws it back down the sideline.

Key Points

- To gain an edge and progress toward the partner's end zone, a player must deliver a more powerful throw that travels farther or move laterally more quickly (under fatigue) to get to the ball sooner, preventing it from bouncing down the floor and thus setting up sooner for the return throw.

- Players always let the incoming ball hit the floor at least once; they should not try to catch it in the air if they arrive early.

- This is an extremely fatiguing drill. Players' heart rates will reach maximum. Lactate accumulation is full body.

Tip-In

Purpose

To condition skating mobility, footwork, quickness, speed endurance, and anaerobic conditioning

Skills Used

Forward and backward skating with puckhandling, stopping and starting, transition from forward to backward while facing play, shooting, hand-eye coordination, and tip-ins

Procedure

1. Each drill uses one goalie, one defensive player, and one forward. The defensive player starts in the middle of the ice at the blue line. The forward begins in the middle of the slot.

2. Set up two piles of pucks toward the boards inside the blue line. Make sure all pucks in the slot and behind the net are cleared.

3. On the whistle, the defensive player sprints over to one pile of pucks, drags a puck back to the center of the ice, and aims a low and controlled slap shot for the forward to tip.

4. On the starting whistle, the forward begins by skating backward around the net to the middle of the net. At that point, he or she must open up at the hips and turn forward to keep facing the play. The forward's objective is to move around the net and back into the slot quickly, to travel as close as possible to the back of the net, and to watch the defensive player at all times.

5. The defensive player alternates sides until he or she has taken six point shots (three coming off each side). The forward alternates direction of travel around the net, always jumping up into the midslot position.

Key Points

- If the forward is much quicker than the defensive player, move the pucks in from the boards (less distance for the defensive player to skate).

- If the defensive player is getting a shot away before the forward reaches the midslot position, make sure the pucks are right over at the boards and add a coach for the defensive player to move around.

Hockey

- After each tip-in, make sure the forward *starts* backward, not turning from the slot to skate forward toward the net and then turning backward around it. The movement is immediately backward from the stationary slot position to midway around the net. Then the player turns forward and jumps out and up into the slot as efficiently as possible.

Walking Hockey Stride Lunge With Contact

Purpose

To condition stride power, leg strength, dynamic hip and groin flexibility, proprioception, core stability, and single-leg dynamic balance

Skills Used

Hockey striding and keeping balance during contact

Procedure

1. Athletes work out in groups of three—one lunging and two walking alongside and providing contact.

2. The lunge pattern is a long stride with a controlled descent. The player lunges out with the left leg at an angle similar to his or her hockey stride, approximately 45 degrees, by outwardly rotating at the hip. The player lands with the left foot out at the same angle so the knee is in line with the foot (this also places the player in T-start position so the next lunge moves back across the floor at 45 degrees).

3. Rather than pushing back to the start position, the player *pushes off* with the right foot, strides through to an upright position, and pauses to check balance. When balance is solid, the player strides off to the opposite side, landing with the right foot. The player continues lunging left and right down the floor.

4. Once the player can lunge under control with good balance, add contact. Two teammates walk alongside, adding light contact at various locations and random times, including the arms and shoulders at the starting and the landing positions.

5. The lunger must fire the appropriate muscles to counteract the contact and maintain solid balance and a controlled lunge. The lunger should ward off contact to the arms.

6. The next progression is lunging with the eyes closed, still receiving random light contact.

Key Point

The player should initially open the eyes just before landing and progress to having the eyes closed throughout the entire sequence.

The efficacy of a hockey conditioning program is determined not only by physiological testing but, more important, by improvement in game performance. Skill rehearsal, individual tactics, and segments of team systems must be integrated with conditioning for optimal player development and game readiness.

Hockey

SOCCER

Vern Gambetta

The primary goal of all soccer drills is to simulate the physiological, biomechanical, and psychological demands of the game. The basic paradigm for designing and implementing drills is based on three main criteria: the demands of the sport, the demands of the position, and the qualities of the individual athlete.

Sport Demands

Drills and conditioning (as you'll read in chapter 13) should meet the specific demands of the game of soccer. Soccer is a skill-dominant game that requires quick starts and quick stops executed in a state of fatigue. The game calls for a constant interplay of force production and force reduction. Most of the injuries and performance errors occur during the force-reduction phase of stopping and kicking. Consequently, drills that emphasize speed, speed endurance, and power production are most effective for soccer players.

Notational analysis reveals some telling statistics about the game that have direct implications on how to design drills that condition for soccer. Less than 2 percent of the total distance covered by a player during a match is with the ball. Each match requires 1,000 to 1,200 bouts of action, which include walking, running, sprinting, jumping, planting, and cutting. All require quick changes of direction as well as precise execution of game skills. About 16 percent of movement is backward or sideways. Sprints average about 15 meters in length and generally occur about once every 90 seconds.

Position Demands

Although players are designated by positions in modern soccer, it is better to think of a series of interchanging roles that change with the ebb and flow of the game. Each position has unique demands as well as overlapping responsibilities.

- Forward—acceleration ability, explosiveness, and skill
- Midfield—skill, high level of specific fitness, and agility
- Defender—explosiveness, agility, and power
- Goalkeeper—reaction speed, agility, and explosive power

Qualities of the Individual Athlete

What are the physical qualities of the individual player relative to the demands of soccer and the position? Every player is different. The toughest challenge is designing effective drills that meet the demands of the individual player in a team context. Evaluate each player relative to the following parameters:

- Work capacity
- Strength and power
- Speed

- Coordination and skill
- Flexibility
- Body composition

It is important to consider the player's developmental level. The demands on the young player who is still trying to master the intricacies of the game from a technical and tactical viewpoint are quite different from the demands on the mature professional player.

The following conditioning drills and exercises are divided into three categories that help define their purpose. The goal of all the drills is to prepare to play. Soccer practice and individual skill work will address the skill component.

- General—drills composed of generic movements that emphasize fundamental movement skills. These are often done without the ball but, as in the "Leg Circuit" below, can also be done with ball touches.
- Special—drills that imitate specific movements of the game, usually without the ball. If the ball is involved, it is with an individual player and not in a team situation (see "Carolina Shuttle," page 254).
- Specific—drills that incorporate the actual movements of the game, with the ball (see "Gates Workout," page 255).

Skill level in a skill-dominant sport such as soccer will obviously have a significant impact on ability to play the game. Without mastery of skill, all aspects of conditioning are for naught. At the same time, deficiency in any component of conditioning will cause skill to erode quickly. A proper conditioning base will create a favorable learning environment, which will enable players to attain a higher level of skill development.

Leg Circuit

Purpose
To work on fundamental movement skills and develop strength endurance

Skills Used
Executing quality touches on the ball (during active recovery) while fatigued

Equipment
- One ball per player
- Box or bench 12 to 15 inches high
- Timer

Procedure
The circuit consists of 30 seconds of exercise and 30 seconds of active recovery involving contact with the ball. The goal is to perform as many repetitions of each exercise as possible during the 30-second work period.

- Body-weight squat

Soccer

(continued)

- Active recovery—play solo with the ball at the feet
- Body-weight lunge
- Active recovery—one-touch pass with a partner
- Body-weight step-up
- Active recovery—volley with a partner
- Body-weight jump squat

Key Points

Do this workout twice a week with two days of recovery between sessions during the off-season to develop strength endurance.

- Week #1—three circuits with three minutes of rest between circuits
- Week #2—three circuits with two minutes of rest between circuits
- Week #3—three circuits with no rest between circuits
- Weeks #4 through #6—When the player can do three circuits without stopping, add one circuit each week. In the sixth week of the progression, the player can perform six circuits without stopping.

For the high school player or developing player, the first three weeks are sufficient. The college and professional player should follow the full six-week progression. For the developing player who does not have the skill to execute quality touches on the ball, do not include the ball.

Carolina Shuttle

Purpose

To develop speed endurance as well as the ability to stop and change direction

Skills Used

Stopping and changing direction

Equipment Needed

- Six 12-inch cones
- A stopwatch

Procedure

1. Set 12-inch cones in a line spaced at 0, 5, 10, 15, 20, and 25 yards.
2. Players run the cones in a shuttle fashion (5 yards and back, 10 yards and back, and so on), attempting to achieve the following target times:

- Basic level—complete all shuttles in 40 seconds with 20 seconds of rest after each shuttle.
- Intermediate level—complete the first 5 or 6 shuttles in 35 seconds with 25 seconds of rest between each shuttle. Run the last 4 or 5 (to complete a set of 10) in 40 seconds with 20 seconds of rest after each shuttle.
- Highest level—complete all shuttles in 35 seconds with 25 seconds of rest after each shuttle.

Soccer

Key Points

- Emphasize the mechanics of stopping and starting. Although this is a conditioning drill, players must never compromise good technique.
- If you add the ball, remember that energy cost rises significantly, so be sure to adjust the volume of the work.
- This drill is appropriate throughout the training year. In the early season and midseason, it is an effective team conditioning activity. Group players by position with specific goals for each position group.

Variations

- Alternate one shuttle run without the ball and one shuttle run dribbling the ball around the cone.
- Alternate one shuttle run without the ball and one shuttle run stopping and turning the ball at the cone.

Gates Workout

Purpose

To work speed endurance into curved running and to couple that with quality passes

Skills Used

Accelerating, changing body position, and one-touch passing

Equipment Needed

- Two cones, one for the start of the flagged course and one for the finish
- Six corner flags (three pairs). Flags within each pair are placed 5 yards apart to form the gates. Each pair of flags is positioned about 10 yards from the pair closest to it.
- One ball

Procedure

1. Players line up in two lines (a line of starters and a line of receivers). Starter #1 (at the starting line) passes the ball to receiver #1 (on the receiving line). Starter #1 then immediately accelerates through the flagged course to the finish cone. After crossing the finish line, starter #1 jogs to the end of the receiving line.
2. Once receiver #1 receives the ball from starter #1, he or she immediately passes the ball back to the starting line (to starter #2) and sprints 10 yards before jogging to the end of the starting line.
3. Starter #2 passes the ball as soon as he or she receives it to continue the process.

Key Points

- Players accelerate through the flags.
- Players jog back to the receiving line.
- Players in the receiving line should be moving constantly—no standing!

(continued)

Soccer

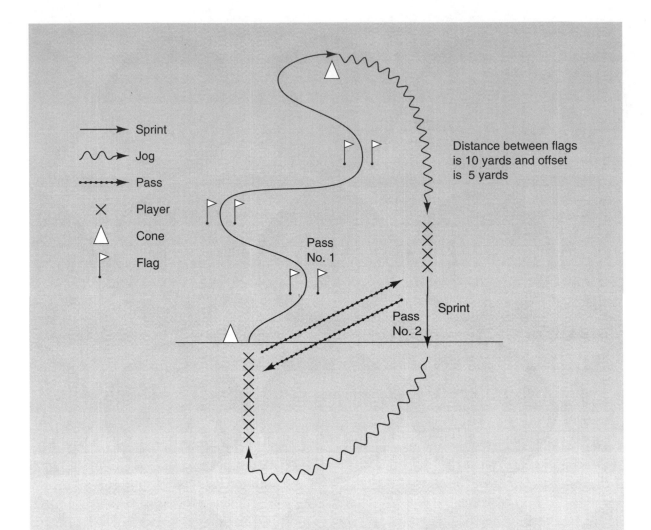

Sprint
Jog
Pass
× **Player**
△ **Cone**
⚐ **Flag**

Distance between flags
is 10 yards and offset
is 5 yards

Pass No. 1

Pass No. 2

Sprint

Variations

- Execute for a set number of repetitions: 6 to 8 repetitions for developing players, 8 to 10 repetitions for high school players, and 12 to 15 repetitions for college or professional players.
- Execute for a set time and keep track of how many repetitions players attain in the prescribed time. Developing players perform the workout for 3 minutes, high school players for 5 to 8 minutes, college and professional players for 8 to 10 minutes.

TENNIS   E. Paul Roetert and Barrett Bugg

In a French Open Final, Sergei Bruguera and Jim Courier battled for over five hours. Postmatch analysis revealed that a total of only 15 minutes of actual tennis—involving sprinting and constant shot adjustment with the feet—was played during that time span! That is, within the obvious aerobic component of a match of tennis (in this case, five hours), the sport also requires explosive bursts of quickness and power. Due to enhanced technology and increased knowledge about how to properly execute strength training and conditioning for tennis, the game now demands more and better agility than ever before.

Here are some common tennis statistics that help a coach develop effective conditioning drills for the sport:

- Players are allowed 25 seconds between points.
- Players are allowed 90 seconds on a changeover.
- An average point on clay courts lasts 10 seconds.
- An average point on hard courts lasts 5.2 seconds.
- An average point on grass courts lasts 2.8 seconds.
- The average proportion of effective playing time versus non-playing time is 35 percent to 65 percent.
- The average distance run per stroke is four meters.
- The average number of directional changes per point is four.

Although improving strength and conditioning involves intensity, duration, frequency, mode, and progression, tennis drills focus most directly on intensity and duration. Intensity is essential because of the anaerobic demands of the sport. The duration of each tennis point is typically very short; training should reflect this sport-specific characteristic. Following are some sample drills focusing on these training variables.

Box Drill

Purpose
To develop anaerobic capacity, first-step quickness, agility, split-step timing, balance, and good posture

Skills Used
Acceleration, deceleration, change of direction, and unpredictable movement

Procedure
1. Mark off a square or rectangular area that is large enough to allow the athlete to move two to six steps in every direction from the middle.
2. The player starts in the middle of the box while a coach stands outside of the box ready to supply a directional signal.

3. The coach signals which direction the player should move by pointing high toward one of the rear corners of the box or low toward one of the near corners of the box.

4. Upon the signal, the player runs to the specified corner, touches it with the foot, returns to the starting position in the middle of the box, and performs a split step (similar to the technique skiers use to turn, a split step is an unweighting technique in which the athlete quickly bends the knees to take the weight off the feet for a split second) before the next signal is given. The coach should supply the next signal when the player is two to four inches off the ground in order to assure minimal, but manageable, response time.

5. The player repeats two to five sets of the drill either based on time (5 to 10 seconds) or number of repetitions (5 to 10) using a 1:2 work-to-rest ratio and taking no more than 25 seconds for recovery.

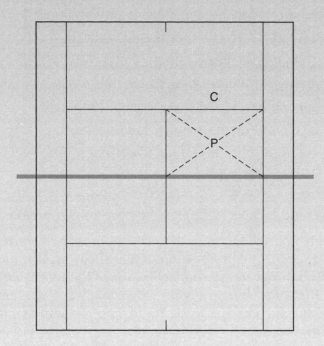

Key Points

A split step must be performed each time the player reaches the middle of the box. The next signal should be given based on the athlete's individual response time capabilities. For instance, if a player cannot respond in time, then the signal should be given while he or she is higher off the ground (before landing) during the split step.

Variations

- Attach rubber tubing to the player's waist or hips at various angles to increase resistance.
- Vary the surface for the drill (grass, clay, hard surface, or sand) to improve agility.
- Add a straight-ahead movement to mimic the retrieval of a drop shot.

Triangle Drill

Purpose

To develop hip mobility, anaerobic capacity, first-step quickness, agility, split-step timing, and balance

Skills Used

Acceleration, deceleration, change of direction, unpredictable movement, vertical jumping and landing

Procedure

1. Set up a triangle big enough to allow the player to move one to four steps in each prescribed direction. The wide portion (bottom) of the triangle should represent the room needed for forehand and backhand volleys, while the point (top) of the triangle should allow room for overhead shots.

2. One player stands in the middle of the triangle. A coach standing to the side signals the point of the triangle the player should move toward. The coach points low to either side for a low forehand or backhand volley and points straight up for an overhead.

3. Upon the signal, the player runs to the specified corner, performs the specified action, returns to the starting position, and does a split step before the next signal is given. The coach should supply the next signal when the player is two to four inches off the ground in order to assure minimal, but manageable, response time.

4. The athlete repeats two to five sets either for time (15 to 20 seconds) or number of repetitions (5 to 15) using a 1:2 work-to-rest ratio and taking no more than 25 seconds for recovery.

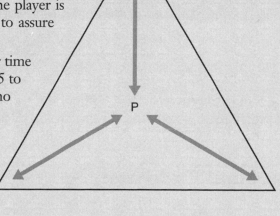

Key Points

- Emphasize that a drop step (such as a football quarterback uses after the snap) is preferred over backpedaling to most efficiently and effectively get back for the overhead.

- Encourage athletes to get low on the volleys. Performing a shoulder-high, hip-high, or knee-high volley is not the goal here; rather players should position the racket so low that it is nearly touching the ground. Patrick Rafter and Jana Novotna are known for getting incredibly low like this for volleys.

Variations

- Attach rubber tubing to the player's waist or hips at various angles to increase resistance.
- Vary the surface for the drill (grass, clay, hard surface, or sand) to improve agility.
- Add a straight-ahead movement to mimic the retrieval of a drop shot.

Step Off, Split, and React

Purpose

To develop first-step quickness, agility, split-step timing, and balance

Skills Used

Acceleration, deceleration, and the recovery step

Procedure

1. The athlete starts by standing on an 18- to 24-inch high bench or wood box. A coach stands to the side ready to signal.

2. As the athlete steps off the bench and is in the air, the coach points quickly to the athlete's forehand or backhand side.

3. The athlete lands with a split step and quickly explodes in the designated direction for two to five steps.

4. He or she then recovers back to the split-step point with proper footwork.

5. The athlete performs three sets of two to six repetitions.

Key Points

- Perform this drill on an appropriately soft surface (not cement).

- This drill is intended for intermediate to advanced athletes who have developed trunk and leg strength. Good posture and a quiet landing are essential requirements for performing this drill.

- Heavy athletes may want to limit pounding activities such as these to avoid lower-body joint injuries.

Variations

Use a lightweight vest on the upper body or a rubber tubing cord attached at the waist to add resistance. A sport cord can also supply an overspeed training stimulus.

Forehand-Backhand

Purpose

To develop first-step quickness, high-intensity movement training, response time, and heightened awareness during high-intensity training

Skills Used

Acceleration, deceleration, agility, the recovery step, weight transfer, and split-step timing as well as tennis-related skills such as unit turning, loading, and racket preparation

Procedure

1. Set up two cones or place tape approximately two to five steps from where the player will be starting. These will serve as the lateral limits for the drill.

2. A coach or partner stands five feet in front of and facing the player to provide the movement signal by pointing in the intended direction.

3. When the player is in the ready stance, the coach points quickly to the athlete's forehand or backhand side.

4. The athlete quickly explodes in the designated direction for two to five steps and correctly completes the shadowing of the shot.

5. He or she then recovers back to the starting point with proper footwork and split steps before the next signal is given.

6. The athlete performs two to three sets of 4 to 10 movements. The work-to-rest ratio should be 1:2 and the athlete should rarely take more than 25 seconds rest.

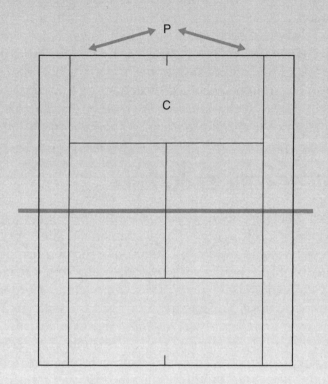

Key Points

- The coach should give the next signal just before the athlete touches the ground during the split step.
- The player should concentrate on proper technique for best results.

Variations

- Use rubber tubing attached to the player's waist or hips at various angles.
- Vary the surface for the drill (grass, clay, hard surface, or sand) to improve agility.
- Have the player start the drill with his or her eyes closed, responding to an aural stimulus.
- Encourage the player to move at an angle to cut the ball off instead of moving directly to the side.

VOLLEYBALL 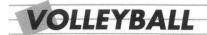 Courtney Carter

Volleyball is a game of skills and strategies. One skill is the ability to place the ball in the desired location, with the right height, direction, and speed. An athlete must be able to time the approach and jump to attack or block the ball. The athlete must also be able to react to the opponent's placement of the ball and move quickly in the correct direction. These are the skills that players work on during practices, scrimmages, and games. Without a doubt, the best and most specific way to become a better volleyball player is to play volleyball. The primary objective of the volleyball strength and conditioning program is to develop explosive power and agility and to improve volleyball-specific endurance.

The mode of training included in a strength and conditioning program must match the physical adaptations that are specific to volleyball. By first performing a needs analysis, the coach can design a conditioning program that uses the relevant energy systems, movement patterns, and power.

Volleyball-Specific Endurance

To develop a better understanding of endurance as it relates to volleyball, it is helpful to look closely at how energy is supplied. The energy source that players use depends on the intensity and duration of the exercise. Examining the energy requirements of the sport reveals that the average play in volleyball lasts about 6 seconds, followed by 14 seconds of rest, not including timeouts or player substitutions. This analysis underscores the need for volleyball players to focus on maximum-intensity efforts by performing short, quick drills followed by adequate recovery. Conversely, the practice of using short rest periods between drills to "push through" the pain threshold is counterproductive to developing maximum performance potential. Without adequate recovery, maximum efforts are not possible, and the training is no longer specific to volleyball. Furthermore, swimming or bicycling for long distances does not duplicate what the athlete needs to play volleyball. This kind of training causes an athlete's muscle tissue to take on aerobic characteristics, which are counterproductive to developing the explosive, powerful muscle contractions that volleyball requires.

Agility

When designing a volleyball conditioning program, consider the specific types of movements needed to play the sport. Essentially, a volleyball player needs to be able to attack, block, and dig effectively for an entire game. To get in the proper position to carry out these tasks, the player must be able to execute the basic motor skills of changing direction, starting, stopping, shuffling, and jumping. Therefore, agility drills specific to volleyball should be part of the program.

In setting up an agility program for volleyball, remember that the court is about 30 feet by 30 feet. Doing sprint drills that incorporate only straight-ahead running is not particularly helpful to volleyball players. The average number of steps taken in any one direction during a match is two to three. What is important is being able to start, stop, and change direction quickly. A volleyball player must be able to move forward, backward, and side to side, and to execute front-to-side angles and back-to-side angles. Being able to move quickly from a horizontal plane to jump into a vertical plane is also important. This horizontal to vertical movement must be executed regardless of the initial direction of movement. The size of the court and the types of movements used in playing the sport clearly illustrate the importance of including a variety of movements and footwork skills in a volleyball program.

Power and Explosiveness

After agility, the next important element in a conditioning program for volleyball is power or explosiveness. Although speed is not a concern in volleyball, the ability to accelerate is essential. The more powerful the athlete, the faster he or she can accelerate. The superior volleyball athlete can go from having no movement to maximum speed in two or three steps. This comes from the ability to accelerate quickly. Volleyball is also a game of deceleration. Players should have the ability to stop on a dime and change direction quickly.

Newton's second law states that force = mass $\times$ acceleration. Therefore, the greater the force, the greater the acceleration. Furthermore, the development of power is as important for agility as it is for jumping. Both eccentric contractions (stretching of a muscle) and concentric contractions (shortening of a muscle) occur when executing many sports skills that require a maximum rate of force development. An eccentric contraction followed by a concentric contraction is known as the stretch-shortening cycle. When an athlete jumps or changes direction, an eccentric contraction, or stretch, occurs in the muscles of the hips, knees, and ankles. When the muscle is stretched, elastic energy builds up in it. The muscle then fights to return to its normal resting length, similar to the way a stretched rubber band pulls back to its original size. If the muscles shorten immediately after the stretch, greater force and power can be generated.

Conditioning drills for volleyball players are divided into these two categories: power development and agility. Both types of movement require explosiveness and use the stretch-shortening cycle. The downward movement when executing a jump stretches the muscles and tendons of the hips, knees, and ankles. This causes elastic energy to build up in these muscles. If the direction of the jump is reversed quickly, a greater force is generated, thus enabling the body to go higher. Agility also uses the stretch-shortening cycle. As an athlete stops quickly to change directions, the same muscles are stretched (in the hips, knees, and ankles). Again, elastic energy builds up in these muscles. If the athlete changes direction quickly a greater force is generated, enabling the body to accelerate faster.

The volleyball conditioning program uses the split-routine method of training. This simply means that the program is split into working different types of exercise movements on alternating days. The split routine allows the body to recover and rebuild from one type of exercise movement while the player works on a different type of exercise movement. With the split routine, at least two full days of recovery occur between similar exercise movements. The split routine used in this conditioning program is divided into plyometric (power) drills and agility drills.

Volleyball

Before beginning a plyometric program, athletes must learn to land properly. This is accomplished by doing a series of landing drills followed by a series of box drills. The purpose of the landing drills is to develop proper jumping and landing technique and prepare the body for more intense power drills. The first landing drill that players perform is the drop jump. After athletes learn to land correctly, they perform a series of box drills. The box-drill routine continues to emphasize proper landing and begins to develop explosive vertical and lateral movements.

Drop Jump

Purpose

To strengthen the legs and hips and learn how to land

Skills Used

Proper neuromuscular landing and jumping

Procedure

1. The athlete stands on a plyometric box with feet parallel and about hip-width apart.
2. He or she steps off the box, landing on the balls of both feet.
3. Upon landing, the athlete flexes the knees and hips and holds the position for a five-second count.
4. He or she then relaxes the legs and immediately gets on the box for the next repetition.
5. The athlete completes five repetitions.

Key Point

Start with a 24-inch high box and gradually increase the height of the box (up to 36 inches) as strength increases.

Depth Jump

Purpose

To develop explosive vertical movements

Skills Used

Proper landing and jumping technique

Procedure

1. The athlete stands on top of a box with feet hip-width apart.
2. He or she steps off the box, lands on both feet, and immediately jumps as high as possible.
3. The athlete swings both arms straight up while jumping as if making a block or attacking.
4. He or she does five jumps.

Key Points

• When landing, the body should flex at the knees to absorb the weight.

- The athlete must not stay on the ground; he or she must jump up as quickly as possible.
- Make sure the landing surface is firm, yet has some resiliency (carpet, rubber flooring, etc.).

Variation

Have the athlete jump to a target overhead to assure maximum-effort jumps.

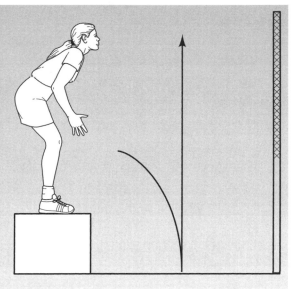

Shuffle Transition

Purpose

To develop footwork patterns and improve agility

Skills Used

Proper backpedal and shuffle technique

Procedure

1. Set up 7 to 10 cones three yards apart in a zigzag pattern.
2. The athlete stands in a two-point stance with knees slightly bent, torso upright, and head up.
3. He or she backpedals diagonally behind the first cone.
4. The athlete then shifts feet and shuffle steps to the side of the next cone.
5. He or she squares the body and makes a bumping action with the arms.
6. The athlete repeats the same footwork pattern throughout the rest of the cones.

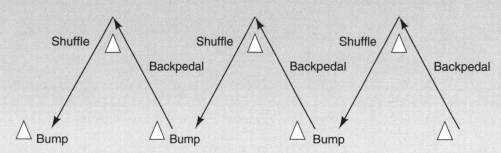

Key Points

- The athlete should stay low throughout the drill.
- The shoulders must be over the feet on the backpedal movement.
- The athlete should eliminate false steps when making the transition from one movement to the next.

Zigzag

Purpose
To improve footwork and quickness

Skills Used
Maintaining proper position throughout continuous changes of direction

Procedure
1. The athlete stands facing a row of 10 cones that have been placed one yard apart.
2. He or she steps with the right foot diagonally forward to the right of the first cone and then slides the left foot to the right foot.
3. Taking the next step, the athlete leads with the left foot to the left side of the next cone and then slides the right foot to the left foot.
4. He or she zigzags through all the cones.

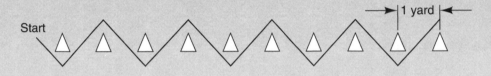

Key Points
- Movement is quick and explosive.
- The hips and shoulders are kept square.
- Both feet should go around each cone.
- The athlete pushes off with the outside foot.

Variation
Have the athlete perform this drill while holding a medicine ball with the arms extended up to ensure proper passing position.

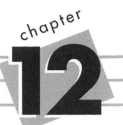

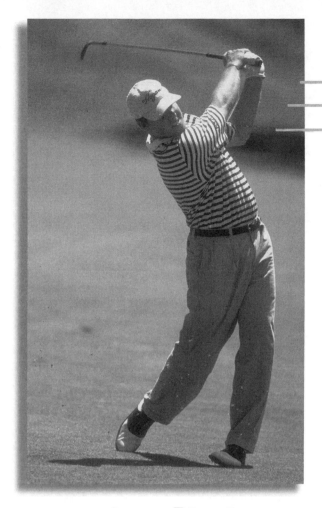

chapter 12

Periodizing Training for Peak Performance

Tudor O. Bompa

*I*t is well known that organized people are more productive than others. This holds true in sports training; an athlete who plans a program well is more efficient in his or her conditioning. An effective plan, which normally translates into better performance, strongly depends on *periodization*.

The term itself is derived from *period*, which in this case refers to a particular phase of training. But the periodization concept is more than that; it includes the following two aspects of a training program:

- Periodization of the annual plan, or how to divide the annual plan into smaller phases that are easier to manage
- Periodization of the motor abilities (strength, speed, and endurance), or how to manipulate a sequence of training methods and concepts to produce a sport-specific quality such as power, power endurance, or muscular endurance

Anyone using periodization will feel its benefits. First, it provides a better, more effective way of arranging the annual plan, in which training loads and stress alter from phase to phase. Similarly, periodization builds specific emphasis on volume (quantity) and intensity (quality, speed, and power) of training into each phase (see pages 278 to 280). By varying the intensity of stress and emphasizing physical, technical, tactical, and psychological training elements during preparatory and competitive phases, the athlete facilitates better peaking and more consistent performance during the competitive phase.

Many athletes have benefited from periodization. Canadian sprinters and track cyclists, for instance, never broke a world record and were not even visible on the world sports scene before applying periodization in the 1980s and 1990s. Since their exposure to periodized training, especially the periodization of strength, they have been ranked among the best in the world, breaking world and Olympic records. Many rowers, tennis players, swimmers, and triathletes from other countries have also noticed dramatic improvements from using this method of planning. The application of periodization to team sports has also been effective. Several U.S. college football teams that used periodization have climbed from the bottom of their league standings to the top.

PERIODIZATION OF THE ANNUAL PLAN

Figure 12.1 illustrates the structure of an annual plan with only one peak, or single periodization, where peak performance is planned to be achieved at the time of the national championships (NC).

Most team sports and some seasonal individual sports such as skiing, rowing, triathlon, and cycling use the one-peak cycle, or mono-cycle. Other sports such as track and field and swimming use a two-peak annual plan, often called a bicycle or double periodization, which has two separate cycles, one for each peak. For track and field, the two cycles are the indoor and outdoor competitions.

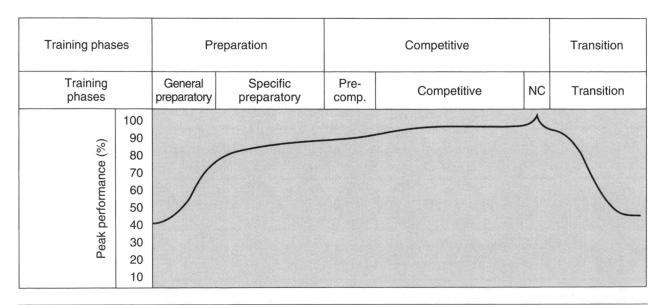

Figure 12.1   Annual plan for periodization.

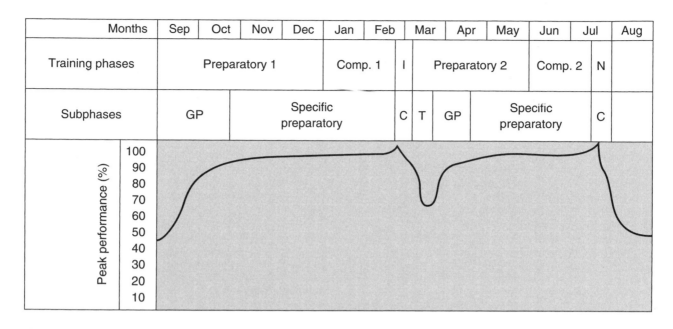

Months	Sep	Oct	Nov	Dec	Jan	Feb	Mar	Apr	May	Jun	Jul	Aug
Training phases	Preparatory 1				Comp. 1		I	Preparatory 2			Comp. 2	N
Subphases	GP		Specific preparatory				C	T	GP	Specific preparatory		C

Figure 12.2 Structure of a bi-cycle applicable in track and field.

Figure 12.2 illustrates such a plan. Note the difference in the peaking curve between a mono-cycle and a bi-cycle.

As exemplified by figure 12.2, a bi-cycle annual plan has two main peaks: the first in late February or early March, the indoor championships (IC), and the second in late July, the national championships (NC). The dates of the two major competitions dictate the length of training phases and subphases. Thus, preparatory 1 is longer than preparatory 2, and the two competitive phases are of almost equal length. For the same reason, the general preparatory (GP) and the specific preparatory phases (SP) are longer for the first cycle than the second cycle. Between the first and second cycles is a two-week transition (T) phase, whereas after the national championships in July a four- or five-week transition occurs.

Other sports such as gymnastics, wrestling, and martial arts have three main competitions per year. This plan is a tri-cycle, or triple periodization. As seen in figure 12.3, the proximity of the three main competitions results in shorter training phases and subphases. Note also that the curve of peaking has more abrupt increases and decreases; the athlete must shift abruptly from GP to SP to peak at the desired times of the year.

In figure 12.3, the months of the year are numbered rather than named. This is simply because the main peaks of the sports using tri-cycles do not occur in the same months.

Equally visible is the shortness of training time before each peak. The longest preparatory time (P1) is in the first cycle. The other two preparatory periods are shorter, especially in the third cycle (P3). These conditions also dictate that the general preparatory (GP1, GP2, and GP3) subphases become shorter as the athlete advances through the cycles, especially in the third cycle. This brief analysis shows that a good performance in all three peaks is possible only if solid physical training is achieved through both general and specific (SP1, SP2, and SP3) physical preparation at the beginning of each cycle, especially the first.

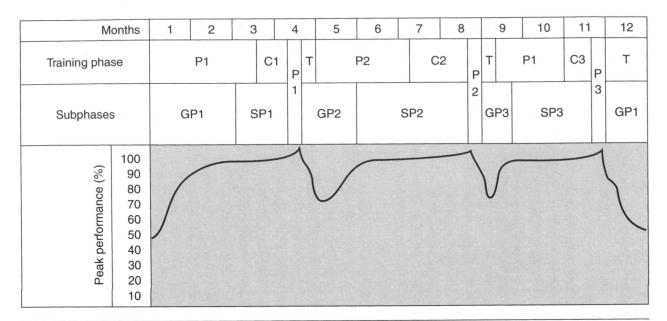

Figure 12.3   Tri-cycle with three peaks.

Selective Periodization

Training programs for junior athletes often duplicate those of elite athletes. Yet, in most cases, those using the programs of successful athletes fail to analyze whether junior athletes are ready for a multipeak plan or whether they can tolerate the high-intensity training that accompanies the training programs of elite athletes.

Irrespective of whether an athlete competes in a multipeak sport or a single-peak sport, the following types of annual plans must be considered.

- A mono-cycle is strongly advisable for junior athletes. The advantage is that it has long preparatory phases free from the stress of competition. This allows the coach to concentrate on developing skills and building a strong foundation of physical training.

- A bi-cycle is suggested for national-class athletes, individuals who can qualify for national championships. Even in this situation, the preparatory phase should be as long as possible to allow time to train the fundamentals.

- A tri-cycle and a multipeak plan are recommended only for advanced or international-class athletes. It is assumed that these athletes have a solid foundation and a background that allows them to handle with greater ease an annual plan with three or more peaks.

Although the duration of training phases depends on the schedule of competitions, table 12.1 provides a guideline for the distribution of weeks per training phase.

Characteristics of Annual Plan Training Phases

Irrespective of the number of peaks or cycles in an annual plan, all have three standard phases: preparatory, competitive, and transition.

Table 12.1 Distribution of Weeks for Various Types of Annual Plans

Annual plan (weeks)		Preparatory (weeks)	Competitive (weeks)	Transition (weeks)
Mono-cycle	52	32 or more	10–15	5
Bi-cycle	26	13 or more	5–10	3–4
Tri-cycle	17–18	8 or more	3–5	2–3

Preparatory Phase

The *preparatory phase* is of enormous importance to the entire year of training. During this period, the general framework of physical, technical, tactical, and psychological preparation is developed for the competitive phase. Inadequate training performed during this period will cause repercussions during the competitive phase, which no form of training can remedy. A significant amount of training, based especially on increased volume (quantity of work), will in the long run result in a relatively low level of fatigue after training and may enhance recovery. Therefore, throughout the preparatory phase, and especially during the initial part, a high volume of training is essential to cause adequate body adaptation to the specifics of training.

In general terms, the objectives of training in this phase are the following:

- To acquire and improve general physical training
- To improve the motor abilities required by the sport
- To develop specific psychological qualities
- To develop, improve, or perfect technique
- To familiarize athletes with the basic strategic maneuvers to be employed in subsequent phases

The preparatory phase should last between three and six months depending on the climate, the characteristics of the sport, and the type of annual plan employed. For individual sports such as track and field, rowing, and winter sports, the duration should be between one and two times as long as that of the competitive phase. For team sports it may be shorter but should not be less than two to three months.

The preparatory phase is divided into two subphases: general and specific preparation. The *general preparatory* subphase has the objectives of developing working capacity and general physical condition, improving technical elements, and teaching basic game strategy. The foremost objective, however, should be to develop a high level of physical conditioning that will facilitate future training and performance.

The *specific preparatory*, or the second part of the preparatory phase, represents a transition toward the competitive season. Though the objectives of training are similar to those of the general subphase, the character of training becomes more specific. Although the volume of training is still high, most work (70 to 80 percent) is directed toward the specific exercises related to the skills or technical patterns of the sport. Toward the end of this subphase, the volume tends to drop progressively, allowing an increase in the intensity or quality of training. For sports in which intensity is an important attribute, such as sprinting, jumping, and team sports, the volume of training must be decreased to allow the coach to concentrate on sport-specific training.

Competitive Phase

The *competitive phase* has among its main tasks the perfecting of all training factors; this enables athletes to improve their abilities and thus compete successfully in the main competition or championship meet. Among the general objectives of the competitive phase are the following:

- To improve motor abilities and psychological qualities according to the specifics of the sport
- To perfect and consolidate technique
- To perfect tactical maneuvers and gain competitive experience

During the competitive phase, which for team sports includes precompetitive or exhibition games, the goal is to improve performance from game to game and, obviously, to qualify for the playoffs for the major competition of the year.

Before the playoffs or championship competition, a short *taper*, or *unloading phase*, occurs. The goal of the taper is to facilitate peak performance, the best performance of the year.

Let us examine the specifics of tapering for two types of sports: speed-power sports (team sports, many of the track and field events, martial arts, etc.) and endurance sports (most swimming events, triathlon, cross-country skiing, rowing, canoeing, etc.). For each of the two types of sports, we will analyze the last two weeks before the major championships of the year.

As illustrated by figure 12.4, in the first week the volume of training is reduced by approximately 50 percent of previous levels. Intensity is reduced slightly and progressively over the two-week phase. Intensity may have one peak in the first

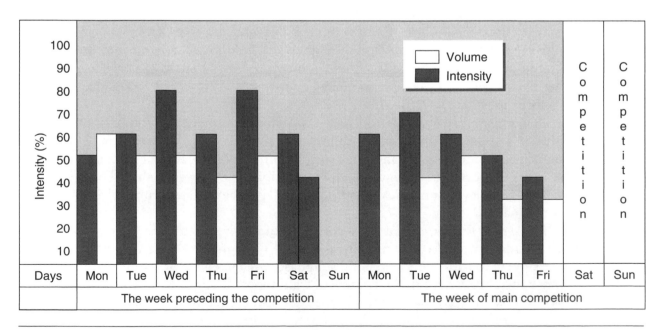

Figure 12.4 Dynamics of volume and intensity for unloading phase in speed-power sports.

part of the second week, on Tuesday, although it will not be of high intensity. Obviously, repetitions or drills of high intensity may be performed on any of the days, bearing in mind the following: The number of repetitions or drills should be much lower than during a normal week, and the rest interval should be longer than normal to eliminate the possibility of accumulating fatigue before the championships begin.

Figure 12.5 illustrates the tapering strategy of a sport where endurance is the most important physical ability. Unlike speed-power sports, in which intensity of training must be maintained, endurance sports require the participant to guard against doing too much training at high intensity, which is the most fatiguing element. Throughout the two weeks of tapering, therefore, intensity must be progressively reduced. The volume of training, though decreased as well, remains slightly higher. In this way, the athlete preserves his or her fitness level while removing the fatigue of high-intensity training because intensity drops below 40 percent.

Transition Phase

After months of stressful training and many competitions or games, the *transition phase* is a welcome change for athletes and coaches alike. The objective of transition is to remove fatigue from both the body and mind, to relax psychologically, and to regenerate biologically before a new annual plan starts. During transition, however, the athlete must maintain an acceptable level of physical training, about 40 or 50 percent of the level of the competition phase. If this amount of training is not performed, detraining of most of the qualities developed during the year occurs, in the form of protein degradation and an inability to recruit the same number of muscle fibers. Consequently, the rate of strength loss may be as much as 3 or 4 percent in the first week, with even greater losses in the following weeks.

When strength decreases, so does speed because speed and quickness rely heavily on the force of muscle contraction. Inactivity also affects endurance ca-

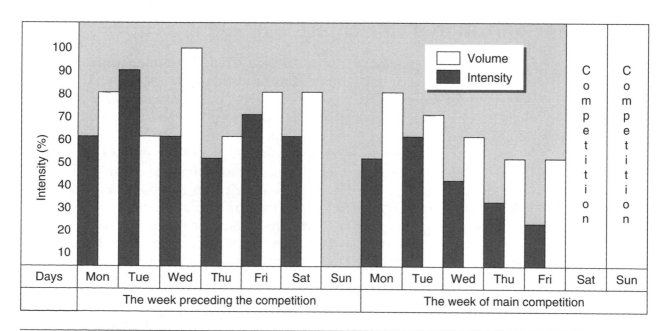

Figure 12.5 Dynamics of volume and intensity for unloading phase in endurance sports.

pacity. A loss of some 7 percent occurs in the first two weeks (a 30 percent decrease in the level of hemoglobin and a loss of up to 50 percent of mitochondria volume).

To avoid excessive biological degeneration, the athlete must maintain two to four workouts per week. Informal and relaxed training can be the norm.

PERIODIZATION OF MOTOR ABILITIES

One of the key elements in the success of periodization is how the main motor abilities such as strength, speed, and endurance are trained during the annual plan.

In several sports, the benefits of periodization of motor abilities are not yet recognized and therefore not applied. For instance, I have seen football players working on maximum speed from February on without building any base, without doing any tempo running to develop an anaerobic-aerobic foundation. Without a proper base, the athlete will reach a plateau in maximum speed training. In addition, maximum nervous system stimulation, which occurs in maximum speed training, cannot be maintained for long without fatiguing the central nervous system (CNS). A well-developed periodization of speed, as shown in figure 12.6, will eliminate such problems.

Figure 12.6 illustrates the periodization of main motor abilities. A brief explanation of the periodization of strength, endurance, and speed will define the sequence and training methods employed in each phase. Adherence to the periodization sequence of specific phases develops the necessary combination of abilities for each sport. All but a few sports require a certain combination of motor abilities. Developing the correct mixture, through periodizing motor abilities, is the secret to achieving the best specific conditioning for each sport.

Figure 12.6 refers to a mono-cycle annual plan. It is easy to apply the same concept to a bi- or tri-cycle. The same sequence, with more condensed phases, is repeated as many times as the number of competitive phases in a plan.

Periodization of Strength

During the training phases of the annual plan, strength-training plans and methods vary depending on the requirements of a given sport. Although the critical ingredient for many sports is power, for others muscular endurance is the key element. Power, or the ability to apply force in the shortest time, is a combination of speed or quickness and strength. Football, baseball, most other team sports, martial arts, sprinting, jumping, throwing, and so forth are all sports in which the level of power has a strong impact on final performance.

Muscular endurance, on the other hand, refers to the ability to apply force against a lower resistance for a long period. Athletes in most swimming events, rowing, canoeing, triathlon, cross-country skiing, and so forth benefit from improving muscular endurance to the highest level realistically possible. Let us briefly examine the specific training phases and methods of the periodization of strength.

Anatomical Adaptation

Following a transition phase, when athletes usually do little strength training, it is scientifically and methodologically sound to begin a strength program aimed

Phases	Preparatory		Competitive		Transition
Subphases	General preparatory	Specific preparatory	Precompetitive	Main competitions	Transition
Strength	Anatomical adaptation	Maximum strength	Conversion: • Power • Muscular endurance • or both	Maintenance C	Compensation
Endurance	Aerobic endurance	• Aerobic endurance • Specific endurance	Specific endurance		Aerobic endurance
Speed	Aerobic and anaerobic endurance	• Specific speed • Alactic • Lactic • Speed endurance	• Specific speed • Agility • Reaction time • Speed endurance		Play and games

Figure 12.6 Periodization of motor abilities.

at adapting the anatomy to a new strength program. The main objective of the anatomical adaptation phase is to involve most muscle groups, thus preparing the muscles, ligaments, tendons, and joints to endure the subsequent long, strenuous phases of training. A general strength program, using many exercises (9 to 12) performed comfortably without pushing too hard, is desirable. Apply the following to help achieve the objectives of this first phase: a load of 40 to 60 percent of the athlete's maximum, 8 to 12 repetitions in two or three sets, performed at a low to medium rate, with a rest interval of one to one-and-a-half minutes between exercises, over 4 to 6 weeks. Longer periods of anatomical adaptation (8 to 12 weeks) should certainly be considered for junior athletes and those without a strong background in strength training.

Maximum Strength Phase

The level of maximum strength affects both types of strength—power and muscular endurance. The athlete cannot reach a high standard of power without achieving a high level of maximum strength. Because power is the product of speed and maximum strength, it is logical to develop maximum strength first and then convert it into power. During the maximum strength phase, then, the goal is to develop maximum strength to the highest level the athlete is capable of reaching. The duration of this phase (one to three months) is a function of the sport's events and the athlete's needs. This phase may be quite long, perhaps three months, for a shot-putter or football player, whereas an ice hockey player may allocate only one month for the development of this type of strength.

Conversion Phase

To meet the needs and characteristics of the sport or event, maximum strength must be converted into sport-specific qualities such as power, muscular endurance, or both. Through the application of the appropriate training method for the type of strength sought and the use of training methods specific to the selected sport, maximum strength is gradually transformed into power or muscular endurance. Throughout the conversion phase (one to two months), the athlete must maintain a certain level of maximum strength. Otherwise, power may decline slightly toward the end of the competitive phase.

Although the maximum strength phase is specific to the preparatory phase, the duration of the conversion period begins toward the end of the preparatory phase and continues into the beginning of the competitive phase (precompetitive phase).

Maintenance Phase

As the term suggests, the main objective of strength training for this phase is to maintain the standards achieved in the previous phases. Again, the program followed during this phase is a function of the specific requirements of the sport. The ratio between maximum strength, power, and muscular endurance must reflect such requirements. For instance, a shot-putter and a lineman in football may plan two sessions for maximum strength and two for power, whereas a jumper may consider one for maximum strength and three for power. A baseball player, a wide receiver in football, or a 100-meter swimmer may plan one session for maximum strength, two for power, and one for muscular endurance. A 1,500-meter swimmer may dedicate the entire strength program to building muscular endurance.

The athlete should dedicate two to four sessions each week to maintaining the required strength, depending on his or her level of performance and the role that strength plays in the skills and performance of the particular sport. Considering the objectives of the competitive phase, the time allocated to the maintenance of strength is secondary. The coach, therefore, must develop an efficient and specific maintenance program. Two to a maximum of four exercises involving the prime movers (the muscles performing the technical skills) should maintain strength levels.

Cessation (C) Phase

The strength-training program ends five to seven days before the main competition so that all energy is available to achieve a good performance.

Compensation Phase

This phase completes the annual plan and coincides with the transition phase from the present to the next annual plan. The objectives of the transition phase are to remove fatigue and replenish exhausted energies. An informal strength-training program, therefore, should have the goal of involving muscle groups other than the prime movers in order to build the weaker muscles that are not often trained.

Periodization of Endurance

During an annual training plan, endurance is developed in several phases. For an annual plan with one peak, endurance training is accomplished in three main phases: (1) aerobic endurance, (2) aerobic and specific endurance, and (3) specific endurance.

Each of the suggested phases has specific training objectives. *Aerobic endurance* is developed throughout the transition phase and early preparation phase (one to three months). Although each sport may require a slight alteration, the athlete could achieve the goals of aerobic endurance through the uniform and steady-state method, with moderate to medium intensity. As a general consequence of such a program, the athlete's working capacity and cardiorespiratory system progressively improve. As the athlete adjusts to training, he or she must elevate the workload, especially the volume (quantity) of training.

Aerobic endurance and specific endurance play an extremely important role in achieving the objectives set for endurance training. Throughout this phase, which represents a transition from aerobic endurance to a type of endurance specific to each sport, aerobic endurance is still emphasized. Elements of anaerobic activity specific to the sport are introduced. Particularly in team sports, the rhythm of activity and the pace of specific drills become progressively sport specific. Intensive training specific to the competitive phase may fail unless the foundations of endurance are solidly developed during the second phase. The prevailing methods are uniform, alternating, and long and medium interval training (toward the end of this phase). The volume of training reaches the highest levels during the aerobic phase and the aerobic and specific endurance phases of the annual plan.

Specific endurance coincides with the competitive phase. The selection of the appropriate methods depends strictly on the demands of the sport and the needs of the athlete. For many sports, however, the intensity of training must be emphasized so strongly that it often exceeds racing intensity. The alternation of various types of intensities should facilitate a good recovery between training sessions, leading to a good peak for the final competition.

Periodization of Speed

Training for periodization of speed depends on the characteristics of the sport, the athlete's level of performance, and the competition schedule. Training for team-sport athletes will therefore be different from that for sprinters. The first group of athletes usually follows a mono-cycle annual plan, whereas sprinters, who in most cases participate in both indoor and outdoor seasons, follow a bi-cycle plan.

Whether for individual or team sports, the periodization of speed may follow several training subphases. *Aerobic and anaerobic endurance* should be considered the training base for the phases that follow it. Whether through tempo running for sprinters, football players, baseball players, and basketball players or through steady-state training for athletes in other sports, this first phase is necessary for building a solid aerobic foundation for speed training. Training progressively incorporates activities that are more specific to the particular sport. At the beginning of the phase, fartlek (speed play) is used to build a strong aerobic base. Later, various types of interval training and repetition training, which are one step closer to specific speed, are added.

Alactic speed and anaerobic endurance training become more intensive, event specific, refined, and specialized as the competition phase approaches. Specificity of training prevails in methods and specific exercises. Maximum velocity for sprinters, wide receivers, basketball players, and similar athletes is emphasized, progressing from 10 to 15 meters to 30 to 60 meters.

Specific speed could incorporate some or all of the speed components (alactic, lactic, and speed endurance), depending on the specifics of the sport. Drills for the development of agility and reaction time are also introduced.

Specific speed, agility, and reaction time require specific methods and drills that are designed to work toward the goal of developing specific speed and refining related abilities such as agility and reaction time.

During the competitive phase, the intensity of training is elevated through specific training methods and participation in competitions. Although exercises specific to the chosen sport prevail, general ways of training, including games and play for fun, relaxation, and active rest, should also be incorporated. A correct ratio between these two groups of exercises will lower stress and strain in training. Many sprinters and team-sport athletes are prone to injuries because of high-intensity training; alternation between various means and intensities is an important training element.

DYNAMICS OF THE VOLUME AND INTENSITY OF TRAINING

The volume and intensity of training play an important role in the loading strategy of training during the annual plan, as well as being crucial elements to consider for peaking purposes.

The *volume* of training is the quantitative element of training, which includes the duration of activity; the distance covered or weight lifted in a training session; and the number of repetitions of an exercise, skill, or drill. The volume also refers to the sum of work performed in a given training phase. Thus, an athlete may perform 24 training sessions in August and 21 in October. The same athlete may run 80 kilometers per week in April and only 72 kilometers per week in July. In both examples, the volume of training is higher in the first month.

The quantity of work, or the volume of training, is an important element to train in all sports, especially in sports in which endurance is the key physical quality. High volume is an important training ingredient, especially during the preparatory phase when the foundation of strong conditioning is built. As the competitive phase approaches, the volume of training decreases more visibly for speed-power sports such as sprinting, jumping, throwing, martial arts, football, and baseball. For endurance sports such as distance events in track, swimming, cross country, rowing, road racing in cycling, and triathlon the volume of training is still high during the competitive phase because aerobic endurance must be constantly emphasized to maintain good performance.

The *intensity* of training, on the other hand, represents the qualitative component of the work performed in a given period. It usually refers to how fast an action is performed (speed), the power or strength displayed in training or competition, and the psychological stress experienced by the athlete while competing or performing a difficult skill or routine.

Both the volume and intensity of training have specific dynamics during the main phases of the annual plan. The following two examples illustrate the dynamics of volume and intensity in endurance and speed-power sports.

Figure 12.7 illustrates the dynamics of volume (aerobic endurance) and intensity (lactic-acid training) used in training for a 400- or 800-meter swimming event. Peak performance is scheduled for the winter and summer nationals. On the left of figure 12.7 is the kilometrage per week. The dynamics of the aerobic endurance (volume) and lactic-acid (intensity) training change according to the phase. In the early preparatory phases (P1 and P2), the volume of training increases in steps every three to four weeks, alternating with a lower volume, with the goal of removing fatigue, regenerating the body, and relaxing the mind. Toward the end of the preparatory and early part of the competitive phases (C1 and C2), the volume stabilizes around 100 to 105 kilometers per week. As the main competitions approach and the taper for the nationals begins, the volume of training decreases progressively to 50 kilometers per week. These less fatiguing conditions promote removal of fatigue, regeneration of the body, and relaxation of the mind so the athlete can achieve peak performance.

Since the 400-meter or 800-meter event is one in which the proportions of aerobic and anaerobic lactic acid are about 85 percent and 15 percent, the kilometrage of lactic-acid training is quite low. Even in the hardest months, December, January, May, and June, the height of lactic-acid training is not above 20 kilometers per week. Training designed to tolerate lactic-acid buildup is not to be neglected, however, in most months of the year.

Figure 12.8 illustrates the dynamics of volume and intensity for a speed-power sport such as football. The same approach is possible for any other speed-power sport, but the dates of competitions might change. The dynamics of volume and intensity for a football team are far different from those for the swimmer in the previous example. In football, both volume and intensity are measured by hours per week. The types of training done for volume are tempo running (200 to 600

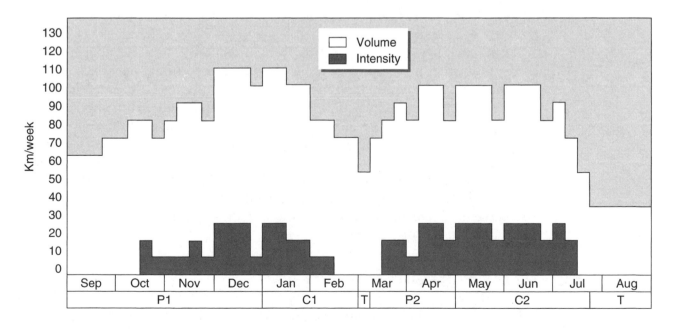

Figure 12.7 Dynamics of volume and intensity for training for a 400- or 800-meter swimming event.

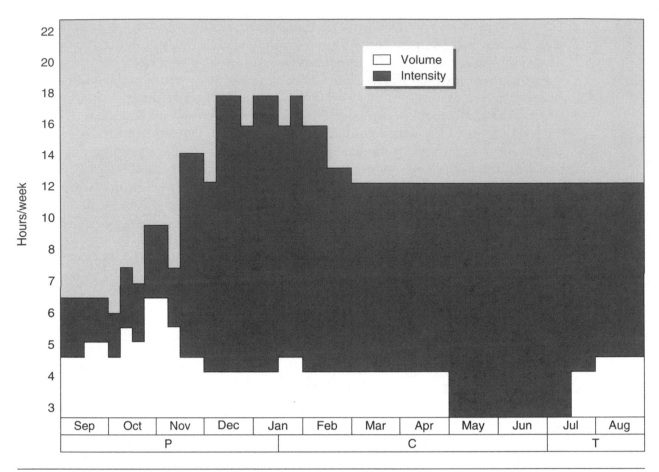

Figure 12.8 Dynamics of volume and intensity for a college football team.

meters with repetitions at 60 to 70 percent of maximum velocity for that distance), strength training using lower loads (below 80 percent of 1RM), and technical drills of low intensity. For intensity, on the other hand, training includes technical and tactical drills performed with high velocity and quickness, speed training, and power and strength training with loads over 80 percent of 1RM.

During the early preparatory phase (P), most work may be done independently by the individual player, anywhere between 10 and 16 hours per week. Tempo training is used to build an anaerobic-aerobic endurance base. Repetitions of 400 meters at 60 percent (i.e., 8 × 400 meters) and then 600 meters at 60 percent (i.e., 6–8 × 600 meters) are successful in building this base. As June approaches, tempo running is performed at shorter distances (i.e., 10–12 × 200 meters at 70 percent and 12–15 × 80–100 meters at 70 percent). From July on, players must work on position-specific maximum speed: 40 to 80 meters for wide receivers and 20 to 40 meters for players at other positions (i.e., 8–12 × 50 meters at 95 to 100 percent of maximum). Strength training must follow the periodization of strength discussed in this chapter.

INTEGRATED PERIODIZATION

Periodization, as the key element in successful planning and training, is not limited in application to how to cycle an annual plan or how to sequence the development of motor abilities for a given sport. Periodization also incorporates nutrition and mental and psychological training.

Sport psychologists, physiologists, and nutritionists often develop their training plans and programs without considering the planning-periodization process or the specific objectives in each phase of training. Mental and psychological training focuses on the athlete, often in connection with the competitive environment. This is also true for nutrition programs. Seldom are the sport scientists in these disciplines aware that athletes and coaches need their help throughout the annual or long-term training process, not just before competitions.

Integrated periodization represents the process of combining all components of training and matching them to the periodization of motor abilities. The periodization of the motor abilities dictates the diet and psychological skills best suited for a given training phase. An instructor, therefore, should learn what kind of diet and which psychological skills are best for training aerobic endurance, maximum strength, or any combination of such abilities. Armed with such information, the coach will be able to improve athletes' abilities and, as a result, their performance.

Figure 12.9 illustrates a model of integrated periodization for a sport in which speed and power are the dominant abilities. In the top of the chart are the months, training phases, and subphases. Because training dates differ among sports, the months of the plan are numbered rather than named.

Because this model of integrated periodization refers to a sport in which speed and power are the dominant abilities, the figure refers only to the periodization of speed, strength, mental and psychological attributes, and nutrition. Under normal conditions, the periodization of nutrition would also incorporate the periodization of training supplements.

Both psychological training and nutrition are periodized according to the periodization of strength because strength training represents a vital quality for all speed-power sports. Therefore, for each of the strength-training phases, the corresponding psychological techniques to employ and the primary nutrients necessary to supply the body with the fuel needed in training are given. To establish integrated periodization, use the following process: (1) define the periodization of motor abilities, (2) select the psychological technique to support the physical endeavors, and (3) produce the diet necessary to energize the body.

SUMMARY

The fundamental concept for good annual planning is periodization, which is especially useful in structuring the phases of motor abilities and maximizing training efforts. The periodization of strength, speed, and endurance represents the manipulation of different training phases with specific goals, organized in a specific sequence, with the ultimate goal of creating sport-specific adaptation. When this adaptation is complete, the athlete will be physiologically equipped to produce better sport-specific performances.

A good understanding of periodization will assist the coach in producing better annual plans and training programs. The schedule of games or competitions guides the timing of training phases. The coach should also integrate the periodization of nutrition and psychological training into the plan.

Months	1	2	3	4	5	6	7	8	9	10	11	12
Training phases	Preparatory					Competitive					NC	Trans
Subphases	General		Specific		Pre-competition	Official/league competitions						Trans
Speed	• Anaerobic/ aerobic, endurance		• Maximum speed short • Maintain anaerobic endurance	• Maximum speed short • Maximum speed medium • Maximum speed long		All in sport-specific proportion					Unloading	Play/fun
Strength	Anatomical adaptation	Maximum strength	Power	Maximum strength	Conversion	Maintenance						Compensation
Mental/ psychological	• Evaluate skills • Learn new skills • Quiet setting	• Mental skills to attain training objectives • Visualization • Imagery • Relaxation • Energy management			• Mental rehearsal • Energize • Positive self-talk • Visioning • Focus plans • Simulation • Coping	• Mental skills to cope with specific opponents • Stress management/relaxation • Energizing • Focus plans • Mental rehearsal • Motivational positive thinking/optimism • Positive thinking/optimism					Cessation	• Active rest • Regenerate, de-stress
Nutrition	Balanced diet	High protein	High carbs	High protein	High carbs	Fluctuates according to the schedule of competition					High carbs	Balanced diet

Figure 12.9 Integrated periodization for a speed–power sport.

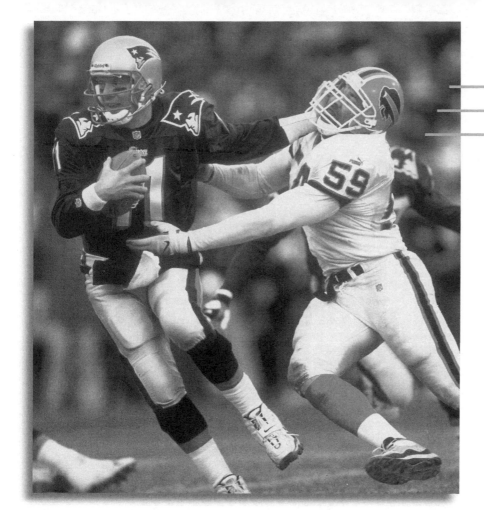

chapter 3

Designing Periodized Training Programs

In the previous chapter, Tudor Bompa provided the principles and a prototype of an annual conditioning program. This chapter now takes the generic principles of periodization and identifies the specific considerations coaches should make when designing workouts and programs for their particular sport. As with the sport-specific drills provided in chapter 11, nine sports are sampled in this chapter: baseball, basketball, football, golf, hockey, soccer, tennis, track and cross country, and volleyball.

Every coach must have an organized conditioning plan that takes into account the sport's competition schedule and the events athletes need to be in peak condition for. By clearly defining the seasons and the phases within each season, coaches can design a conditioning plan that ensures that athletes will peak when they need to peak.

The first part of each sport section in this chapter covers the overall framework of an annual periodized training plan. From there, many of the contributors design and share some specific workout plans that combine some of the drills introduced in chapter 11 with other key training methods athletes need for all-around sport-specific conditioning.

Some sports, including most team sports with seasons that culminate in a championship game or series, have one peak per year (*mono-cycle* programs). Other sports, such as some track and field events that have both an indoor and outdoor championship, have two peaks in a year (*bi-cycle* programs). Some individual sports, such as golf or tennis, may have several peaks throughout the year but, depending on the athlete's individual goals, the coach and athlete may decide to focus on a specific major tournament or championship. And while most of the following programs follow Bompa's basic examples in the previous chapter, the breakdown of seasons and phases may differ slightly from sport to sport to allow for specific application to the particular sport being discussed.

You'll see that each of the sample annual plans work to establish a base level of fitness, sport-specific skill training, strategic development, and the conversion of base strength into functional power and speed, all within the context of peaking at the proper time during the competition phase.

BASEBALL   Fernando Montes

In professional baseball today, players must participate in some type of year-round physical training program. Designing and monitoring such a training program is a monumental task. A major complication is that only during spring training are all the players on a team physically in one location. They spend the rest of the year playing at their respective locations, and after the season ends they return to their hometowns throughout the United States, Latin America, Canada, Japan, and Australia. As a coach of a professional team, I can tell you that there are many things a coach must keep in mind when designing a training program.

Eight months of traveling with, living with, and training players during a strenuous season has given me knowledge and insight about the physical and mental stress to which players are subjected. Baseball presents a unique situation for the strength and conditioning coach. A marathon season that demands peak performance day after day makes managing the grueling physical and mental stress associated with this game a challenge. The season starts in February and ends in late October, with only the month of November off. Proper preparation is necessary to endure this season and stay healthy. However, high school and collegiate players also endure long seasons and often play fall ball as well as spring ball. The high school, collegiate, and professional player needs a well-constructed year-round training protocol that includes strength training, cardiovascular conditioning, and mobility and agility training, as well as other types of individually tailored sport-specific training.

The program itself must be simple, safe, and interchangeable. It must be simple because many programs have limited equipment and facilities. It must be safe

Table 13.1 Baseball Periodization Model

Month	Nov	Dec	Jan	Feb	Mar	April	May	June	July	Aug	Sep	Oct
Phase	Transition	Preparation		Precompetitive		Competitive						
	Off-season			Spring training		In-season						Postseason
Focus	Anatomical adaptation		Max. strength	Conversion to power		Maintenance		Power		Power endurance		

because supervision will be limited. It must be familiar to all players in the organization, regardless of location or level of play. It is therefore important to design a program that the athlete can use successfully, no matter what the location, weather, or facilities.

This section provides guidance for creating such a training plan based on over 15 years of experience training professional and collegiate athletes. Keep in mind that the ability to adapt and adjust is the most critical element in the philosophy. Without built-in flexibility on a daily, weekly, and yearly basis, even "perfect" programs fall short of expectations. As you will see, the basic core program is consistent throughout the year.

The exercise variations are by design, sometimes for variety, other times because of facility availability, or the lack of it, on the road. The periodization structure of the year-round program will change according to the time of year. The program is designed around four training periods: off-season, spring training, in-season, and postseason (see table 13.1). Each must have specific goals and expectations. Remember, you must be able to adjust during any of these programs. As you will see, no perfect training program exists; however, it is possible to create an effective training program. Establish one that is safe, has scientific basis and is specific to the goals of the sport and the individual.

Off-Season

The off-season program allows each player to recover from the long season and prepare for the upcoming one. The player needs to recover during the month of November, not only physically, but mentally; thus, during this first month of the off-season the athlete is given a rest period. The rest of the off-season, from December to February, is designed to retool the body and get it ready to play. The 18- to 22-week off-season program is broken down into four phases: anatomical adaptation, strength, conversion, and power. The off-season ends with explosive power exercises specific to individual positions.

Off-Season Subphases

- Anatomical adaptation phase—four to five weeks
- Strength phase—four to five weeks
- Conversion phase—three to four weeks
- Explosive power phase—three to four weeks
- Download phase—every fourth or fifth week (circuit training)

Note that three major holidays occur during the off-season. Therefore, it makes sense to provide flexibility in the program to allow the athlete to enjoy this time off with family and friends. I like to include active rest days during this time in which athletes have the flexibility to engage in several different exercises that simply keep them active. Design your program around these major events to avoid lost training days.

The basic structure of the off-season program centers around a one- to two-hour workout per day. We work with a four-day split routine; Monday and Thursday we focus on the upper-body lifts and exercises, and Tuesday and Friday we focus on the lower-body exercises (see table 13.2). We do basic aerobic conditioning six days a week and add in mobility, agility, and skill work three to four times a week as we get closer to in-season (during the conversion and explosive power phases).

Table 13.2   Off-Season Program (Four-Day Split)

Upper-body exercises	Lower-body exercises	Special exercises
Chest	Quads	Physio ball movements
Back	Calves	Balance movements
Shoulders	Trunk	Stott-Pilates training
Arms (triceps and biceps)	Hamstrings	
Forearm, wrist, fingers	Rotational movements	
Shoulder-specific exercises		

Anatomical adaptation phase		Strength phase		Conversion phase		Power phase	
Reps	20-15-12-10	Reps	8-6-4, 6-4-3	Reps	6-5-4	Reps	4-3-2
Sets	4 or 5	Sets	4 or 5	Sets	3 or 4	Sets	4 or 5

Off-Season Workout in Anatomical Adaptation Phase

Upper body		Lower body	
Dumbbell incline press	4 × 15	Safe squat	4 × 15
Seated row	4 × 15	Calf raise	3 × 15
Dumbbell shoulder shrugs	4 × 15	Seated leg curls	4 × 15
Triceps push-downs	4 × 15	Good mornings	4 × 10
EZ-bar curls	4 × 15	Step-ups	3 × 10
Medicine ball push-ups	3 × 10	Shuttle 2000	4 × 10
Dumbbell row	3 × 10	Dumbbell lunge	3 × 10
Dumbbell shoulder front and lateral raise	3 × 10	Plate twist	4 × 10
Cable French press	3 × 10		
Towel pull-ups	3 × 10		

A professional baseball club may include as many as 150 players. This fact, coupled with the challenge of working at various locations with differing equipment, creates a unique situation for training. The program must be flexible but consistent in structure and simple in application.

Spring Training

During this period from February through March (six to eight weeks), the focus changes from physical preparation to baseball fundamentals and skills in preparation for the upcoming season. The strength and conditioning coach must strike a balance in providing a training program that prepares the athlete for the season without producing an overtraining effect. For this reason we build in one to two days of active rest per week into this phase. The player lifts twice a week, does general conditioning and mobility and agility work two to three times per week, and works on baseball skills daily. Workouts last from 30 to 45 minutes.

A typical spring training week might be set up as shown here:

- Monday—upper-body lifting
- Tuesday—conditioning and sprint work
- Wednesday—agility work (outdoor)
- Thursday—lower-body lifting
- Friday—off day
- Saturday—agility (indoor)
- Sunday—conditioning (pool)

One way to work in this training with a large team is to divide the team into training groups (see table 13.3).

Table 13.3　Spring Training Group Assignments

	Mon	Tues	Wed	Thurs	Fri	Sat	Sun
Group 1	Off	Lift	Agility	Condition	Lift	Agility	Condition
Group 2	Condition	Off	Lift	Agility	Condition	Lift	Agility
Group 3	Agility	Condition	Off	Lift	Agility	Cond	Lift
Group 4	Lift	Agility	Cond	Off	Lift	Agility	Cond
Group 5	Condition	Lift	Agility	Cond	Off	Lift	Agility
Catchers	Agility	Condition	Lift	Agility	Condition	Off	Lift
Infielders	Lift	Agility	Condition	Lift	Agility	Condition	Off
Outfielders	Off	Lift	Agility	Cond	Lift	Agility	Condition

(Groups 1-5 are pitchers)

Note: Adjustments are made with group and individual programs as they start to play games in March. During the last two weeks of spring, pitchers are moved into their in-season routine.

Baseball

In-Season

The in-season program from April to October (for professional players) is designed to maintain the physical strength the athlete needs to be ready to play every day (or every fifth day if a starting pitcher) and recover quickly afterward. The best way to judge a training program is not by how strong the player is but by how well he plays late in the season and deep into the playoffs.

The program must be flexible enough that the strength and conditioning coach can adjust for the demands of daily baseball competition, the conditions of travel, and the ability of players to focus on the work at hand during physical and emotional stress. The players' focus is now on playing every night. Distractions are numerous, so the ability to motivate athletes is important.

It's good to break the in-season into two phases—the first and second halves of the season. Total training time each day (outside of games) should be between 30 and 45 minutes long. Athletes should lift twice per week during the in-season, perform a conditioning routine two to three times per week, and do mobility and agility drills once or twice a week. Skill work is included in playing games.

The following sections provide some samples of how to break down in-season weekly workouts for pitchers and players.

Starting Pitchers

The following breakdown is based on a five-man starting rotation:

- Game day—postgame shoulder exercises and 15-minute bike workout
- Day 1—lifting and 45 minutes of conditioning workout
- Day 2—side bullpen work and hard conditioning day (85 to 98 percent target heart rate). Simulated six- or seven-inning game (heart-rate baseball game)
- Day 3—heavy lifting day and moderate conditioning day (75 to 85 percent target heart rate)
- Day 4—optional day (no assigned training)
- Day 5—game day

Relievers and Situation Pitchers

Relievers do all lifting after the game, adjusted by game activity and game usage. Use a split routine or individualized program that will meet the needs of each pitcher, considering age, injury, and physical limitations that prevent any type of normal training. Consider the same variables when designing a conditioning program.

For example, the workweek of a reliever might look like this:

- Monday—pitch one inning, lift postgame (upper body)
- Tuesday—cardiovascular postgame workout for 30 to 45 minutes (80 to 85 percent target heart rate)
- Wednesday—no work (team travel day)
- Thursday—pitch to four batters, lift postgame (lower body)
- Friday—no postgame work

- Saturday—cardiovascular postgame workout for 30 to 45 minutes (80 to 85 percent target heart rate)
- Sunday—no work (team travel day)

Position Players

In setting up a program for position players, the strength and conditioning coach must consider that they perform every day and that each position has particular needs and physical stresses.

For example, a position player's program for a week might look like this:

- Monday—lift postgame (upper body)
- Tuesday—agility (pre- or postgame)
- Wednesday—conditioning or treadmill sprints
- Thursday—off (team travel day)
- Friday—no work
- Saturday—lift postgame (lower body)
- Sunday—optional day

Assign specific in-season exercises by considering the athlete's preference, medical limitations, and, when on the road, the availability of equipment and facilities. Players perform forearms and special exercises on either lifting days or conditioning days. Table 13.4 shows an example of an in-season workout.

Table 13.4   In-Season Workout

Maintenance phase		Lower body		Upper body	
Reps	6-4-3	Quads	8-6-4-4-4	Chest	8-6-4-4
Sets	2–4	Calf raise	3 × 8–10	Back	3–4 × 6
		Hamstrings	4 × 6–8	Shoulder	3–4 × 6
		Low back	3 × 8–10	Triceps	3–4 × 6
		Step-ups	3 × 6–8	Biceps	3–4 × 6

Postseason

Lifting is optional during this phase. Players who choose to lift will perform a 10- to 12-exercise circuit routine, consisting of 15 to 20 seconds of work and 30 seconds of rest. The pitchers, both starters and relievers, continue with their weekly routines. The position players have endured the long season, playing over 150 games on average. The adjustment in their program is a welcome change.

BASKETBALL

Bill Foran

A year-round training program for basketball has four distinct seasons: preseason, in-season, postseason, and off-season. Every level from middle school through the NBA can use this sequence, varying the length of each season as needed to take into account the respective major championships and tournaments. Table 13.5 illustrates the training year for NBA, collegiate, and high school players.

Table 13.5   Annual Schedules

NBA Annual Schedule

Jan	Feb	Mar	April	May	June	July	Aug	Sep	Oct	Nov	Dec
In-season				Playoffs	*Post-season	Off-season			Pre-season	In-season	

*Postseason can start anytime between mid-April and mid-June.

College Annual Schedule

Jan	Feb	Mar	April	May	June	July	Aug	Sep	Oct	Nov	Dec
In-season		Tourn-ament	*Post-season	Off-season						Pre-season	In-season

*Postseason can start anytime in March.

High School Annual Schedule

Jan	Feb	Mar	April	May	June	July	Aug	Sep	Oct	Nov	Dec
In-season		Tourn-ament	*Post-season	Off-season						Pre-season	In-season

*Postseason can start anytime in March.

Off-Season

The off-season is the time for basketball players to become better players. They can improve their skills, speed, agility, jumping ability, strength, power, quickness, flexibility, and conditioning. To develop all these components, athletes need a well-rounded program that incorporates skill development, weight training, agility drills, conditioning, stretching, jumping plyometrics, quick-feet plyometrics, and medicine ball work.

The first four weeks of the off-season can be devoted to basic weight training and general conditioning to start the process of building a new strength and conditioning base. The next 12 to 16 weeks of the off-season training program emphasize the periodization phases of hypertrophy, basic strength, and building strength and power. Each component of off-season training listed in table 13.6

Table 13.6 Off-Season Training Schedule

Monday	Tuesday	Wednesday	Thursday	Friday
Skill development	Skill development	Skill development	Skill development	Skill development
Weight training (upper body)	Quick-feet plyometrics	Medicine ball work	Weight training (upper body)	Quick-feet plyometrics
Agility drills	Jumping plyometrics		Agility drills	Jumping plyometrics
Conditioning	Weight training (lower body)		Conditioning	Weight training (lower body)
Stretching	Stretching		Stretching	Stretching

Basketball

progresses from high volume, low intensity to higher intensity, lower volume. Repetitions should be 8 to 12 for the hypertrophy phase, 6 to 8 for the basic stregth phase, and to 4 to 6 for the strength and power phase.

With so many components involved in developing a basketball player, workouts must be efficient. The following one-week off-season training schedule includes all the components of a total program.

Each workout starts with some aspect of skill development—shooting, dribbling, ballhandling, passing, or other skills. As shown in table 13.6, the Monday and Thursday workouts include upper-body weight training, agility drills, sport-specific conditioning, and flexibility. The Tuesday and Friday workouts include lower-body weight training, jumping plyometrics, quick-feet plyometrics, and flexibility. Wednesday is the recovery day with only medicine ball work after skill development.

Weight training is the key to developing a solid strength base. Athletes with a solid strength base benefit the most from plyometrics (both quick-feet and jumping plyometrics) and agility drills.

The following sections offer an example of a weight-training program that works the total body, split into two routines that the athlete performs on different days. One routine works the upper body, and the other works the lower body.

Upper-Body Day

To build a strong and balanced upper body, this program uses an equal number of pressing movements and pulling movements, four of each in the standard program. For time efficiency, each pressing movement is followed by a pulling movement and then a rest period. (These are commonly called supersets.) A beginner's program, dropping the incline press and seated row, could start with three pressing movements and three pulling movements. The abdominal work should be three to five sets of a variety of crunches, leg raises, and twisting crunches.

Two to four sets

- Bench press
- Lat pull
- Military press
- Shrugs

Two to three sets

- Incline press
- Seated row
- Triceps press-down
- Arm curl

One to two sets

- Rotator-cuff work
- Wrist curls

And three to five sets of abdominal work.

Lower-Body Day

This is the more important day of weight training because it concentrates on the power center of the body, the muscles involved in running, jumping, and moving quickly in all directions. The hang cleans, high pulls, and squats are excellent exercises for developing the power center but can be dangerous if the athlete uses poor technique. The lunges and step-ups are important because they work each leg independently. Most basketball players have a strength imbalance in the legs that independent work with each leg can eliminate. The leg extension, leg curl, calf raise, and dorsiflexion can be done as a four-exercise minicircuit for time efficiency.

Three to four sets

- Hang cleans or high pulls
- Squats or leg presses

One to two sets

- Lunges
- Step-ups

Two sets

- Leg extensions
- Leg curls
- Calf raises (seated and standing)
- Dorsiflexion

And three to five sets of lower-back work.

Preseason

The preseason is the two- to four-week period from the start of practice until the first game. The first 7 to 10 days may have two practices per day. This is the time to introduce the in-season weight training program.

In-Season

The basketball season is when players use the strength, power, quickness, speed, agility, and conditioning that they developed in the off-season. A solid in-season program will maintain the improvements developed in the off-season. Intense, quality basketball practices will eliminate the need for extra conditioning, jumping plyometrics, and agility drills. The players who are not getting playing time in games may need extra conditioning to maintain their fitness. The extra conditioning can include agility drills, on-court conditioning, quick-feet plyometrics, and medicine ball work (see chapter 11, pages 224 to 229).

To maintain their strength and power throughout the season, basketball players need to be involved in a quality, in-season weight-training program. Players should perform in-season weight training twice a week. The program should involve the total body, and be time efficient and able to be modified according to the needs of the individual athlete.

The program illustrated in table 13.7 uses five minicircuits with three or four exercises in each. In the first minicircuit, for example, the player performs a pushing movement (bench press), a pulling movement (lat pull), and a leg exercise (squats) and then rests for two minutes before repeating the sequence at a higher weight. After two or three sets of the first minicircuit, the athlete moves to the next circuit. A total-body program can be accomplished in a short time with minicircuits.

Table 13.7   In-Season Weight Training Program

Minicircuit 1 (2 or 3 sets)	Minicircuit 2 (2 or 3 sets)	Minicircuit 3 (2 sets)	Minicircuit 4 (1 or 2 sets)	Minicircuit 5 (2 or 3 sets)
Bench presses	Military presses	Triceps press-downs	Calf raises	Ab work
Lat pulls	Shrugs	Arm curls	Dorsiflexion	Low-back work
Squats	Lunges or step-ups	Leg extensions	Rotator-cuff work	
		Leg curls	Wrist curls	

Postseason

The postseason is a two- to four-week period of active rest. Athletes recover from a long season and prepare for a productive off-season.

DISTANCE RUNNING   Jack Daniels

The first step in designing a training program for distance runners is to look at the overall season that lies ahead, including all competitions, and determine how many weeks are available for training, how much time is available (within each week), and what performance achievements (goals) are realistic. Besides these broad considerations, give considerable thought to some specific factors, such as the

- current level of fitness,
- primary event or events being trained for,
- expected conditions during the most important competitions at the end of the season,
- individual strengths and weaknesses,
- types of training that are of particular interest to the individual involved, and
- intermediate goals or competitions along the way to the season-ending goal.

After the various factors that influence the training program for the season are spelled out, it is possible to lay out the program itself. One of the more important considerations in designing a training program for distance runners is that it should be specific to each individual. Generic programs set up for a group of runners seldom work well for the individual members of the group.

Phases of Training

Before writing out workouts, divide the season into a number of training phases. The approach I prefer is to identify four phases of training, with the first phase set aside for injury prevention and foundation work. For runners, this initial phase is for easy running, stretching, and strengthening. This phase can be referred to as a foundation and injury-prevention (FI) phase of training. The remaining three phases of training are then identified as early quality (EQ), transition quality (TQ), and final quality (FQ), respectively. The ideal amount of time to spend in each of these four phases would be about six weeks. Figure 13.1 shows how the four phases of training are laid out.

If 24 weeks are available for a season of training, each of the four phases may well receive 6 weeks of attention. Some coaches and runners may feel that more attention should be given to phase I and less to other phases, based on individual strengths and weaknesses and time available. Still, 24 weeks provide ample time to make solid preparation for any competition.

Often, 24 weeks are not available, and a runner or coach may have to deal with a season that is considerably shorter than this ideal model. Figure 13.2 provides a way to deal with this dilemma. In this figure are the four 6-week training phases, progressing from left (foundation and injury prevention) to the far right (final quality training). Each phase has six numbers associated with it. These numbers indicate an order of priority that the runner or coach can use to determine how much time to allocate for each phase of training if less than the ideal 24 weeks are available. For example, if only 3 weeks are available for an entire season, all three

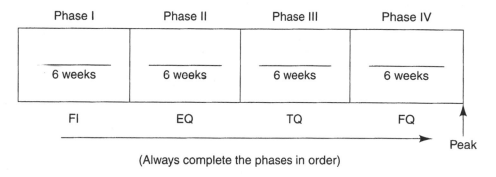

Figure 13.1   Sample plan for setting up a 24-week training program. Insert the dates (into the four boxes) to train in each phase starting with the peak performance date and working backwards.

	Phase I		Phase II		Phase III		Phase IV	
1	2	3	10	11	12	7	8	9	4	5	6
13			18			14			17		
	21			19			15			22	
		23			20			16			24

FI   EQ   TQ   FQ

(Always complete the phases in order)

Figure 13.2   Priority weekly numbering system to determine the number of weeks of training per phase according to the number of weeks available for training.
Adapted from Daniels, J. June 1993. "World's best peaking program." *Runner's World* 28 (6): 43.

weeks should be made up of foundation and injury-prevention (FI) training. If 12 weeks are available, each phase would receive 4 weeks of attention, as shown in the various four phases of training. Note, for example, that if only 9 weeks are available, phase II is completely ignored. It is better to place a fair bit of emphasis on fewer phases of training than to put a little emphasis on all types of training.

Note that regardless of how many weeks the coach or runner arrives at for any phase (or that lower priority numbers may be assigned to phase IV than to phase III, for example), the runner performs the assigned weeks of training for each phase in order. That is, a runner performs the assigned training at level I before going on to the next phase, does all assigned weeks of phase II before doing any weeks assigned to phase III, and so forth.

Phase IV

As figure 13.2 shows, the runner will always begin by spending some time on phase I training. Despite this and regardless of how much time the runner will devote to phase II, III, or IV, the coach or runner should first consider phase IV training. I suggest this because phase IV training prepares the runner for optimum performance and the other phases should be set up to prepare the runner for this all-important final phase.

Some considerations for phase IV include the following:

- Work on specific strengths (speed, endurance, etc.).
- Include workouts that are favorites or are particularly satisfying.
- Train during the time of day that is appropriate for the upcoming important competitions.
- In the case of major competitions, train in the same time zone and climate as the events for which the runner is preparing.
- Always be sensitive to the needs of the specific goal race or races. For example, a smaller amount of faster training is usually more applicable to racing a good 1,500-meter race, whereas less intense work is better when preparing for a marathon.

Phase III

Once the specifics of phase IV have been worked out, place major emphasis on the type of training in the earlier phases that will prepare the runner for phase IV. In general, phase III is the most demanding phase of training, regardless of the event or events the runner is training for. By this time, the runner has had enough time to build a solid foundation (in the initial foundation and injury-prevention phase) and also to get involved with some early quality training in phase II.

Another characteristic of phase III is that event-specific training is extremely important. For example, a 1,500-meter runner will become highly involved in longer repetition training, which is more anaerobic in nature but develops speed and ease of movement at race pace. On the other hand, runners who mainly race distances of 5,000 and 10,000 meters will become more involved in longer intervals. Although some of the same type of training may have already taken place in phase II and may continue into phase IV, phase III will usually feature greater emphasis on these specific types of training.

Phase II

Just as the training emphasis in phase IV determines the training to be performed in phase III, so should phase III training dictate what goes into phase II. For example, if phase III will heavily emphasize fast running, then some faster running should be introduced in phase II. The training sequence should follow a logical progression from what the runner is currently doing to what will come next. The specific decisions fall largely into the category of coaching philosophy. What suits one coach's method of operation may not fit as well into another coach's way of doing things. The main point here is that the runner should follow a logical path from the beginning to the end of a season of training.

Coaches and runners should remember that phase II is the first phase in which quality training occurs (something other than just steady easy runs and possibly some strides—20- to 40-second runs using a light, quick turnover at a speed that is about equal to current mile pace). These early quality workouts should not be excessively demanding, but they should provide a springboard on which the runner can build future quality training. For example, I generally like to start repetition training during phase II because reps are relatively fast but, because of their brevity and the long recovery between runs, not particularly stressful. Then during the following phase III training, harder intervals can be introduced. Though the speed of these phase III intervals is actually less demanding than the reps that they followed, they stress the aerobic system more than phase II intervals because they are longer and allow for less rest between them. In other words, phase II is a good time to work on running mechanics. Phase III can then be used to increase the stress put on the entire aerobic system.

Phase I

This initial phase is set aside to build a foundation through easy runs, strengthening routines, and stretching. This phase is crucial to help an athlete prevent injury when workouts get more intense in phases II, III and IV.

Note that more than one type of quality training goes into each phase of training. So, for example, although reps may receive primary emphasis in a particular phase, other quality workouts will also occur. The section that follows should clarify this concept.

Individual Weeks of Training Within Phases II, III, and IV

During each phase of training it is a good idea to include two or even three quality days of training. My preferred method of handling this is to identify a type of training that will receive *primary* emphasis and another type of training that will receive *secondary* emphasis. There may even be a third type of training, *maintenance training*, during some weeks. I place the training of primary emphasis early in the week, as the first quality session of the week, and the secondary emphasis workout second in the week. If three quality sessions occur in the same week, the third session is either another primary session or a maintenance session. Of course, if a day of competition occurs within any week of training, it should replace a workout.

Figure 13.3, a and b, shows a number of quality days in each week of training. All other days are listed as E (easy days of training). It is important to clarify the meaning of "easy." In a general sense, easy refers to the intensity of running on that particular day. For a marathon runner accustomed to running 120 miles each week, an easy day may involve two runs, each lasting over an hour. But the intensity of these runs is easy. For someone else, an easy day may be one easy run of just 30 minutes or no running at all (no running can certainly be viewed as an easy day). It is often desirable to include a few strides in the middle or at the end of most easy runs. Strides are 20- to 40-second runs performed at about current mile pace using a light, quick leg turnover. Strides are not sprints and should not resemble all-out running.

Weeks Without Competition

Figure 13.3, a and b, presents three approaches to a weekly training schedule. Weeks 1 and 2 show a primary day, a secondary day, and a second primary day

Distance Running

Training Plan—Weeks Without Competition

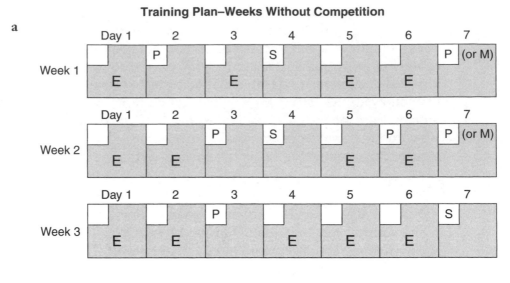

E = easy day of running
P = primary quality emphasis
S = secondary quality emphasis
M = maintenance quality emphasis

Training Plan—Weeks With Competition

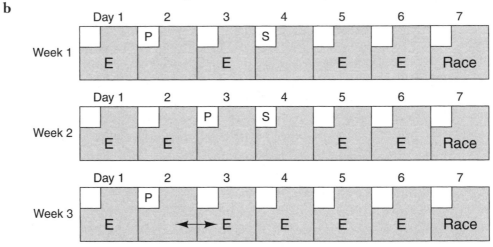

Figure 13.3   Careful planning will ensure that appropriate emphasis is placed on each type of training.

(which could also be a third type of training, or a maintenance day). In week 1 the first two quality days have an easy day between them. The week 2 example shows the first two quality days coming back to back, with no recovery day in between. An advantage of back-to-back quality days is that runners tend not to overdo the primary day, knowing the next day will also be of high quality. Being too enthusiastic is a common fault of young runners, so the back-to-back system is often a good approach for them. Back-to-back quality days are also desirable when the runner competed on the previous weekend and needs an extra day of recovery before getting into another quality training session. Back-to-back quality days offer the additional advantage of simulating competitions in which preliminary events are held on one day and finals on the next.

Week 3 in figure 13.3a includes just two quality days. This approach is good when the quality days are particularly strenuous. It can also be used as a relatively easy week between weeks that include three quality days each. In other words, it is sometimes an excellent scheme to alternate either a week 1 or week 2 schedule with a week 3 schedule, throughout the season.

Weeks That Include Competition

Week 3 in figure 13.3b shows three different schedules for weeks during which a race occurs at the end of the week (the order of days could be arranged to accommodate a race on any day of the week). Weeks 1 and 2 both involve two quality training days in the week leading up to a competition. As discussed earlier, the only difference is whether to schedule the two quality days back to back or to separate them with an easy day. Again, this may be dictated by the severity of the previous week's competition or training or the rigor of the back-to-back days.

Figure 13.3b shows just one quality day before race day. This quality training day could just as well be on day 2 as day 3, depending mainly on how many easy days are desired before the week-ending race. It is noteworthy that the initial quality day of each week is designated as a primary quality session. In the week 3 plan, the one quality day may be of any type; the main concern is that whatever training is performed on that day does nothing to detract from the upcoming race. The week 3 plan is usually the preferred approach to season-ending competitions.

Putting It All Together

A big advantage of the scheme presented here is that the runner can follow the same weekly approach throughout the season. Only the type of training that receives *primary*, *secondary*, and *maintenance* emphasis changes. For example, the following is my preferred approach to a general training program for most distance runners.

Phase I

- Primary emphasis = easy runs
- Secondary emphasis = strength training
- Maintenance emphasis = flexibility training

Phase II

- Primary emphasis = repetitions
- Secondary emphasis = threshold training
- Maintenance emphasis = long, steady runs

Phase III

- Primary emphasis = intervals
- Secondary emphasis = repetitions
- Maintenance emphasis = threshold training

Distance Running

Phase IV

- Primary emphasis = threshold training
- Secondary emphasis = repetitions (of a reduced nature)
- Maintenance emphasis = intervals (of a reduced nature)

The preceding scheme is not suited to all runners. Those training for a marathon will not do as much repetition work but will do more threshold training. Runners mainly interested in racing 1,500 meters or the mile will do less threshold running and more repetitions. Although coaching philosophies vary, the model presented here can be used with adjustments to fit almost any situation. The main concern should be to design a program that will address the needs of each athlete. And, for the coach's benefit, the program can always answer the question, "What is the purpose of today's workout?"

FOOTBALL

Kent Johnston

An annual conditioning program for football aims to improve each athlete's on-field performance throughout the season by improving explosiveness in both the upper and lower body. As Tudor Bompa noted in the previous chapter, breaking up the year into phases gives a coach a method of structuring a complete workout plan based on the needs and goals of the players on a team.

No two athletes are the same. In a perfect training world, coaches would create individual programs for every athlete. Unfortunately, time constraints at the high school and college levels can work against coaches trying to get the best out of their athletes. The truly innovative coach recognizes this and makes the best of the situation, adapting a conditioning program to fit his team and athletes while remaining true to the end goal of the program.

One tried-and-true method of structuring an annual plan is to divide the year into three types of phases: transition, off-season, and in-season phases (see table 13.8).

Table 13.8   Football Periodization Model

Month	Dec	Jan	Feb	Mar	April	May	June	July	Aug	Sep	Oct	Nov
Phase	Transition	Off-season							Transition	In-season		
Focus	Active rest	Alternate base an development focus each month, starting with base building in January						Peak	Contact	Maintenance		

Transition

Transition phases provide athletes with a way to recover while staying active. Most athletes take short breaks from training at the end of their season. These breaks are necessary physical and mental respites from the game and training; however, athletes should not lose all the conditioning they have gained. Athletes may want to do some activities such as basketball, racquetball, swimming, or tennis on a noncompetitive basis before moving into the anatomical adaptation phase.

The primary objective of the anatomical adaptation transition phase is to enhance each athlete's general condition. Before specific explosiveness training for football can be trained, the athlete must have a respectable cardiovascular fitness level, including a good aerobic base. The program shown in table 13.9 is for athletes in average to above-average condition.

Engaging in vigorous strength training without properly adapting the tendons and ligaments can cause injuries to muscle attachments and joints. Circuit training, emphasizing a full range of motion in all lifts, and increasing the number of repetitions per set can condition tendons and ligaments. Later, in the off-season, athletes will begin to develop acceleration, speed, and agility while maintaining solid position-specific football skills.

During the transition from off-season to in-season, athletes gradually prepare for and readjust to the demands of in-season training and competition.

Football

Table 13.9   Sample Anatomical Adaptation Transition Workouts

Week	Day	Warm-up	Jumps	Agility	Weight training	Running drills	Conditioning
Week 1	Monday and Thursday	Jog 2 min. 2 sets of 30-yd. drills -skipping -lateral shuffle -carioca -backward run Stretch	2 × 10 squat jumps	2 × 20-yd. shuttle from 3-point stance. 2 min. rest	**Perform 3 circuits (50% 1RM)** -10 body-weight squats -10 push-ups -10 crunches - 5 pull-ups -10 hyperextensions -8 walking lunges -6 dips -10 barbell curls -10 dumbbell lateral raises	2 × 10 yd. butt kickers 2 × 10 yd. high knees	6 × 60 yd. build ups 6 × 50 yd. strides
	Tuesday and Friday	Stationary bike 3 to 5 min.	3 × 3 standing long jumps	3 × four-corner drill. 1 min. rest	**Perform 3 circuits (50% 1RM)** -8 squats or leg presses -8 bench presses -8 incline sit-ups -8 hyperextensions -8 upright rows -8 leg curls -8 lat pull-downs -8 narrow grip bench presses -8 calf raises	None	Stationary bike 30 min.
Week 2	Monday and Thursday	Jog 2 min. 2 sets of 30-yd. drills -skipping -lateral shuffle -carioca -backward run Stretch	3 × 10 squat jumps	2 × 200-yd. shuttle from 3-point stance. 2 min. rest	**Perform 3 circuits (50% 1RM)** -10 body-weight squats -10 push-ups -10 crunches - 5 pull-ups -10 hyperextensions -8 walking lunges -6 dips -10 barbell curls -10 dumbbell lateral raises	3 × 10 yd. butt kickers 3 × 10 yd. high knees	6 × 60 yd. buildups 8 × 50 yd. strides
	Tuesday and Friday	Stationary bike 3 to 5 min.	4 × 3 standing long jumps	3 × four-corner drill. 1 min. rest	**Perform 4 circuits (55% 1RM)** -8 squats or leg presses -8 bench presses -8 incline sit-ups -8 hyperextensions -8 upright rows -8 leg curls -8 lat pull-downs -8 tricep press-downs -8 calf raises	None	Stationary bike 30 min.

Football

Off-Season

Strength training during the off-season, what we call "force training," is best divided into two- or three-week cycles incorporating five distinct lifting methods:

1. The **dynamic method** uses the relationship between force and velocity to improve starting strength and acceleration using submaximal weights. With this method athletes bench press 8 to 10 sets of 3 reps at 60 percent of 1RM and squat 10 to 12 sets of 2 at 50 to 70 percent of 1RM.

2. The **maximal-intensity method** involves overcoming maximum resistance—the most weight an athlete can lift for 1 to 5 reps at 80 to 100 percent of 1RM. It is especially important to warm-up properly before these maximum lifts.

3. **Isometric exercises and the functional method** are for more advanced players. This method involves attaching large chains or surgical tubing as additional resistance to lifting apparatus. The athlete then lifts the apparatus until the mini-max is achieved and holds one to three seconds or to failure. Like the maximal-intensity method, these exercises develop absolute strength.

4. The **repetition method** increases the excitability of the central nervous system. Athletes complete to failure 1 to 3 sets of 6 (barbell) to 10 (dumbbell) reps.

5. The **conjugate method** is combined with the maximal-intensity method to help perfect classical lifting form and increase coordination and special strength in weaker muscle groups. The athlete or coach selects the appropriate bar exercise that is closest in nature to the classical lift the athlete is performing (clean and jerk, snatch, bench, squat, or dead lift).

Off-season force training is best guided by the following five principles:

1. Every workout is performed with maximum effort. This is not to be confused with maximum intensity—lifting the maximum for one to five repetition sets. Rather, maximum effort is performing each repetition explosively each time, even if the athlete is lifting to failure.

2. Divide training into typical two- or three-week cycles on maximum intensity days. One workout a week will require 100 percent intensity.

3. Change the core exercise(s) used on the maximum intensity day every two- to three-week cycle to prevent overtraining.

4. Follow every four to six weeks of maximum intensity training with two to three weeks of repetition method training to improve power endurance, build muscularity, and prevent overtraining the maximum intensity group.

5. Once a week use the dynamic method to emphasize bar speed and acceleration. The dynamic method should include upper and lower body exercises.

Table 13.10 (see page 304) shows one way to structure six weeks of off-season workouts using a three-workouts-per-week schedule. Some coaches prefer a four-workouts-per-week schedule, especially if they work with more advanced players.

In-Season

Once the regular season starts, the emphasis shifts from the strength and conditioning program to actual practice and improvement of live game skills. The job of the strength and conditioning coach is to maintain the levels achieved during

Football

Table 13.10   Sample Off-Season Workouts

Week	Monday	Tuesday	Wednesday	Thursday	Friday
1-3	4 × 5 squats (last three sets to failure) 3 × 10 lunges (with weight) 2 × 8 leg curls 10 × 3 bench presses (50%, 52.5%, 55% 1RM by week) 4 × 5 rows 3 × 10 dips 10 × weighted sit-ups 10 × crunch pull-downs 10 × weighted crunches 10 × weighted leg raises	Position-specific work	4 × 5 clean high pulls (last three sets to failure) 2 × 10 reverse leg presses 4 × 5 standing military presses 2 × -10 good mornings -10 step-ups -10 hyperextensions -50 body weight squats 3 × 15 calf raises 2 × 10 neck exercises	Position-specific work	4 × 5 bench presses (last three sets to failure) Push-ups to exhaustion 10 × front-plate raises 10 × straight-arm side raises 10 × negative chin-ups 10 × bent flies 12 × 2 box squats (50%, 52.5%, 55% 1RM by week) 3 × 8 glute-ham raises or leg curls 10 × weighted sit-ups 10 × 1/2 sit-ups 10 × start at top of sit-up and slowly resist into down position 10 × sit-ups with no weights 20 × scissor kicks
4-6	5 × 3 leg presses 3 × 10 leg extensions or hack squats 3 × 10 lunges 10 × 3 bench presses (57.5%, 60%, 62.5% 1RM by week) 5 × 3 rows Medicine ball circuit -10 sit-ups off chest -10 overhead sit-ups -10 Russian twists -10 leg raises with ball -10 knee-ups with ball -10 overhead push (isometric)	Position-specific work	5 × 3 dumbbell cleans and presses 3 × 8 clean shrugs 3 × 10 plyometric push-ups 2 × -10 reverse hyperextensions -10 abdominal plate rotations -10 abductors -50 body weight squats 3 × 10 calf raises 2 × 8 neck exercises	Position-specific work	5 × 3 dumbbell cleans and presses 5 × 3 bench presses to limit 2 × 10 dumbbell incline 10 × upright rows 10 × dumbbell front raises 50 × push-outs 10 × negative pull-ups 12 × 2 box squats (57.5%, 60%, 62.5% 1RM by week) 3 × 10 glute-ham raises 10 × weighted sit-ups 10 × 1/2 sit-ups 10 × start at top of sit-up and slowly resist into down position 10 × sit-ups with no weights 20 × scissor kicks

the off-season conditioning workout period. Coaches at every level must adjust their manner of thinking in order to do the following:

- Improve actual sport skill traits
- Perfect fundamentals and techniques of the sport
- Allow for game simulated conditioning
- Maintain power, maximum strength, and power endurance

It is vital that an in-season strength and conditioning program focus on maintaining the maximum strength levels gained during the off-season and on high power or force velocity outputs.

GOLF

Pete Draovitch

As discussed in chapter 11, a delicate balance must exist between posture, motor learning, strength, flexibility, balance, and conditioning to produce a successful, consistent golf swing. The percentage of each component may be based on age, gender, physical status, period of season, or skill level. Science has made it possible to manipulate training programs so that athletes receive the appropriate mix of these components to peak at the right time in the competitive season.

Designing an annual program for conditioning for golf begins with breaking down the year into seasons. Seasons are typically broken down into three specific training periods—preseason, in-season, and off-season. Because golf is played globally year-round, many of today's competitive golfers may find it difficult to identify an off-season in which they are not playing. Still it is important to plan for an off-season, or a building time in the season, in order to ensure peak condition for certain tournaments later in the annual plan.

Although volume and intensity may vary between the specific training seasons, it's important to address all of the fitness components required in the golf swing during each training season. During the off-season, weight training and conditioning may take precedence over skill training. As the athlete approaches the time when he or she wishes to peak, however, strength training and power training will take a back seat to developing and sharpening skills for the important competitive events. For example, an athlete may use the medicine ball to develop trunk stability during the off-season, work on motor learning during the preseason, and train for explosive power during the in-season. During the three competitive seasons, the variables of volume and intensity are changed by manipulating either the resistance, the speed of the activity, or the time or number of repetitions during each workout. Without exception, the athlete's health and well-being are paramount.

Research has shown that the amount of compressive force placed on the spine during a golf swing, regardless of skill level, is about eight times body weight. Therefore, because golf is a sport that can cause either traumatic or overuse injuries, each training session must consider the fitness of the athlete's body at the time. Good players tend to practice often and sometimes grind more at the range than they should. Many times during the year, then, the program should be adjusted for changes in the way the athlete is feeling or the way the body is reacting to the skill training sessions that have taken place.

Debate may rage over whether golf is a sport or a skill, but from a force standpoint, golf certainly qualifies as a sport. Consider the enormous amount of force to which the spine is subjected. Because golfers must practice every single type and distance of shot, a tremendous amount of skill training takes place within the sport. Let's put to rest the idea of golf fitness. Coaches do not refer to football fitness or basketball fitness. There is sport-specific conditioning and training for those sports, and there is sport-specific training for golf.

Most professional golfers strive to play their best competitive golf in the four major tournaments (Masters, U.S. Open, British Open, PGA Championship) and probably one or two other events they view as important during the year; the examples in this section are structured on this model. You can adapt the

Golf

information in this chapter, however, to your particular circumstances and goals—winning the club championship, winning the high school county championship, or winning that 50-cent Nassau off your most competitive friend.

To satisfy off-season, preseason, and in-season training needs, break down the year according to the climate in which you live. In areas of the country that feature a harsh winter, this is straightforward. In states such as Florida, California, and Arizona, which tend to have playable weather year round, it's sometimes hard to establish distinct training seasons because athletes can work on their skills at any time of year. The advent of indoor driving ranges, practice nets, practice putting greens, and large basements allows athletes to work on skills year round even in colder climates, but the weather will dictate whether they can be out on a golf course.

One way to break down an annual program follows:

- Off-season—November through February
- Preseason—March
- Competitive season, or in-season—April through October

Off-Season

November can be a month in which athletes establish strength and an aerobic base by working out four days a week. Volume of training is higher and intensity is lower to accommodate increased workloads and reduce the stress being placed on the body.

In December, after athletes have established the strength and aerobic base, the program can begin to be periodized with more attention paid to volume and less to intensity.

In January and February, it is time to incorporate true periodization. Increase the percentages of weight lifted and move from high volume and low intensity to high intensity and low volume. A player should reach peak strength at the end of February.

Preseason

In preseason a player works out three days per week instead of four. Increase the intensity and decrease the volume at this time because athletes are beginning to prepare for the season.

In-Season

During this period, set up three periodized programs in order to reach maximum intensity and decreased volume at or about June 1, near the end of the school season. Another periodized program takes place between June 1 and August 31, corresponding to end of the summer events in the amateur ranks. A third periodized program occurs from September 1 through October 31, which corresponds to the fall season that occurs in some states.

In the beginning part of the in-season periodized programs, at least for the first two weeks, a player may work out as many as three times per week (see table 13.11). The first day after finishing a weekly competition should be the hardest day of work and should include strength training, flexibility, balance, and some postural activities. The second day of the week may emphasize explosive training at the appropriate progressive levels, and the third day may stress postural training. Some events are set up so that athletes play early one day and late the next. If that's the case, a player will want to work-out early the third day of the week so that he or she will have almost a full day to recover before the event. Note also that the third day of working out should not be extremely stressful. It is meant only to activate the trunk musculature in either a weight-bearing or non-weight-bearing position, depending on the number of balls hit, injury status, or the amount of work needed to keep the player functioning at an acceptable level.

Table 13.11   Sample In-Season Training Week

Day of week	Competitive golfer	Recreational golfer
Day 1 (first day after tournament)	Weight-room work	Weight-room work Explosive training
Day 2 (one to two days before next tournament)	Explosive training	Posture training Stabilization ball and tubing
Day 3 (day after playing morning round)	Posture training Stabilization ball and tubing	

Depending on the player's level of fitness and the time available, he or she should train using one of the four weekly workout schedules shown in table 13.12. Level 1 workouts are perfect for beginning golfers who have just started training, whereas Level IV workout weeks are geared for the competitive player. If an athlete plans to train year-round, it might be best to start training at Level I, progress through Levels II and III, and end the season with Level IV.

Table 13.12   Weekly Workout Schedules

Level I	Off-season	In-season
Flexibility	3–5 × week (10 min.)	3 × week (6 min.)
Strength training	3 × week (10 min.)	2 × week (8 min.)
Lower body	2 × 20 reps	1 × 20 reps
Upper body	1 × 15 reps	1 × 15 reps
Trunk (day 1/day 2)	Time/reps	Time/reps
Balance	3 × week (5 min.)	2 × week (5 min.)
Skill training	2 × week (5 min.)	2 × week (5 min.)

(continued)

Golf

Table 13.12 (continued)

Level II	Off-season	In-season
Flexibility	3–5 × week (12 min.)	3 × week (10 min.)
Strength training	3 × week (15 min.)	2 × week (8 min.)
Lower body	3 × 20 reps	2 × 20 reps
Upper body	2 × 15 reps	1 × 15 reps
Trunk (day 1/day 2)	Time/reps	Time/reps
Balance	3 × week (5 min.)	2 × week (5 min.)
Skill training	2 × week (5 min.)	2 × week (5 min.)
Level III	**Off-season**	**In-season**
Flexibility	4–5 × week (12 min.)	4 × week (12 min.)
Strength training	3–4 × week (15–20 min.)	2 × week (12 min.)
Lower body	3 × 20 reps	2 × 20 reps
Upper body	2 × 15 reps	2 × 15 reps
Trunk (day 1/day 2)	Time/2 reps	Time/2 reps
Balance	4 × week (5 min.)	2 × week (5 min.)
Skill training	3 × week (5 min.)	4 × week (3–5 min.)
Level IV	**Off-season**	**In-season**
Flexibility	5–7 × week (15 min.)	5 × week (12 min.)
Strength training	3–4 × week (20–25 min.)	2 × week (12–15 min.)
Balance	4 × week (5–7 min.)	2 × week (5 min.)
Skill training	4 × week (5–7 min.)	2 × week (3–5 min.)

Golf

HOCKEY 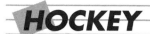 Peter Twist

Various sport-specific factors affect program development for hockey. Many of the biomechanical, physiological, and technical considerations of hockey are detailed in chapter 11 (pages 247 to 251). Other general influences in the professional and amateur hockey environment include game schedule and schedule density. Tables 13.13 and 13.14 illustrate typical variations in training.

Teams in the NHL play almost every second night with long road trips. The volume of training on practice days and the opportunity for recovery are much less than that available in other leagues. Minor professional and college league teams schedule most games around the weekend, the former to draw fans and the latter out of respect for class schedules. A minor professional league team often plays three games in three nights—Friday, Saturday, and Sunday—with four days between games. College hockey teams usually play Friday and Saturday; Sunday is a rest day followed by four good practice days. The college schedule provides an optimal weekly schedule for quality practices, quality workouts, and adequate recovery time between games.

At the NHL level, players occasionally do strength training the morning of games and always do postgame workouts, sometimes to accelerate recovery but more often to fit in enough workouts while allowing adequate recovery time before the next game.

Table 13.13 Continuum of Change Throughout the Year

Phase	Postseason	Off-season	Preseason	Pre-camp	In-season
Focus	Recovery	Build base	Specificity	Taper	Maintenance
Sample time period	April 15–May 9	May 10–July 4	July 5–Aug 29	Aug 30–Sept 5	To April or May
Length	3½ weeks	8 weeks	8 weeks	1 week	About 8 months
Theme	R and R	Grab the lead	Intensity wins	Peak to compete	Teamwork
Key components:	Unloading Rest and recovery Regeneration Use variety and cross-training to maintain fitness and strength (outside the rink and weight room). Upgrade flexibility with micro-Stretching.	Aerobic capacity ($\dot{V}O_2$max) Strength base Muscle mass Flexibility Perform break-in workouts for anaerobic power, speed, agility and quickness, plyometrics, and speed endurance. Also work on balance, proprioception and athleticism.	Anaerobic systems Explosive power Speed Agility Quickness Plyometrics Speed endurance Read-and-react skills On-ice skills Also work on aerobic capacity, strength, balance, proprioception, and athleticism.	Taper to camp Refuel for camp On-ice timing Speed endurance Cross-training Flexibility	Maintain all, together as a team. Also work on individual weaknesses (specific focus for each individual). Emphasize recovery and regeneration more than building.

During the season, injuries, trades, demotions, and call-ups all alter conditioning requirements. On the long road trips experienced by the western teams, players become accustomed to the travel-play-travel-play circus, continually moving to the next city. Conditioning is a greater challenge on the road because less time is available and no team facility is at hand. Thus, teams feel added pressure to schedule high-quality workouts when at home.

Each league has a different off-season, as does each team, depending on the amount of playoff success achieved. College seasons finish by March, and professional teams missing the playoffs finish in April, leaving four and a half months for the out-of-season training phase. Teams that go to the championship, however, finish in mid-June, leaving them with only two and a half months—and that period must allow for postseason recovery and the entire conditioning phase!

All levels of hockey—high school, college, and pro—emphasize leg and speed-center strength training. Players at the high school and college levels, however, are younger and consequently physically immature; thus they have a greater need for upper-body strength and hypertrophy programs. These athletes are usually still building their foundations. This is a fact that coaches should keep in mind when designing programs for them (see table 13.13 on page 309 and table 13.14 below).

Table 13.14 Frequency Per Week

	Sept Testing	Oct	Nov	Dec	Jan Retesting	Feb	Mar	April Postseason	May	June	July	Aug
On-ice	7	6	6	6	6	6	6	0	0	0	1 or 2	4 or 5
Continuous aerobic	1	1	1	1	1	1	1	0	2	2	1	1
Aerobic interval	1	1	1	0	0	1	1	0	1	2	1	0
Anaerobic sprints	1	1	1	1	1	1	1	0	1	1	3	3
Strength and power	3	3	3	2	2	2	3	3	5	5	4	4
Speed, agility, and quickness	1	2	1	2	1	2	1	0	1	1	3	3
Flexibility	3	3	3	2	2	3	3	3	3	3	3	3
Balance and and proprioception	2	2	2	1	1	2	2	0	1	1	2	2
Cross-training*	0	0	0	0	0	0	0	3	2	1	1	0

*Cross-training activities: 2-on-2 basketball; 3-on-3 soccer with small boundaries; 2-on-2 hockey; one zone, high-level singles tennis

Off-Season

The goal during the off-season is to build the foundations of strength, muscle mass, aerobic power, and balanced flexibility. To achieve this, I prescribe both high volume and high intensity but more recovery days for each muscle group. May and June are skewed toward aerobic and strength development. As the players proceed into preseason training (in July and August) they progress to anaerobic intervals, speed agility and quickness, and explosive lifting. Players continue to work on flexibility, balance, and proprioception throughout the summer.

Off-season strength training works the muscles in two groups: (a) chest, shoulders, and triceps, and (b) legs (with hips), back, and biceps. My athletes lift four days per week during this phase, alternating twice for each grouping. Abdominals are the only group worked three times a week. Because many proprioception and balance-oriented core-stability drills link the back and hips with abdominals, I group the abs with legs, hips, and back. (On one day they stand alone as a core workout, with no other lifting that day.)

Players start with the legs, hips, and abs and continue with the back, biceps, and forearms. Athletes perform exercises at extremely high intensity (max overload weight) rather than simply huge volume. Most sets are between 12 and 20 reps total (broken into 2 to 3 sets). One day's workout starts with intense lifting (see chapters 4, 5, and 7 for some specific exercises), then 65 minutes of aerobic intervals on a stationary bike (10-minute warm-up, 10 sets of 2.5 minutes at 95 percent followed by 2.5 minutes at 75 percent, finishing with a 5-minute cooldown) followed by 15 to 20 minutes of stretching (see chapter 3). This lift-bike-stretch sequence is a long workout that can be broken into a two-a-day approach. I prefer that players work with greater intensity on their work days than most coaches recommend. On the other hand, my players take more frequent high-quality rest periods and more recovery days. Working harder and resting smarter pays greater dividends.

Players build lower-body strength predominately through squat and lunge variations. Exercises to increase core strength include upper and lower abdominals, hips, lower back, and some rotational movements.

The aerobic intervals are designed to drive up $\dot{V}O_2$max and to elevate the lactate threshold. The grueling aerobic training always pushes this boundary.

Flexibility prescription is the opposite end of the continuum—slow and easy stretching, partial range of motion, gentle micro-Stretching©. Micro-Stretching achieves superior long-term flexibility, balances flexibility of muscle groups, and better facilitates recovery from tough workouts.

Preseason

In the main noncompetitive periods, as the player moves from the off-season and into the preseason in midsummer, workouts become more hockey specific. A shift occurs toward anaerobic intervals and high-speed multijoint and single-leg activity. Exercises maximize the transfer of conditioning improvements to on-ice performance. The workouts are denser, with shorter rest periods.

Once players are skating daily and training on the ice, their dryland conditioning must be modified accordingly. The contribution of the legs and anaerobic

Hockey

system must be carefully analyzed. Coaches sometimes recommend frequent leg-strength training and anaerobic intervals all summer for hockey players. What they overlook is that the legs and the anaerobic systems are taxed by upper-body multijoint lifts, circuit training, plyometrics, quickness and agility drills, on-ice practices, game activity or scrimmages, anaerobic intervals, intense running and biking aerobic intervals, and cross-training such as two-on-two basketball and mountain hiking. Younger high school athletes are (or should be) also playing other sports. Coaches must assess all of this to determine the workload on the legs and anaerobic systems, not just count the number of times they type in "leg strength" or "anaerobic sprints" on a player's program.

This preseason workout begins with a 12-minute dynamic warm-up to prepare the body for explosive multidirectional quickness drills, which follow while the athlete is fresh. The quickness drills are more accurately defined as footwork drills than plyometrics (see chapter 6). They are modified to use a smaller vertical component with less impact and more efficient sport movement, but they still harness the neuromuscular mechanisms for explosive action. Single-leg, bilateral, stop-and-start, and lateral movement drills predominate.

To build leg strength, the program uses more single-leg exercises, stride-specific work, crossovers, and higher strength-endurance reps. Additional exercises for the adductors balance out strength in those small muscles. Most sports use a progression to 1RMs and low reps, but during the competitive season hockey players need to exert force repetitively over a 45- to 60-second shift, not lift something once or twice and then rest.

The abdominal work done during this phase of the season should include more exercises done in a standing position. Endless lying curl-ups do little to build strength 360 degrees around the core and have little application for a game in which the core must contribute from an athletic and dynamic position. Include numerous partner drills with torso rotation in which players produce leverage or withstand contact.

Players eat and rest and then return to complete an extremely intense 60 minute bout of anaerobic sprints on a stationary bike. These are without a doubt lactate-tolerance sprints—each sprint is similar to the Wingate bike test with only a 1:1 work-to-rest ratio:

- Warm up for 15 minutes to elevate heart rate
- 12 sets of the following: 60-second full-out sprint followed by 60-second active rest (70 percent)
- Cool down for 11 minutes

In-Season

Most hockey seasons begin in September. The focus is driving up conditioning on the ice, learning team systems, and getting timing down to game intensity. Testing is done in training camp in September to assess the strengths and weaknesses of each player. Testing is repeated in January or early February to check midseason conditioning and to allow enough time to gear up down the stretch for the playoffs. Players strength train three times per week and work the energy systems three times per week (dryland) from September to November, when they are also on the ice daily. Toward the middle of the season, in December and January, the volume and frequency decrease and more emphasis is placed on recovery and regeneration to ease players over the hump of a long season.

Strength training and energy-system work decrease. I prescribe a lower volume and lower frequency of drills and include variety in every workout. This is as much for mental rejuvenation as it is for physical growth and repair. After retesting in late January, conditioning is reemphasized. Maintaining peak output for over 100 games every second night (exhibition, regular season, and playoffs) is an extraordinary task compared with peaking for an Olympic event once every four years. Coaches must monitor players to ascertain their energy level and motivation. Proprioception and flexibility work continue throughout to minimize likelihood of injury.

A good in-season conditioning workout to complete after a practice of quick-feet drills, mobility drills, and regular on-ice practice moves players into the weight room for an anaerobic strength circuit. Exercises are at a fast pace, usually with a one-to-one tempo. I prescribe mainly full-body, closed kinetic-chain multijoint exercises that simulate the on-ice demands of the legs, speed center, and upper body; exercises such as squats, standing chest passes, side-to-side stick handling, jump squats, medicine ball sit-up passes, and cleans into a push press are good choices. These exercises build on the premise that the body must operate as a linked system to produce hockey actions.

Because the circuit is an anaerobic endurance workout, similar to sprint intervals, the athlete who forges through it will be under extreme fatigue with a heart rate very near maximum. If the athlete does not reach this level, he or she is not attacking the workout aggressively enough. No rest is permitted between sets. The athlete should bang off each set.

The reps are moderate to high (2 sets of 10 to 20) because the goal is to build strength endurance on the ice; this is not a hypertrophy phase. The in-season program requires a mix of workouts to maintain mass and absolute strength.

Postseason

After the season, players need an unloading phase to make the transition from the intensity of playoffs to this rest-and-repair phase. For up to four weeks, players maintain a base of strength and fitness through workouts outside the weight room and by cross-training. They should stay away from the rink and the weight room for complete mental, emotional, and physical regeneration. In the example given in table 13.14, players finish competing in March and begin their postseason in April. This is a month for family and friends, for alternative activities, for rest and relaxation. By participating in other sports activities three times a week, micro-Stretching three times per week, and strength training using just body weight as resistance three times a week, athletes will maintain a fitness base into May and thus not start from scratch in a deconditioned state.

Hockey

SOCCER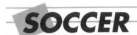

As with most sports, the soccer competition schedule determines the plan for training. Physical training should be part of daily training throughout the year. The various components of training should be distributed throughout each training week and should meet the following three primary objectives:

- Injury prevention—With good coaching and a solid work ethic, a healthy player will improve.
- Performance enhancement—A sound, well-designed training program will improve performance.
- Education—A good program will teach players how the various drills and exercises relate to the game.

To accomplish these objectives, the coach must emphasize three key concepts:

1. Warm up to play. Do not play to warm up.
2. Condition the body to kick and run. Don't kick and run to condition.
3. Condition and prepare the whole body using the kinetic-chain concept.

Failure to understand and use these concepts will predispose players to injury and obstruct their skill development. The body is a linked system in which all parts work together to produce efficient movement.

To prevent injuries, it is important to understand how and when they occur. A significant portion of conditioning must be devoted to injury prevention. Ankle sprains, groin pulls, and knee injuries are prevalent in soccer. All these occur in the force-reduction (eccentric) phase of movement. Therefore, it is necessary to spend considerable time on force reduction, which involves stopping and changing direction. Remedial injury prevention work must be included as part of the warm-up daily and in individual sessions as needed. This is true regardless of the level of development.

All aspects of an effective soccer conditioning program must meet the 3M criteria. Everything must be *manageable*. Can it be accomplished given the facilities, equipment, and personnel available? Facilities and equipment should not be limiting factors. All training should be done on the field. Any activities off the field are supplemental. The results must be *measurable*. Can the work and progress be quantified? The program must be *motivational*. The player and coach must understand the reason for the training and be able to relate it to greater success as a soccer player.

What are the physical qualities of the individual player relative to the demands of soccer and the position? Every player is different. The toughest challenge is designing an effective program that meets the demands of the individual player in a team context. Evaluate each player relative to the following parameters:

- Work capacity
- Strength and power
- Speed
- Coordination and skill

Testing is the highest form of training stress outside the actual game, and thus is useful in determining the individual player's athletic qualities relative to the demands of his or her position and the game. The information collected from testing, along with game performance, provides a coach with a good basis from which to build a soccer program.

Rather than comparing a player against arbitrary norms, compare a player against himself or herself. Be careful not to draw too many conclusions from one series of tests. Only after conducting several tests periodically throughout the training year is it possible to develop an in-depth profile of each player. In most instances, the tests will indicate deficiencies that have already been identified through observation of training and game performance. The following tests give specific numbers that can quantify improvement and serve as motivation, but remember that the ultimate test is the match itself.

Test results are used to develop recommendations for the coaches, who then implement the training prescriptions in daily and weekly training sessions. The goal is to use testing to design individual training programs and make training more specific to the physiological and biomechanical demands of the game. All tests should be electronically timed to ensure accuracy.

10-Meter Start

Use a standing start, first off the right foot (with the right foot forward) and then off the left foot. This tests the ability to accelerate. A deficiency here indicates a lack of strength or poor starting technique. It would be best if the two times were almost the same. That would indicate symmetry between legs, which is desirable in soccer.

20-Meter Fly

The player begins running 20 meters back from the start so that he or she is at top speed during the 20-meter test distance. This test indicates top-end speed and closing speed expressed in meters per second, which is how much distance a player can cover in a particular time. A deficiency here indicates inadequate speed due to lack of power (also indicated on the repetitive jump test) or poor technique.

Illinois Agility Test

The athlete starts by lying prone near the first bottom-corner cone. He or she gets up and sprints to the closest top-corner cone, goes around it, weaves back around the middle cones, sprints to the other top-corner cone, turns around the corner, and sprints to the finish. This tests the ability to change direction and control the center of gravity. It also indicates body awareness, body control, and footwork. A deficiency here indicates a lack of functional core strength and leg strength. A score under 15 seconds is considered good.

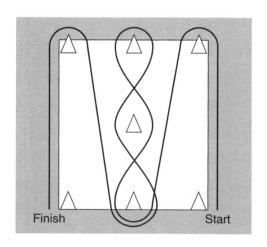

Soccer

50-Meter "Ajax" Shuttle

Establish two lines 10 meters apart. The player begins at line A, runs and touches line B, and plants and returns to line A. The player does this five times for a total of 50 meters. The test indicates the ability to start, stop, restart, and change direction quickly. A deficiency here indicates a lack of functional leg strength and core strength. A score under 10 seconds is considered very good.

Bangsbo "Intermittent Recovery" Beep Test

This is a multistage test to assess the athlete's soccer-specific endurance in terms of use of oxygen. The athlete performs 20-meter running intervals at progressively increasing speeds. At each running speed, the player completes between 7 and 15 repetitions of the 20-meter interval. The player starts each interval when an audiotaped beep sounds (or when the coach blows a whistle) and tries to reach the end of the interval and turn before the next beep (or whistle). The athlete is tested at 20 running speeds. The score for a player who is able to continue running through 8 intervals at the 16th running speed would be reported as 16-8. Bangsbo includes a conversion from the running speed and repetition completed (which actually corresponds to aggregate distance run during the test) to $\dot{V}O_2$max. Early in the test the beeps are spaced out every two to four minutes; as the test progresses the time between the beeps decreases. Each athlete should be able to cover 1,000 meters sprinting between the beeps; this is the minimum standard for readiness to play 90 minutes at the highest level. If an athlete cannot cover this distance (5 × 20 meter intervals), he or she needs to work on developing aerobic work capacity.

Squat Jump

The athlete assumes a stationary squat position with the thighs parallel to the floor and attempts to jump as high as possible. This tests the contractile properties of the muscles, which relate to basic strength and the standing start. The score of this test should be lower than that of the countermovement jump that follows.

Countermovement Jump

The player starts up, quickly squats down, and then jumps as high as possible. This tests the elastic properties of muscle, or basic explosive power. Performance on this test relates to performance in the 20-meter fly. The player should be able to jump higher on this test than on the squat jump test as this is a higher intensity jump.

Repetitive Jump

The player performs as many countermovement jumps as possible in 15 seconds. This test indicates power and power endurance. Performance on this test also relates to performance in the 20-meter fly.

Using hypothetical test results, the following are specific training recommendations that might be made to the coaches:

Player #1

10-meter left	Best: 1.83 sec.	Average: 1.86 sec.
10-meter right	Best: 1.80 sec.	Average: 1.80 sec.
20-meter fly	Best: 2.45 sec.	Average: 2.48 sec.
	Maximum velocity, meters per sec.: 8.16	
Illinois agility	Best: 16.00 sec.	Average: 16.05 sec.
Ajax shuttle	Best: 10.73 sec.	Average: 10.79 sec.
Beep test	Speed/level: 21/4	Distance: 920 m
Squat jump	Height: .464 m	
Countermovement jump	Height: .484 m	
Repetitive jump	Number of jumps: 15 Average height: .414 m	
	Power: 31.16	

Recommendations: Acceleration work twice a week, all short burst with an emphasis on good technique. This player tends to take too long a first step. Work agility on the same day as acceleration, and possibly do some agility work each day. Emphasize quick change of direction and footwork. His 15-second repetitive jump test indicates good power potential, but it does not show up in the speed and agility tests. I also think the need for speed and agility improvement is reflected on the field in this player's inability to gain a step on the opposition.

Player #2

10-meter left	Best: 1.72 sec.	Average: 1.77 sec.
10-meter right	Best: 1.84 sec.	Average: 1.85 sec.
20-meter fly	Best: 2.35 sec.	Average: 2.36 sec.
	Maximum velocity, meters per sec: 8.51	
Illinois agility	Best: 14.60 sec.	Average: 14.65 sec.
Ajax shuttle	Best: 10.00 sec.	Average: 10.05 sec.
Beep test	Speed/level: 21/6	Distance: 1,000 m
Squat jump	Height: .383 m	
Countermovement jump	Height: .394 m	
Repetitive jump	Number of jumps: 14 Average height: .445 m	
	Power: 26.73	

Recommendations: This player needs to work on acceleration. Emphasize correct mechanics! His agility is good, but his endurance is just barely acceptable for a player at this level. Jump tests indicate that he needs to emphasize a plyometric program two times a week. Poor jump results are reflected in his lack of ability to accelerate. Emphasize jumps and hurdle jumps. He should do strength training with emphasis on legs and trunk two times a week.

Soccer

TENNIS   E. Paul Roetert

Only five players have ever won the Grand Slam in tennis (winning all four Grand Slam tournaments in the same year), and it appears that achieving this feat is becoming more difficult. Better competition, more court-surface specialists, and an amazing number of lead-up tournaments make it extremely difficult for players to prepare properly for the Grand Slam events. By the end of 1998, Pete Sampras had won 11 Grand Slam titles and was chasing Roy Emerson's record of 12. Yet Pete decided not to play the Australian Open Championships in January 1999. He was tired and needed a break.

Although some criticized his decision, from a sport science perspective it may have been a wise move. Tennis does not have an official off-season like most other sports; this makes it difficult for players to peak for specific tournaments, recover fully from injuries, and build in any rest periods. This problem is not restricted to the pros—junior and adult players can also participate in tournaments just about every week of the year.

So how can a player prevent injuries, burnout, and poor tournament results related to overplaying? The answer is to design an appropriate periodization training program. As mentioned in the previous chapter, periodization training has been used for many years, mostly in Olympic sports such as weightlifting, swimming, and track and field. It is a method for organizing the training activities of an athlete to minimize the chances of overtraining and optimize the chances of achieving peak performance. Coaches and players must balance competition, rest, practice, and physical training throughout the year. Table 13.15 and figure 13.4 show an example of how to manipulate these four components depending on where the player is in the cycle. First, because tennis does not have official seasons, they must be created. Each of the four "seasons" makes up a cycle. In a full year the player may go through three or four cycles.

Table 13.15   Periodization Phases

	Phase I Preparation	Phase II Precompetitive	Phase III Competitive	Phase IV Active rest
Goal	Firm base fitness level	Tennis-specific training	Physiological peak	Recovery
Fitness training	Mostly aerobic; 20–40 minutes continuous	Anaerobic/ aerobic mix	Tennis-specific drills; short, explosive	Light fitness training, especially in other sports
Strength training	2–3 sets; high repetitions, 12–15	2–4 sets; lower repetitions, 8–10	Circuit training, 1–2 sets; 12–15 repetitions	3 sets; 8–10 repetitions (optional 3–7 day rest depending on athlete's needs)

The percentages in figure 13.4 refer to the relative amount of time to spend on each of the four components. The percentages are just guidelines. For optimum benefit each of the "seasons" should last about three or four weeks. Notice that even in the active rest phase the player will play some tennis—very little initially, but the amount steadily increases throughout the period. During the first few days of the active rest period, the player will play no tennis. As the period goes on, the rest days will steadily decrease and the other components will increase. Introducing seasons to the player's games increases the likelihood of the player remaining injury free and enhancing his or her performance.

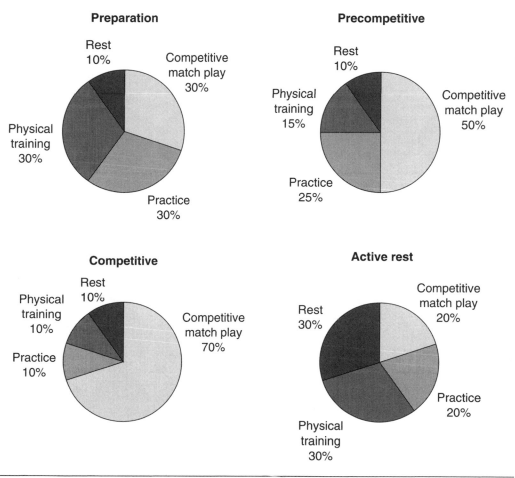

Figure 13.4 Sample distribution of time spent on each training component during each of the four phases.

Keep in mind that a program should be designed for the individual. Each player has different genes, a different tournament schedule, and a different fitness level. Many players will need to take a short break after two or three tournaments. Furthermore, it makes a big difference whether a player (a) loses in the first round or makes it to the finals, (b) has a short or long match, (c) travels a long way to get to the tournament, or (d) must deal with extreme environmental conditions. Figure 13.5 illustrates programs for players at the junior, collegiate, and professional levels.

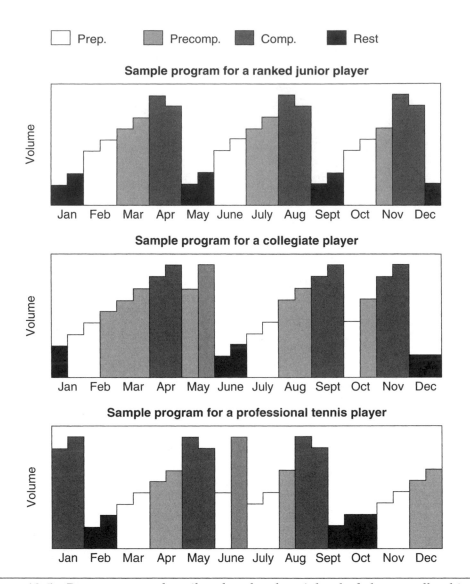

Figure 13.5   Programs must be tailored to the player's level of play as well as his or her individual characteristics and circumstances.

The most important (and difficult) component of preparing a proper periodization training program is scheduling a time to rest the body. One way to structure a periodization schedule is to choose tournaments that carry the most significance and then build a training program based on performance peaks for those events. To obtain the best results, control the following five variables:

1. Volume or duration—the amount of work performed or how long the player trains

2. Intensity—how hard the player trains

3. Frequency—how often the player trains

4. Specificity—how similar the training is to the demands of the sport

5. Variation—how much the player varies the training

Depending on the training phase of the year—preparation, precompetition, competition, and active rest—the training program will change to allow for the particular goal of that phase (strength improvement, increased power, and maintenance). The following program example for a week in the competition phase of training provides a guide. Keep in mind that individual differences are responsible for the most significant changes to the program. For instance, just as the goals of a lineman and a defensive back in football differ, so too do the goals of a baseliner and a serve and volleyer differ.

Some proponents of strength and conditioning programs feel that periodization is not possible in tennis because the sport doesn't have an off-season. But by applying the programs and exercises outlined here and figuring out when to use them, the athlete and coach can determine how best to build the athlete's periodized program.

The sample in-season training programs shown in table 13.16 are for use during the competitive phase. Athletes should perform these circuits three times per week.

Table 13.16 In-Season Strength Training Programs

Program 1		Program 2		Program 3	
Squats	2 × 12	Step-ups	2 × 12	Lunges	2 × 15
Bench press	2 × 12	Push-ups	2 × 12	Chest press	2 × 15
Seated row	2 × 12	Biceps curl	2 × 12	Bent-over row	2 × 15
Sit-ups	2 × 12	Lat pull-downs	2 × 12	Medicine ball ab work	2 × 15
Back extensions	2 × 12	Swiss ball trunk work	2 × 12	Lower-back work	2 × 15
Trunk rotations	2 × 12	Light plyometric work if no tennis that day		Hamstring work	2 × 15
Calf raise	2 × 12			Leg extensions	2 × 15
Dorsiflexion	2 × 12			Calf raises	2 × 15

VOLLEYBALL   Courtney Carter

The strength and conditioning program for volleyball changes throughout the year depending on the game and practice schedule. Volleyball has two basic types of strength and conditioning programs: in-season and off-season. The two off-season periods are the summer program and the winter program. There are also two in-season periods: the fall season and a much shorter spring season.

Beginning in January, the first segment of the annual cycle begins with a transition period immediately following the regular in-season. The winter program begins in late January and continues through February. The spring in-season then begins in March and continues through April.

The second segment of the annual cycle begins with another transition consisting of active rest throughout May. The summer program then begins in early June and continues through July. The regular in-season program begins on the week that two-a-days start in August and continues for the remainder of the year.

Regardless of the level of the athlete, the strength and conditioning program for volleyball must focus on ground-based, multiplane, multijoint movements that specifically match the biomechanical needs of the volleyball athlete. This type of program will develop the strength and explosive power that athletes need to improve performance. See table 13.17 for an example.

Coaches must handle athletes with little or no lifting experience differently than they do advanced lifters. The primary difference in the program is the skill level required to complete the workouts. A program for beginners, such as high school athletes, includes no explosive lifting or conditioning in the base phase. The explosive lifts are broken into parts and performed as strength lifts. They are introduced later as explosive lifts in the strength phase. Furthermore, a beginner's program does not include a peak phase.

An intermediate program, or perhaps a college athlete's program, is more technical than the beginner's program. The primary difference is that the intensity is greater and the athletes perform more explosive lifts.

The advanced program for professionals includes the most technical moves, more plyometric exercises, snatch movements, and more overhead lifts. As part of the base phase, the advanced program uses the circuit, an extremely intense workout consisting of nine exercises. The athlete performs three sets of 10 repetitions at 60 percent of 1RM with approximately one minute of rest between sets. The athlete must be physically prepared for the intensity that the circuit requires. The professional, or most advanced program, requires the athlete to possess solid technique in all lifts and conditioning drills.

Off-Season

The primary objective of the off-season is to bring athletes to a peak of strength and conditioning. This is accomplished by a series of three phases totaling eight weeks featuring variations in training loads and exercises. Each phase has certain objectives and procedures that lay the foundation for the next phase. The cycle typically begins with the base phase, progresses to the strength phase, and ends with the peak phase. The base phase includes the highest volume of training

Table 13.17   Volleyball Strength and Conditioning Program Basics

	Primary focus	Average length of workout	Target results
January	Active rest (cross-training) and winter program	Varies, but usually 90–120 min.	Recover and build lean body mass, improve technique, and maintain sport skills
February	Winter program	90–120 minutes	Develop strength and explosive power, develop agility, and maintain sport skills
March	Spring in-season	30 min.	Maintain strength and explosive power
April	Spring in-season	30 min.	Maintain strength and explosive power
May	Recovery through active rest to prepare for summer program	Varies	Prepare mentally and physically for summer program
June	Summer program	120 min.	Build lean body mass, increase work and power capacity, improve technique on explosive lifts, and maintain sport skills
July	Summer program	120 min.	Maximize strength and explosive power, develop agility, and maintain sport skills
August	In-season program	30–45 min.	Maintain strength and explosive power
September	In-season program	30–45 min.	Maintain strength and explosive power
October	In-season program	30–45 min.	Maintain strength and explosive power
November	In-season program	30–45 min.	Maintain strength and explosive power
December	In-season program	30–45 min.	Maintain strength and explosive power

Allow a period of complete rest after the season ends.

Volleyball

coupled with the lowest intensity. The peak phase has the opposite characteristics—the least volume with the highest intensity. The summer program and the winter program are the two off-season programs for volleyball. The winter program, being just six weeks long, accomplishes only the base phase of training before the spring season begins.

The off-season strength and conditioning program for volleyball uses the split-routine method of training, which works exercises on alternating days. This efficient method of training allows at least two full days of recovery between types of exercise movements. The split routine used with this program is divided by explosive lifts and strength lifts and by plyometric drills and agility drills.

Base Phase

The primary objectives of the base phase are to build lean body mass, increase work and power capacity, improve technique on the explosive lifts, and maintain sport skills. Doing high-volume workouts (three sets of 10 repetitions) increases the work capacity and prepares the body for the higher intensity workouts of the later phases. Some single-jointed exercises are included in the base phase to stimulate muscle growth. In performing the explosive lifts, players should concentrate on proper technique. The conditioning drills in this phase have the objective of maintaining volleyball-specific endurance and preparing the body for more intense drills in the following plyometric and agility phases.

Strength Phase

The primary objective of the strength phase is to build on the base phase by decreasing the volume and increasing the intensity of the strength workout (three sets of 5 repetitions) and increasing the volume of the conditioning workout. During this phase, the objectives are to develop maximum strength and explosive power, to develop agility, and to maintain sport skills. The core of the strength program is squats and hang cleans. Players do no more than three explosive lifts in one workout and only a few single-jointed exercises at the end of the workout to maintain muscle size.

Peak Phase

The final phase of the off-season program is the peak phase, which emphasizes doing a higher volume of volleyball-specific plyometric and agility drills. The strength program focuses on explosive lifts to produce peak explosive power. Single-jointed exercises are dropped completely from the program to avoid overtraining. Table 13.18 shows a typical off-season (summer) strength and conditioning program for volleyball. In each phase, players do plyometric drills after the strength workouts on Mondays and Thursdays and do agility drills before the strength workouts on Tuesdays and Fridays.

In-Season

The primary objective of the in-season strength and conditioning program for volleyball is to maintain the strength and conditioning levels that players attained during the off-season. The emphasis shifts to improving sport skills and knowledge of volleyball strategies and tactics (see chapter 11). Players do the maintenance program two days per week, typically in the morning, as distant from practice time as possible. This schedule ensures that the athletes are rested for both the morning strength workout and the afternoon practice. The exercises included in the in-season program (table 13.19) are combined to include both strength and explosive exercises in both workouts. Players do no conditioning outside practice during the in-season. The two days of lifting vary from week to week depending on the game schedule.

Transition

The transition phases throughout a season offer athletes a necessary physical and mental break from volleyball and the usual workout routine, while still keeping the athletes active through other activities such as swimming, jogging, tennis, racquetball, and so forth on a noncompetitive basis.

Table 13.8　Off-Season Strength Training

Monday and Thursday (for all phases)

Snatch squat	2 × 5
Rack or hang clean	3 × 5
Squat jump	3 × 5
Trunk twists	2 × 5
Abdominals	

Tuesday and Friday

	Base phase weeks			Strength phase weeks			Peak phase weeks	
	1	**2**	**3**	**4**	**5**	**6**	**7**	**8**
Squat	2 × 10	3 × 10	3 × 10	3 × 5	3 × 5	3 × 5	3 × 5	3 × 5
Romanian dead lift	—	—	—	2 × 10	2 × 10	2 × 10	2 × 10	2 × 10
Leg curl	2 × 10	3 × 10	3 × 10	—	—	—	—	—
Leg extension	2 × 10	3 × 10	3 × 10	—	—	—	—	—
Bench press or jammer press	2 × 10	3 × 10	3 × 10	3 × 5	3 ×5	3 × 5	3 × 5	3 × 5
Shoulder press	2 × 10	3 × 10	3 × 10	—	—	—	—	—
Triceps extension	2 × 10	3 × 10	3 × 10	2 × 10	2 × 10	2 ×10	—	—
Low lat pull	2 × 10	3 × 10	3 × 10	—	—	—	—	—
Bent-over row	—	—	—	2 × 10	2 × 10	2 × 10	2 × 10	2 × 10
Lat pull-downs or pull-ups	2 × 10	3 × 10	3 × 10	2 × 10	2 × 10	2 × 10	2 × 10	2 × 10
Biceps curl	2 × 10	3 × 10	3 × 10	2 × 10	2 × 10	2 × 10	—	—

Table 13.19　In-Season Program

Snatch squat	2 × 5
Hang clean	2 × 5
Trunk twists	2 × 5
Squat	2 × 5
Jammer press or bench press	3 × 5
Pull-ups	2 × 10
Abdominals	—

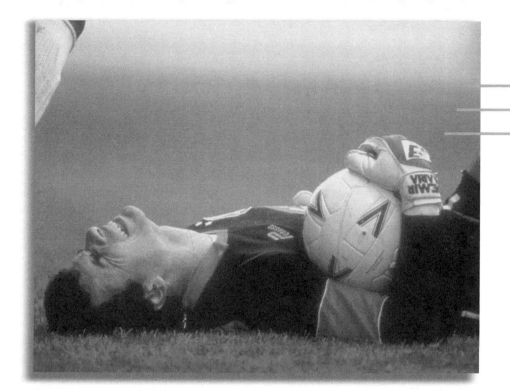

chapter 14

Restoring Performance After Injury

Todd S. Ellenbecker

*T*he purpose of this chapter is to discuss the integral components of high-performance sports training that occur during the critical stage in an athlete's recovery following injury. Specifically, the chapter focuses on the activities that bridge the gap between formal clinical rehabilitation and commencement of normal competitive activities. This critical period, which typically begins once the athlete has been cleared medically for a return to his or hcr sport and ends on successful reattainment of maximal-level performance, truly dictates the success of the surgical procedure or rehabilitation program.

Communication between the individuals responsible for returning an athlete to full activity is essential. The integrated approach contained in this chapter relies on open channels of communication between the physician, physical therapist, athletic trainer, strength and conditioning professional, coach, parent, and athlete. With all those levels of interaction, it is easy to see why communication is important.

Recent advances in surgical and rehabilitative techniques have allowed fast recovery for athletes from injuries that 10 or 15 years ago would have ended careers. Perhaps the best example is the use of arthroscopy for surgical exploration and treatment of the knee, shoulder, and elbow joints. It is not uncommon for an athlete to have his or her knee scoped and return for play at the highest level in three or four weeks. Although some prominent athletes have returned within one or two weeks following arthroscopic knee surgery, such returns are often below previous performance levels and may be temporary and somewhat risky.

Communication between the player and the surgeon, physical therapist, and athletic trainer is needed early in the rehabilitation process to ensure a fast and expedient recovery. Following the initial stages of healing and recovery after injury, however, the team approach becomes evident as the athlete begins to integrate some functional activity into rehabilitation under the guidance of many sports medicine professionals, coaches, and ancillary personnel.

One critical example of communication is the relay of information between the coach and player to the sports medicine team regarding the specific demands and expectations that will be placed on the player, as well as optimal timing for the athlete's return to activity. The honest exchange of information between the athlete and the sports medicine team regarding pain levels and symptoms of instability or weakness is critical for the successful integration of all the input from the sports performance team.

How can communication be optimized between professionals? One suggestion beyond verbal communication or staff meetings is using written reports or tests to measure the athlete's progress and status following surgery or injury (see table 14.1). This information helps to ensure clear, concise understanding of the status of the healing in the operative or injured tissues that is imperative for successful program development. Assurance that the bone is completely healed, that the ligament is not torn, that the joint is not unstable, and so forth is a prerequisite for postrehabilitation training and return to full activity.

Table 14.1   Reports to Facilitate Communication

Region or factor	Test or report
Bone	X ray, bone scan, MRI, or arthrogram
Tendon	MRI, arthrogram, operative report
Ligament	MRI, arthrogram, KT-1000, stress X ray, operative report
Muscle	MRI
Range of motion	Goniometric measurements, flexibility tests
Strength	Isokinetic testing, manual muscle testing
Function	Functional tests such as vertical jump, horizontal jump, push-up, sit-up, 20-yard dash, etc.

COMPONENTS OF THE POSTREHABILITATION PROGRAM

Virtually all the conditioning components discussed earlier in this text are important to the postrehabilitation training program, including frequency, duration, volume, intensity, rest, and recovery. Several of these components need specific mention regarding their application in this phase of training. Overlying all these components are the concepts of pain- and symptom-free training. Although these may be important considerations in all types of training, they are particularly critical when the athlete is most vulnerable to reinjury. The athlete must perform all training activities at a level at which he or she feels no pain. Any activity that re-creates symptoms similar to the injury or in the recently injured region must be modified or discontinued.

Intensity and Pain

The concept of "no pain, no gain" clearly does not apply in this phase of training. The athlete must perform training at a frequency, duration, and intensity that does not create pain or mimic the symptoms associated with the injury. Using the pain levels in table 14.2 helps sports medicine professionals and coaches constantly monitor the presence of pain and understand the athlete's current condition.

One of the most useful aspects of the pain scale is that it helps prevent an athlete from resuming activity unless he or she can perform it without compensating. Performing a sport or activity with compensation can lead to injury in other areas of the body, cause the development of improper sport biomechanics, and delay the return to optimal performance.

Table 14.2 Pain-Level Classification

Pain level	Description
Level 1	No pain.
Level 2	Mild soreness after activity, usually gone in 24 hours.
Level 3	Mild soreness and stiffness before activity, disappears during warm-up, return of mild soreness after activity.
Level 4	Stiffness before and mild pain during activity, not enough to alter activity. Pain and stiffness do not interfere with ability to use normal sport or activity mechanics.
Level 5	Pain during activity that alters ability to perform and does not allow athlete to use normal sport mechanics. Compensatory mechanics are obvious.
Level 6	Constant pain, even at rest. No performance possible.

Modified from Nirschl & Sobel.

Specificity

After incorporating the component of monitoring pain, the team developing the training program assembles the more traditional components. During this stage, the training program must be specific to the demands of the activity or sport in as many ways as possible. Figure 14.1 demonstrates some of the areas that must be considered in order to develop a specific training program for a sport activity. Knowledge regarding the physiological demands of the activity will assist in determining optimal work-to-rest intervals and the type and amount of muscular loading that should occur. Biomechanical information is also necessary in order to understand the position in which the athlete's joints work and the amount of stabilization, acceleration, and deceleration required during the intended activity.

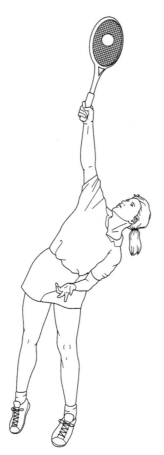

Needs analysis

Exercise movements

- Muscles used

- Joint angles

- Contraction type (eccentric or concentric)

Energy system (metabolism) used

- Estimated contribution from aerobic/anaerobic metabolism

- Work-rest cycles, performance duration, frequencies

Injury prevention

- Most common sites (shoulders, trunk, elbow, knee)

- Player's history of injury

Figure 14.1   Athletic needs and demands for tennis.

Rest and Recovery

Finally, the concept of rest and recovery must be strictly enforced during this stage of training. Many healthy, uninjured athletes can perform every day. During this stage of training, periods of rest longer than what athletes and coaching staff are used to must often be interjected between training and performance sessions. This greater rest interval is often needed to allow muscular recovery and time for the injured tissues to adapt to the return of sport-specific training stresses.

APPLYING FITNESS COMPONENTS IN REHAB

To illustrate the primary fitness components and their application, a more detailed explanation is offered by the specific example of an elite junior tennis player. Breaking down the athlete's sport activity and analyzing its physiological demands can help in developing a program that will ease the athlete's return to activity.

Physiologically, one of the important variables is energy-system utilization. Failure to address the physiological parameters of the athlete in a rehabilitation program will not only delay the functional return but also increase the risk of injury and hurt performance. In tennis, a player performs 300 to 500 acute bursts of activity during an average match. An average point in tennis lasts less than 10 seconds, and a rest of 25 seconds is allowed following each point. During a point, the athlete changes direction an average of 4.2 times and runs, on average, less than 4 meters in any one direction. Professional tennis players run as fast as 18 miles per hour (world-class sprinters reach 22 to 23 miles per hour) and cover over 6 miles in a match.

This sport-specific information assists in developing physiological programming. Based on the time spent in maximal-level exertion (approximately 10 seconds) and rest (25 seconds), a work-to-rest ratio of 1:2 or 1:3 is established. For every unit of work performed, the athlete is able to rest for two or three units. This interval type of activity relies primarily on the anaerobic energy system for the supply of energy during points, yet it demands a superior aerobic base to allow recovery during the rest periods between points. Moreover, a tennis match can last three to five hours, further emphasizing the importance of the aerobic energy system.

Tennis is not the only interval-type sport activity. Sports such as soccer and basketball also fall into this category. Through analysis of the sport, it becomes obvious which training parameters to include. For example, tennis players working on rehabilitation drills or movement training should work at near maximally tolerated levels for short periods of 10 to 15 seconds, with a recovery period of approximately 20 to 30 seconds. Even a simple exercise such as riding a stationary cycle can be made more activity specific for the athlete by having interval riding programs on the bicycle include near maximal periods of cycling followed by submaximal recovery periods specific to the sport. Exercises such as carioca steps and sideways shuffling, often included in postrehabilitation programs, can be adapted to fit this model. Using shorter distances and more frequent directional changes, while adhering to the appropriate work-to-rest interval, is an example of an important modification for the tennis player.

Inclusion of some type of aerobic training in the postrehabilitation program is also important. When aerobic training cannot be totally sport specific—playing tennis for two or three hours would potentially harm or injure the athlete—the aerobic activity must be modified to allow aerobic conditioning to occur. The critical components of aerobic activity include large muscle group activation, repeated and rhythmic movement patterns, performing at 60 to 85 percent of the athlete's maximal heart rate, and maintaining an elevated heart rate or workload at a steady state for at least 20 minutes.

Following a lower-extremity injury, the postrehabilitation program must often use creative methods and strategies to allow aerobic training because running or other weight-bearing movement is inherent in many popular aerobic training activities. Using an upper-body ergometer (UBE) (figure 14.2) can strengthen the upper body and elevate the athlete's heart rate to obtain an acceptable aerobic workout, as can swimming. During the transition to weight-bearing activities following a lower-body injury, athletes can perform extensive aquatic running and sports performance drills, reaping the benefits of reduced body weight while working in the water. Unweighting systems, which allow treadmill running at diminished loads to the lower extremity, are popular but require additional equipment. Allowing the athlete to return to his or her sport without the appropriate aerobic training base leads not only to early fatigue but also to risk of reinjury.

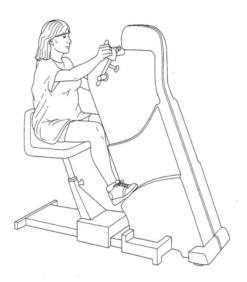

Figure 14.2   An athlete at work on an upper-body ergometer.

ADAPTING REHAB PROGRAMS TO SPECIFIC SPORTS

In addition to physiological variables, the muscular status of the athlete must be addressed by a sport-specific program. Information regarding intensity, duration, rest, and frequency can all be collected by performing a needs analysis and breaking down the athlete's sport activity (refer to figure 14.1). The example of a tennis player or throwing athlete will again be used to develop these concepts. Almost all upper-extremity throwing or racquet sports require explosive yet repetitive muscular activity. Breaking down the throwing motion or tennis serve identifies the important role of both concentric and eccentric muscular activity. Both, therefore, should be stressed in the postrehabilitation program for these athletes.

An additional important factor is the repetitive nature of these sport activities, which often requires a low-resistance, high-repetition program to ensure that local muscular endurance returns to the involved musculature to meet these demands. Figure 14.3 shows how the number of repetitions performed per set relates to muscular development in a repetition-maximum (RM) training program.

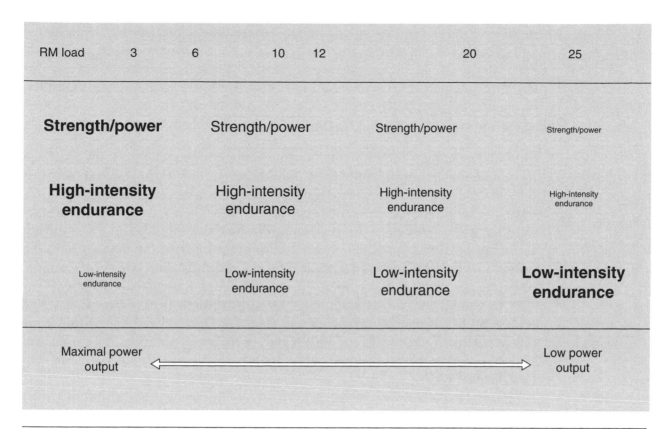

RM load	3	6	10	12	20	25

Strength/power   Strength/power   Strength/power   Strength/power

High-intensity endurance   High-intensity endurance   High-intensity endurance   High-intensity endurance

Low-intensity endurance   Low-intensity endurance   Low-intensity endurance   **Low-intensity endurance**

Maximal power output ⟵————————————⟶ Low power output

Figure 14.3   A theoretical repetition-maximum continuum.

An RM training program is a preferred method of regulating exercise intensity and volume during both performance-enhancement training and rehabilitation. Using the RM system allows for control of both volume and intensity of resistance training. For example, a 10RM load allows an athlete to perform 10 repetitions, encountering significant fatigue by the 9th and 10th repetitions. The athlete is able to perform the 10 repetitions without substitution, compensation, or breaking proper form. When this system is applied to the throwing or racquet-sport athlete in upper-body exercise programming, the athlete typically lifts in a load range between 10RM and 15RM. This develops local muscular endurance and strength and differs from the training program that a less endurance-oriented athlete such as a shot-putter or weightlifter would perform. An RM training program in the 10 to 15 range is often performed during rehabilitation because the loads are far less than those used in a more explosive, power-training program in which only 4 to 8 repetitions are used to achieve fatigue. The athlete must train in the postrehab phase in a pain-free manner and with respect for the healing tissues. The combined benefits of increased endurance training and loads that do not overstress the healing tissues make the use of 10 to 15 repetitions in RM training an appropriate framework during this important phase.

FUNCTIONAL PROGRESSION OF INJURY RECOVERY

A common description for training at this phase in the recovery process is *functional progression*. As stated earlier, exercises for the athlete coming off a rehabilitation program following an injury or surgery must gradually become more functional and specific for the activity and the demands that the athlete will be placing on his or her body. In this section, some specific drills and tests commonly used for the upper and lower extremities are addressed using two sport-specific examples.

Progression for the Upper-Body Athlete

Shoulder injury is a common occurrence among athletes who perform overhead movements. The postrehabilitation training program for this situation involves the use of exercises that further develop and reinforce the principles set forth during rehabilitation and that increase the intensity of performance without risking injury. Knowledge of the specific position of the shoulder and arm during throwing or serving provides critically important information about where the muscles of the shoulder and surrounding regions must function. For example, overhead throwing and serving take place with the shoulder elevated about 90 or 100 degrees (approximately shoulder level). Although it may appear that the release point (throwing) or contact point (serving) is overhead, the shoulder remains essentially in the 90- or 100-degree position of elevation. The overhead appearance is achieved through careful trunk positioning called lateral flexion (see figure 14.4).

Training exercises should be geared to increasing strength and endurance near the position the athlete uses during sport activity. Therefore, using exercises to strengthen the upper back (scapular musculature) and rotator cuff is recommended. These exercises should place the shoulder in the functional position described in this section but not jeopardize the shoulder's supporting structures or tendons. Figure 14.5 contains examples of recommended exercises for baseball and tennis players to increase rotator-cuff strength and endurance for both

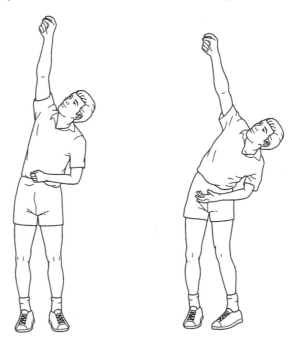

Figure 14.4   The overhead throwing or serving position is not achieved by raising the arm straight up.

1. Side-lying external rotation
Lie on the uninvolved side, with the involved arm bent at 90° and resting at the side. Keeping the elbow of the involved arm bent and fixed against the side of the body, raise the arm into an external rotation. Slowly lower the arm and repeat.

2. Shoulder extension
Lie on the table on the stomach with the involved arm hanging straight to the floor. With thumb pointed outward, raise the arm straight back into extension toward the hip. Slowly lower the arm and repeat.

3. Prone horizontal abduction
Lie on a table on the stomach side with the involved arm hanging straight toward the floor. With the thumb pointed outward, raise the arm out to the side parallel to the floor. Slowly lower the arm and repeat.

4. Supraspinatus-"empty can"
Stand with the elbow straight and the thumb pointed down toward the floor. Raise arm to shoulder level at a 30-degree angle to the body. Slowly lower the arm and repeat.

5. 90/90 external rotation
Lie on the table on the stomach with the shoulder abducted to 90 degrees and the arm supported on the table with the elbow bent at 90 degrees. Keeping the shoulder and elbow fixed, rotate the arm into external rotation, slowly lower to the starting nposition and repeat.

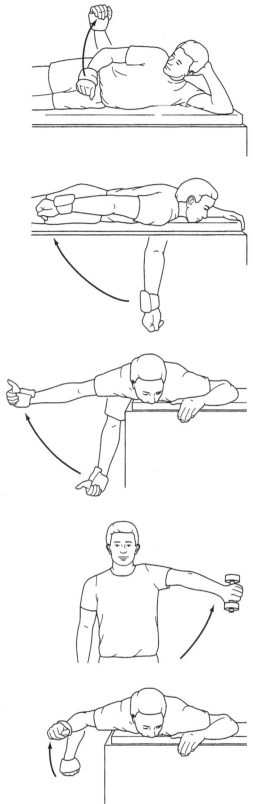

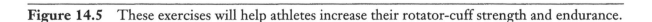

Figure 14.5 These exercises will help athletes increase their rotator-cuff strength and endurance.

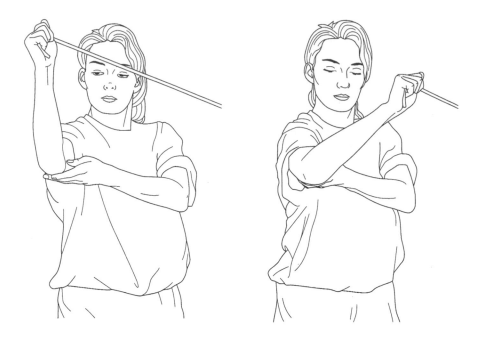

Figure 14.6   A piece of Thera-band can be used to exercise the shoulder musculature both concentrically and eccentrically.

rehabilitation and performance enhancement. Figure 14.6 shows how a piece of Thera-band can be employed to exercise the shoulder musculature both concentrically and eccentrically in a sport-specific way for baseball and tennis players.

The volume of exercise should be high, with performance of three sets of 10 to 15 repetitions traditionally recommended to foster local muscular endurance within the exercising musculature. These exercises target the rotator-cuff musculature to provide a solid strength base in the shoulder. Additional upper-body functional exercises that are often employed include medicine ball tosses using the movement patterns of a chest pass, side throw, forehand toss, and backhand toss. For additional challenge, the individual can perform them seated on a Swiss ball. Doing so will test the individual's balance and increase the amount of trunk muscular activity.

Execution of these training exercises is an important precursor to more aggressive functional activities. Pain-free range of motion and strength in the rehabilitating rotator cuff almost equal to that in the uninjured side are recommended before returning to functional activities and other types of weightlifting. Clinically, therapists and trainers often use a Cybex isokinetic device to measure the strength and muscular balance of the rotator cuff. This type of test can be useful to the sports medicine team in deciding when to return an athlete to aggressive activities following an injury or surgery. If this type of test is not available, the sports medicine team should make sure that the athlete can execute the exercises listed in this section in a pain-free manner as well as move the shoulder and elbow through a full range of motion without symptoms.

Finally, when the return to tennis or throwing activity is indicated, it should take place using an interval program. Table 14.3 lists an interval tennis program used by clinicians for athletes after injury or surgery. A common element in any interval program is that the athlete performs activities only on alternate days. This gives the athlete's arm additional time to recover between events. Of course,

Table 14.3 Interval Tennis Program

Guidelines

- Begin at stage indicated by the therapist or doctor.

- Do not progress or continue the program if joint pain is present.

- Always stretch the shoulder, elbow, and wrist before and after.

- Apply ice after completion of the program.

- Do not use a backboard because it leads to exaggerated muscle work without rest between strokes.

- It is strongly recommended that strokes be evaluated by a USPTA certified teaching professional.

- Play on alternate days, giving the body a recovery day between sessions.

- Perform each stage one to two times before progressing to the next stage. Do not progress to the next phase if pain or excessive fatigue was present during the last outing.

Preliminary stage

- Use a foam ball to perform 20 to 25 forehands and backhands, beginning with ball feeds from the net from a partner.

Stage 1

a. Have a partner feed 20 forehand groundstrokes from the net. Feeds should be looping and waist high.

b. Have a partner feed 20 backhand groundstrokes from the net, looping and waist high.

c. Rest 5 minutes.

d. Execute another 20 forehands and backhands from ball feeds.

Stage 2

a. Begin as in stage 1 above, with the partner feeding 20 forehands and backhands from the net.

b. Rally with a partner from the baseline, hitting controlled groundstrokes, mixing both forehands and backhands for 50 to 60 repetitions.

c. Rest 5 minutes.

d. Repeat step b.

Stage 3

a. Rally groundstrokes from the baseline for 15 minutes.

b. Rest 5 minutes.

c. Hit 10 forehand and backhand volleys, emphasizing a contact point in front of the body.

d. Rally 15 minutes from the baseline.

e. Hit 10 forehand and backhand volleys.

(continued)

Table 14.3   Interval Tennis Program, *continued*

Pre-serve interval (perform prior to stage 4)

a. After stretching with racket in hand, perform a serving motion 10 to 15 times, without a ball.

b. Using a foam ball, hit 10 to 15 serves without concern for performance results (consider only form of racket arm and contact point).

Stage 4

a. Hit 20 minutes of groundstrokes, mixing in volleys using a 70 percent groundstroke/30 percent volley format.

b. Hit 10 serves.

c. Rest 5 minutes.

d. Hit 10 to 15 more serves.

e. Finish with 5 to 10 minutes of groundstrokes.

Stage 5

a. Repeat stages 4a and 4b listed above, increasing the number of serves to 20 to 25 instead of 10 to 15.

b. Before resting, have a partner feed easy short lobs to attempt a controlled overhead smash. Repeat overhead 5 to 10 repetitions.

c. Finish with 5 to 10 minutes of groundstrokes.

Stage 6

- Prior to attempting match play, complete stages 1 to 5 without pain or excess fatigue in the upper extremity. Do not progress from stage to stage if pain develops.

stretching and a proper warm-up precede each stage, and stretching and a proper cool-down follow each stage.

In an interval throwing program for baseball, the intensity of the activity is manipulated primarily through progressive increases in throwing distance. The player throws as little as 30 to 45 feet initially with progression to as much as 120 feet for pitchers and 150 to 180 feet for position players. The rate at which the athlete progresses is individually determined by the presence or absence of symptoms and the degree of injury or disability. Generally, the athlete should complete one to two successful, pain-free trials at each stage before progressing to the next stage. The number of repetitions and the volume of the interval throwing program are increased at each throwing distance as the athlete demonstrates an initial tolerance to that level of activity.

In the interval tennis program presented in table 14.3, the athlete progresses from executing simple groundstrokes from ball feeds, which minimizes impact to the arm and maximizes controlled movements and stroke execution, to rallying with a partner from the baseline. The volume and intensity are gradually increased. Volleys, and eventually serves and overheads, are added. Only after a

Table 14.4 Modification of Traditional Resistive Training Exercises for Athletes Following Shoulder Injury or Surgery

Exercise	Modification(s)
Bench press	Use narrower grip, bring bar only halfway toward chest
Chest fly	Perform in standing position rather than on back, bring hands back only two-thirds of the way to minimize stress on front of the shoulder
Military press	Use incline bench, narrower grip on bar, and raise arms up only to level where elbows are in line with chin
Triceps pullover	Substitute standing triceps press-down with elbows held toward sides
Dip	Substitute standing triceps press-down with elbows held toward sides
Lat pull	Pull toward chest in front only, not behind head or neck

tolerance to forehands and backhands develops are serving and overhead activity attempted because these activities impart greater stress to the shoulder and require a high activation level of the rotator cuff for safe execution.

The interval program format has been applied for other upper-extremity sports such as volleyball and swimming. The basic format includes alternate-day activity and progression from safer, less aggressive movements within a sport to more aggressive and stressful activities. For the athlete who needs additional strength in the upper extremity, traditional upper-body weight-training exercises are often modified following shoulder or arm injury. During this stage of the recovery process, modification of weight exercises is recommended to decrease stress to the rotator cuff and the supporting structures of the shoulder. Table 14.4 lists examples of recommended modifications of traditional upper-body weightlifting movement patterns.

Rotator-cuff exercises and rehabilitation exercises should be continued during the period in which the athlete is performing the interval programs and traditional upper-body weight training. Balance between the rotator-cuff musculature and the surrounding primary-mover musculature including the deltoid, latissimus dorsi, trapezius, and pectorals is critical. The athlete who abandons rotator-cuff and upper-back strengthening exercises following a return to activity risks reinjury and suboptimal performance.

Progression for the Lower-Body Athlete

The postrehabilitation training program for a lower-body athlete such as a runner or basketball player involves all the variables covered in the beginning of this chapter, but it uses different exercise progressions and addresses different concerns. Whereas testing strategies for the upper-body athlete are scarce beyond clinical isokinetic testing, several tests can be used with the lower-body athlete.

These tests can give valuable information to the sport scientist and coach by indicating the athlete's ability to generate and dissipate forces in the lower limbs and to perform lateral movements and changes of direction.

As mentioned earlier, one of the common strategies when working with athletes during this critical stage is to manipulate (minimize) the athlete's body weight by using water exercise or unweighting devices. This allows the athlete to perform a higher volume and intensity of aerobic and anaerobic training while protecting the joint by minimizing impact forces.

During the functional progression, the athlete is gradually challenged by increasing the impact loading on the injured extremity. Using proper footwear, orthotics, and running form is essential not only to enhance performance but also to minimize the effects of compensation on other joints in the lower-extremity kinetic chain. Favoring the right knee, for example, can lead to injury to the right hip or left-lower extremity because of improper impact absorption. It is the responsibility of the sports medicine or sport science professional and coach to monitor the biomechanical form of the individual during all weight-bearing activities. One important example is included in figure 14.7. This figure shows an athlete doing a simple one-leg squat maneuver. In figure 14.7a, the athlete is able to align the lower extremity properly during the execution of the squat while standing on the half-cut foam roller. This roller is often used in the functional progression because it challenges the balance and proprioceptive system of the body more than an exercise performed on flat ground. In figure 14.7b, the athlete is unable to maintain proper alignment, probably because of muscular

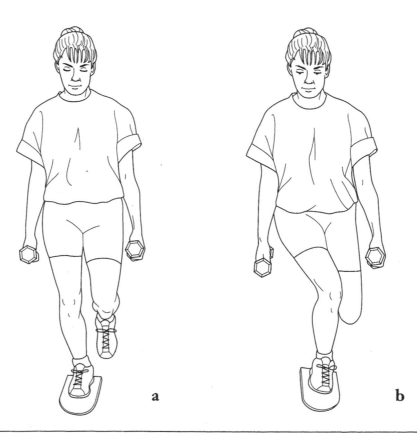

a   b

Figure 14.7   An athlete doing a simple one-leg squat maneuver on a foam roll.

fatigue and inadequate quadriceps and hip stabilization. Proper, pain-free execution of these training exercises is of paramount importance and is the basis for progression of the lower-body athlete during this stage.

Another important adjunct in the progression of the lower-body athlete is the use of functional tests. Several tests that are traditionally applied can be used outside the clinical environment to gauge lower-extremity strength. Typically, tests for the lower extremities have been analyzed relative to the uninjured side. The uninjured extremity forms a good baseline for testing and allows an objective measurement that can guide the progression of exercise during this phase. One example is the vertical jump test. This test has been used as a measure of explosive lower-body strength in fitness tests and in rehabilitation as well. Bilateral symmetry is expected with this test in most athletes. Take care during testing to use the same procedure for each extremity, particularly in whether a step is allowed before the jump. Most vertical jump fitness and rehabilitation testing is done without a step, relying solely on the explosive contraction from a resting position to generate force.

Another test used extensively in rehabilitation is the single-leg hop test. This test involves using the same leg for taking off and landing. This test is helpful in measuring not only gross take-off power and jumping distance but also ability to land and eccentrically absorb the force of body weight. An athlete's hesitancy during testing of the involved extremity is every bit as indicative of his or her ability as the distance jumped. Besides comparing the single-leg hop distance of one extremity to the other, the sports medicine professional can use normative data established by Davies and Zilmer (Ellenbecker 2000) to interpret the results further. Normal healthy male athletes should be able to single-leg hop 80 to 90 percent of body height. Female athletes should attain 70 to 80 percent of body height.

One additional test that can be useful in testing athletes is the hexagon test (see the hexagon drill in chapter 7, page 127 for a description. The advantage of this testing using this drill is that it involves the use of directional changes and cutting movements that are inherent in many sports activities. Table 14.5 lists the normative data for males and females for the hexagon test. Although the test is designed to be performed using both legs, a challenging alternative is to have the athlete perform it on one leg at a time. Comparing performance of the left and right legs is then possible.

Table 14.5   Hexagon Test Norms (in seconds)

Female	Excellent	Good	Average	Needs improvement
Adult	<12.00	12.00–12.10	12.10–12.40	>12.40
Junior	<10.48	10.48–11.70	11.70–12.30	>12.30

Male	Excellent	Good	Average	Needs improvement
Adult	<11.80	11.80–13.00	13.00–13.50	>13.50
Junior	<11.10	11.10–11.80	11.80–12.70	>12.70

Using the tests discussed in this chapter will enable the athlete's progress to be monitored during the postrehabilitation program. Like exercises for the upper extremity, exercises for the lower body often must be modified following specific injuries. Care must be taken not to jeopardize or overstress the ligamentous repair or the patellofemoral joint (kneecap) during exercise in an attempt to challenge the athlete more aggressively. Using the modifications shown in table 14.6 will enable the athlete to perform many of the traditional lower-body exercises safely and in a progressive manner.

Progression beyond the traditional types of resistive exercise listed in table 14.6 is warranted when the athlete can perform these exercises without pain or compensation. Again, knowledge of the athlete's sport or intended activity is essential for setting up work-to-rest cycles and determining the amount of aerobic and anaerobic emphasis in the training program. Exercises that mimic the activity and use elastic cords to produce overload allow the trainer to simulate sport-specific demands. Integration of traditional exercises with balance and proprioceptive challenges such as the use of half-cut foam rolls, trampolines, and balance platforms can further stimulate the injured segment and help prepare the athlete for optimal performance. Research has documented that significant losses in balance and proprioception occur following upper-extremity injuries such as shoulder dislocations and lower-body injuries like ankle sprains and knee-ligament reconstruction.

These sport-specific exercises should be incorporated while maintaining the base of rehabilitation exercises that are geared at reducing injury-specific deficits in muscular strength. Figure 14.8 shows graphically many of the important components outlined in this chapter. Although it is beyond the scope of this chapter to cover all aspects in the pyramid, many of the concepts such as balance, core-

Table 14.6 Modification of Traditional Lower-Extremity Exercises for Athletes Following Injury or Surgery

Exercise	Modification and type of injury indicated
Knee extension	Use "short arc" extension from either 0 degrees (knee straight position) to 30 degrees of bend or flexion, or from 90 degrees of knee bend to 60 degrees of knee bend to protect the kneecap (patella) in athletes recovering from patellofemoral problems.
Knee extension	Use "short arc" extension from 90 degrees of knee flexion to approximately 60 degrees of knee bend to protect the ACL (anterior cruciate ligament) in athletes following ACL injury.
Squat and lunge	Limit the amount of knee bend, keeping the knee bent at less than a 60- to 90-degree angle in athletes recovering from knee injury.
Step-up	Use a 3- to 6-inch step instead of an 8- to 12-inch step to decrease the amount of knee bend and reduce stress to the patellofemoral joint in athletes following knee injury.

stabilization training, and aerobic and anaerobic training are covered elsewhere in this comprehensive text.

TIME GUIDELINES FOR RETURN FOLLOWING INJURY

One of the first things we all realize when dealing with athletes is that individual variation is large. In addition, many factors complicate accurate prediction of recovery time, such as whether the injury was acute or more of a chronic injury stemming from a long history of repeated injuries. The age and underlying fitness level of the athlete are also important factors to consider. Despite these confounding variables, several general guidelines can be given on the average return times following certain types of injuries or surgeries.

In general, three to four weeks are required to return an athlete safely to activity following arthroscopic knee surgery. This is true for most patients who have minor damage to the cartilage and who do not have extensive damage to the surfaces of the femur and patella (kneecap). Following an injury to the ligaments of the knee, specifically the anterior or posterior cruciate ligament, 6 to 12 months are usually required before the athlete can return to sports with cutting and contact. San Francisco 49ers wide receiver Jerry Rice missed most of the season when he tore his anterior cruciate ligament and reinjured his knee, fracturing his kneecap on a reception in the end zone on his return to activity. In sports in which contact or unpredictable activity is common, predicting an appropriate recovery time is even more difficult, as it was with Jerry Rice, who had achieved a full recovery of range of motion and strength in his leg following surgery. Although there are exceptions to every rule, 6 to 12 months are generally required for the reconstructed ligament to heal and mature enough to give the knee stability. Advances in the way surgeries are performed, using less invasive surgical procedures and better instrumentation, are producing faster recoveries.

Four to six weeks are required before an athlete can return to most sports following shoulder arthroscopy, but 6 to 12 months are required when the shoulder is opened and the completely torn rotator cuff is repaired. In cases of tendinitis of the shoulder or elbow as little as two weeks and as much as six to eight weeks are required to return to full activity. An example of an arm injury that requires at least a year of recovery is a tear in the ulnar collateral ligament of the elbow. Chicago Cubs pitcher Kerry Wood missed an entire baseball season following surgery to reconstruct his elbow so that he could throw again at the major-league level. Considered one of the worst injuries that a baseball pitcher could have, it requires a long rehabilitation period.

SUMMARY

In summary, the design and implementation of a training program following injury or surgery requires integral knowledge of the athlete's activity or sport, as well as an integrated exercise and conditioning approach. The use of subpain or subsymptom intensity is important. Careful evaluation of performance mechanics to avoid compensation and reinjury is critical. All the training concepts in this text are important elements in developing a program that will successfully return

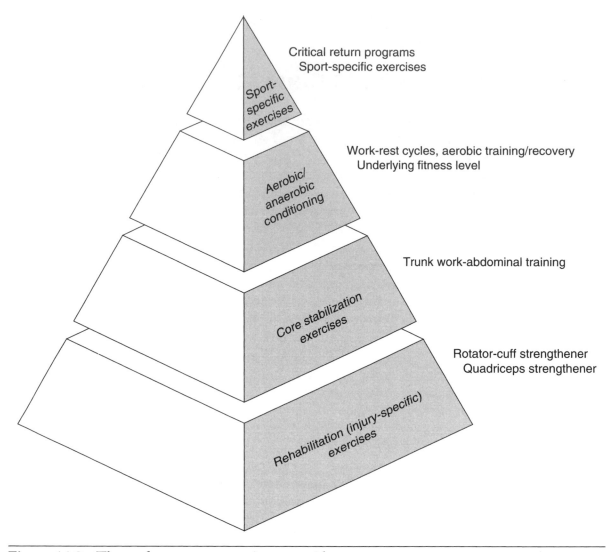

Figure 14.8   The performance-restoration pyramid.

an athlete to activity, whether recreational or professional. Interval return programs and modifications of traditional exercises bridge the gap between formal rehabilitation and functional performance. Finally, a team approach, with open communication among all its members, ensures application of these training concepts in the most efficient and expedient manner.

References and Resources

Abernethy P.J., J. Jurimae, P.A. Logan, A.W. Taylor, and R.E. Thayer. 1994. Acute and chronic response of skeletal muscle to resistance exercise. *Sports Medicine* 17(1):22–38.

Aján T., and L. Baroga. 1988. *Weightlifting: Fitness for all sports*. Budapest: International Weightlifting Federation, Medicina Publishing House.

Alexander, R.Mc. 1968. *Animal Mechanics*. Seattle: University of Washington Press.

Allard, F., and N. Burnett. 1993. Skill in sport. *Canadian Journal of Psychology* 39(2):294–312.

Andrews, J.R., G.L. Harrelson, and K.E. Wilk. 1998. *Physical rehabilitation of the injured athlete*. 2nd ed. Philadelphia: Saunders.

Apostolopoulos, N. 1997. Pubo-adductor syndrome. *Journal of Hockey Conditioning and Player Development* 2(3).

—. 1999. Stretch therapy: A recovery regeneration technique. In *Theory and methodology of training: The key to athletic performance*, ed. T. Bompa. Champaign, IL: Human Kinetics.

Arnold, R.K. 1981. *Developing sport skills: A dynamic interplay of task, learner, and teacher*. Montclair, NJ: Montclair State College.

Baddeley, A.D., and D.J.A. Longman. 1978. The influence of length and frequency of training session on the rate of learning to type. *Ergonomics* 21(8):627–635.

Baechle, T., ed. 2000. *Essentials of strength training and conditioning*. 2nd ed. Champaign, IL: Human Kinetics.

Baker D. 1995. Selecting the appropriate exercises and loads for speed-strength development. *Strength and Conditioning Coach* 3(2):8–16.

Baker G., ed. 1998. *The United States Weightlifting Federation coaching manual*. Vol. 1, *Technique*. Colorado Springs: USWF.

Behm, D.G. 1995. Neuromuscular implications and applications of resistance training. *Journal of Strength and Conditioning Research* 9(4):264–274.

Bloomfoeld, J., T.R. Ackland, and B.C. Elliott. 1994. *Applied anatomy and biomechanics in sport*. Melbourne, Australia: Blackwell Scientific.

Bompa, T.O. 1983. *Theory and methodology of training*. Dubuque, IA: Kendall/Hunt.

—. 1993. *Power training for sport: Plyometrics for maximum power development*. San Bernadino, CA: Borgo Press.

—. 1996. *Periodization of strength—The new wave in strength training*. Toronto: Veritas.

—. 1999a. *Periodization of training for sports*. Champaign, IL: Human Kinetics.

—. 1999b. *Periodization: Theory and methodology of training.* Champaign, IL: Human Kinetics.

Brisson, T.A., and C. Alain. 1996. Optimal movement pattern characteristics are not required as a reference for knowledge of performance. *Research Quarterly for Exercise and Sport* 67(4):458–464.

Chu, D.A. 1983. The link between strength and speed. 1983. *NSCA Journal* 5(2):20–21.

—. 1996. *Explosive strength and power.* Champaign, IL: Human Kinetics.

—. 1998. *Jumping into plyometrics.* 2nd ed. Champaign, IL: Human Kinetics.

Clarke, D., and F. Henry. 1961. Neuromotor specificity and increased speed from strength development. *Research Quarterly* 32:315–325.

Cook, Gray, and Athletic Testing Services. 1998. *The functional movement screen manual.* Danville, VA: Author.

Cyriax, J. 1971. *Textbook of orthopaedic medicine.* 5th ed. Vol. 1, *Diagnosis of soft tissue lesions.* London: Bailliere Tindall & Cassell.

Daniels, J. 1998. Daniels' running formula. Champaign, IL: Human Kinetics.

Daniels, J. N. Oldenridge, F. Nagle, and B. White. 1978. Differences and changes in VO_2 among young runners 10 to 18 years of age. *Medicine and Science in Sports* 13(5) 200-203.

Daniels, J., N. Scardina, J. Hayes, and P. Foley. 1984. Elite and subelite female long distance runners. In *Sport and Elite Performance*, ed. D.M. Landers. Champaign, IL: Human Kinetics.

Davies, D.V., and R.E. Coupland. 1967. *Gray's anatomy: Descriptive and applied.* 34th ed. London: Longmans.

Davis, G.G. 1910. *Applied anatomy: The construction of the human body.* Philadelphia: Lippincott.

Dintiman, G.B. 1964. The effects of various training programs on running speed. *Research Quarterly* 35:456–63.

—. 1966. The relationship between the ratio, leg strength/body weight and running speed. *Bulletin of the Connecticut Association for Health, Physical Education and Recreation* 11:5.

—. 1968 and 1985. A survey of the prevalence, type, and characteristics of supplementary training programs used in major sports to improve running speed. Unpublished work. Virginia Commonwealth University.

—. 1970. *Sprinting speed—Its improvement for major sports competition.* Springfield, IL: Charles C Thomas.

—. 1974. *What research tells the coach about sprinting.* Reston, VA: AAHPERD

—. 1980. The effects of high-speed treadmill training upon stride length, stride rate, and sprinting speed. Unpublished work. Virginia Commonwealth University.

—. 1984. *How to run faster: Step-by-step instructions on how to increase foot speed.* Champaign, IL: Leisure Press.

—. 1985. Sports speed. *Sports Fitness Magazine*, August, 70–73, 92

—. 1987a. A faster athlete is a better athlete. *Sportspeed Magazine* 1, April.

—. 1987b. Speed improvement for football. *Sportspeed Magazine* 2, October.

Dintiman, G. B., G. Coleman, and B. Ward. 1985. Speed improvement for baseball. *Sports Fitness Magazine*, May.

Dintiman, G. B., and L. Isaacs. 1996. *Speed improvement for soccer.* Kill Devil Hills, NC: National Association of Speed and Explosion. Video.

Dintiman, G. B., and J. Unitas. 1982. *The athlete's handbook: How to be a champion in any sport.* Englewood Cliffs, NJ: Prentice-Hall.

Dintiman, G. B., and B. Ward. 1988. *Train America: Achieving championship performance and fitness.* Dubuque, IA: Kendall/Hunt.

Dintiman, G., B. Ward, and T. Tellez. 1997. *Sports speed.* 2nd ed. Champaign, IL: Human Kinetics.

Dirix, A., H.G. Knuttgen, and K.Tittel, eds. 1991. *The Olympic book of sports medicine.* Oxford: Blackwell Scientific.

Drechsler, A.J. 1998. *The weightlifting encyclopedia.* Flushing, NY: A is A Communications.

Drowatzky, J.N., and F.C. Zuccato. 1967. Interrelationships between selected measures of static and dynamic balance. *Research Quarterly for Exercise and Sport* 38(3):509–510.

Ellenbecker, T.S., ed. 2000. *Knee ligament rehabilitation.* 2nd ed. Philadelphia: Churchill Livingstone.

Evans, S., K. Ng, and S. McDowell. 1992. The effect of fatigue on lower limb kinematics in female distance runners. *Research Quarterly for Exercise and Sport* 63(2):A–17.

FitzGerald, M.J.T. 1996. *Neuroanatomy: Basic and clinical.* 3rd ed. London: Saunders.

Fleck, S.J., and W.J. Kraemer. 1997. *Designing resistance training programs.* 2nd ed. Champaign, IL: Human Kinetics.

Fluharty, S., and R. Bahamonde. 1992. Comparison of two arm swings during fitness walking: kinematic parameters. *Research Quarterly for Exercise and Sport 63*(2):A–17.

Fox, E., R. Bowers, and M. Foss. 1993. *The physiological basis for exercise and sport.* 5th ed. Dubuque, IA: Brown.

Fry, A.C., and W.J. Kraemer. 1991. Physical performance characteristics of American collegiate football players. *Journal of Applied Sport Science Research* 5(3):126–138.

—. 1997. Resistance exercise overtraining and overreaching. *Sports Medicine* 23(2):106–129.

Gambetta, V. 1996. A step in the right direction. *Training and Conditioning* 6:52–55.

Gambetta, V., and M. Clark. 1999. Hard core training. *Training and Conditioning* 9:34–40.

Garhammer, J. 1978a. Muscle fiber types and weight training. *Track Technique* 72 (June):2297–2299.

—. 1978b. Muscle fibre types and the specificity concept related to athletic weight training. *Athletica* 5 (December):14–15.

—. 1981–82. Free weight equipment for the development of athletic strength and power. *National Strength and Conditioning Association Journal* 3(6):24–26, 33.

—. 1989. Weight lifting and training. In *Biomechanics of sport,* ed. C.L. Vaughan. Boca Raton, FL: CRC Press.

—. 1993. A review of power output studies of Olympic and powerlifting: Methodology, performance prediction, and evaluation tests. *Journal of Strength and Conditioning Research* 7(2):76–89.

Greisheimer, E.M. 1945. *Physiology and anatomy.* 5th ed. Philadelphia: Lippincott.

Guyton, A.C. 1980. *Textbook of medical physiology.* 6th ed. Philadelphia: Saunders.

Häkkinen, K. 1985. Factors influencing trainability of muscular strength during short term and prolonged training. *National Strength and Conditioning Association Journal* 7(2):32–37.

—. 1988. Effects of the competitive season on physical fitness profiles in elite basketball players. *Journal of Human Movements Studies*, 15(3):119–128.

—. 1989. Neuromuscular and hormonal adaptations during strength and power training: A review. *Journal of Sports Medicine and Physical Fitness* 29(1):9–26.

Häkkinen, K., ed. 1998. *International Conference on Weightlifting and Strength Training conference book*. Lahti: Gummerus Printing.

Harre, D. 1982. *Principles of sports training: Introduction to the theory and methods of training*. Berlin: Sportverlag.

Hartmann, J., and H. Tünnemann. 1989. *Fitness and strength training*. Berlin: Sportverlag.

Hatfield, F.C. 1982. Getting the most from your training reps. *National Strength and Conditioning Association Journal* 4(5):28–29.

—. 1989. *Power: A scientific approach*. Chicago: Contemporary Books.

Hay, J.G., and J.G. Reid. 1988. *Anatomy, mechanics, and human motion*. 2nd ed. Englewood Cliffs, NJ: Prentice Hall.

Haywood, K.M., and N. Getchell. 2001. *Life span motor development*. 3rd ed. Champaign, IL: Human Kinetics.

Henry, F. 1960. Increased response latency for complicated movements and a memory drum theory of neuromotor reaction. *Research Quarterly* 31:448–458.

Herman, D. 1976. The effects of depth jumping on vertical jumping and sprinting speed. Master's thesis, Ithaca College.

Hochmuth, G. 1984. *Biomechanics of athletic movement*. 4th ed. Berlin: Sportverlag.

Hoffman, J.R., G. Tenenbaum, C.M. Maresh, and W.J. Kraemer. 1996. Relationship between athletic performance tests and playing time in elite college basketball players. *Journal of Strength and Conditioning Research* 10(2):67–71.

Hoffman, M.D., L.M. Sheldahl, and W.J. Kraemer. 1988. Therapeutic exercise. In *Rehabilitation medicine: Principles and practice*. 3rd ed. Ed. JA. DeLisa and B.M. Gans. Philadelphia: Lippincott-Raven.

Hollinshead, W.H., and D.B. Jenkins. 1981. *Functional anatomy of the limbs and back*. 5th ed. Philadelphia: Saunders.

Ippolito, E., Perugia, L., and Postacchini, F. 1986. *The tendons; biology-pathology-clinical aspects*. Milano: Editrice Kurtis.

Jones, L. 1991a. *USWF coaching accreditation course: Club coach manual*. Colorado Springs: USWF.

—. 1991b. *USWF coaching accreditation course: Senior coach manual*. Colorado Springs: USWF.

Jones, M. 1990. *Strength training*. Birmingham: British Amateur Athletic Board.

Jones, N.L., N. McCartney, and A.J. McComas, eds. 1986. *Human muscle power*. Champaign, IL: Human Kinetics.

Kemp, M. 1995. Weight training for speed-strength. *Modern Athlete and Coach* 33(2):3–8.

Komi, P.V. 1979. Neuromuscular performance: Factors influencing force and speed production. *Scandinavian Journal of Sports Science* 1(1):2–15.

—. 1986. Training of muscle strength and power: Interaction of neuromotoric, hypertrophic, and mechanical factors. *International Journal of Sports Medicine* 7 (Supplement):10–15.

Komi, P.V., ed. 1992. *Strength and power in sport*. Oxford: Blackwell Scientific.

Kraemer, W.J. 1997. A series of studies: The physiological basis for strength training in American football: Fact over philosophy. *Journal of Strength and Conditioning Research* 11(3):131–142.

Kraemer, W.J., and J.A. Bush. 1998. Factors affecting the acute neuromuscular responses to resistance exercise. In *American College of Sports Medicine resource manual for guidelines for exercise, testing and prescription*. 3rd ed. Baltimore: Williams and Wilkins.

Kraemer, W.J., N.D. Duncan, and F.S. Harman. 1998. Physiologic basis for strength training in the prevention of and rehabilitation from injury. In *Rehabilitation in sports medicine*. Ed. P.K. Canavan. Stamford, CT: Appleton and Lange.

Kraemer W.J., N.D. Duncan, and J.S. Volek. 1998. Resistance training and elite athletes: Adaptations and program considerations. *Journal of Orthopaedic and Sports Physical Therapy* 28(2):110–119.

Kraemer, W.J., S.J. Fleck, and W.J. Evans. 1996. Strength and power training: Physiological mechanisms of adaptation. In *Exercise and sport sciences reviews*. Vol. 24. Ed. J.O. Holloszy. Baltimore: Williams and Wilkins.

Kraemer, W.J. and A.C. Fry. 1995. Strength testing: Development and evaluation of methodology. In *Physiological assessment of human fitness*. Ed. P. Maud and C. Foster. Champaign, IL: Human Kinetics.

Kraemer, W.J., and F.S. Harman. 1998. Conditioning: Building strength. In *Manual of sports medicine*. Ed. M.R. Safran, D.B. McKeag, and S.P. Van Camp. Philadelphia: Lippincott-Raven.

Kraemer, W.J., and L.P. Koziris. 1994. Olympic weightlifting and power lifting. In *Physiology and nutrition for competitive sport*. Ed. D.R. Lamb, H.G. Knuttgen, and R. Murray. Carmel, IN: Cooper.

Kraemer, W.J. and B.A. Nindl. 1998. Factors involved with overtraining for strength and power. Chap. 4 in *Overtraining in athletic conditioning*. Champaign, IL: Human Kinetics.

Kraemer, W.J., J. Patton, S.E. Gordon, E.A Harman, M.R. Deschenes, K. Reynolds, R.U. Newton, N.T. Triplett, and J.E. Dziados. 1995. Compatibility of high intensity strength and endurance training on hormonal and skeletal muscle adaptations. *Journal of Applied Physiology* 78(3):976–989.

Lathan, H.H. 1989. Physiological aspects of the training for muscle power. *World Weightlifting* 89(2):45–48.

Lawson, Gerald. 1997. *World record breakers in track & field athletics*. Champaign, IL: Human Kinetics.

Liebenson, Craig, ed. 1996. *Rehabilitation of the spine: a practitioner's manual*. Baltimore: Williams & Wilkins.

Lotter, W.S. 1959. Interrelationships among reaction times and speeds of movement in different limbs. *Research Quarterly for Exercise and Sport* 31(2):147–155.

Luhtanen, P., and P.V. Komi. 1978. Mechanical factors influencing running speed. In *Biomechanics*. Vl-B, 23–29. Ed. E. Asmussen and E. Joargensen. Baltimore: Baltimore University Press.

Lyttle, A. 1994. Maximizing power development: A summary of training methods. *Strength and Conditioning Coach* 2(3):16–19.

Mateyev, L. 1972. *Periodisierang des sprotichen training*. German translation. Berlin: Berles and Wernitz.

Matuszewski, W. 1985a. Rehabilitative regeneration in sports. *Sports*, January.

Matuszewski, W. 1985b. Rehabilitative regeneration in sports, part two. *Sports*, June.

McCall, G.E., W.C. Byrnes, S.J. Fleck, A. Dickinson, and W.J. Kraemer. 1999. Acute and chronic hormonal responses to resistance training designed to promote muscle hypertrophy. *Canadian Journal of Applied Physiology* 24(1):96–107.

McGraw, M.B. 1989. *The neuromuscular maturation of the human infant.* London: MacKeith Press.

McKeon, R. 1941. *The basic works of Aristotle.* New York: Random House.

Medvedyev, A. 1988. Several basics on the methods of training. *Soviet Sports Reviews* 22(4):203–206.

Mendryk, S. 1959. Reaction time, movement time, and task specificity relationships at ages 12, 22, and 48 years. *Research Quarterly for Exercise and Sport* 31(2):156–162.

Miller, B.F., and C.B. Keane. 1987. *Encyclopedia and dictionary of medicine, nursing, and allied health.* 4th ed. Philadelphia: Saunders.

Morrissey, M.C., E.A. Harman, and M.J. Johnson. 1995. Resistance training modes: Specificity and effectiveness. *Medicine and Science in Sports and Exercise* 27(5):648–660.

National Strength and Conditioning Association. 1993a. Position statement: Explosive exercises and training. *National Strength and Conditioning Association Journal* 15(3):6.

—. 1993b. Position statement: Explosive/plyometric exercises. *National Strength and Conditioning Association Journal* 15(3):16.

National Strength and Conditioning Association, T.J. Chandler, and M.H. Stone. 1991. The squat exercise in athletic conditioning: A position statement and review of the literature. *National Strength and Conditioning Association Journal* 13(5):51–60.

Newton, R.U. 1997. Expression and development of maximal muscle power (PhD thesis, Southern Cross University). Lismore, NSW: Optimal Kinetics Pty. Ltd.

Newton, R.U., and W.J. Kraemer. 1994. Developing explosive muscular power: Implications for a mixed methods training strategy. *Strength and Conditioning* 16(5): 20–31.

Newton, R.U., W.J. Kraemer, and K. Häkkinen. 1999. Effects of ballistic training on preseason preparation of elite volleyball players. *Medicine and Science in Sports and Exercise* 31(2):323–330.

Polquin C., and I. King. 1992. Theory and methodology of strength training. *Sports Coach* 16–18.

Radcliffe, J. 1999. Getting into position. *Training and Conditioning* 9:38–47.

Ritzdorf, W. 1999. Strength and power training in sport. In *Training in sport*, ed. B. Elliott Chichester: Wiley.

Roetert, E.P., and T.S. Ellenbecker. 1998. *Complete conditioning for tennis.* Champaign, IL: Human Kinetics.

Roman, R.A., and M.S. Shakirzyanov. 1978. *The snatch, the clean and jerk.* Moscow: Fizkultura i Sport.

Schmidt, R.A, and T.D. Lee. 1998. *Motor control and learning.* 3rd ed. Champaign, IL: Human Kinetics.

Schmidt, R.A., and C.A. Wrisberg. 1999. *Motor learning and performance.* 2nd ed. Champaign, IL: Human Kinetics.

Schmidtbleicher, D. 1985a. Strength training (part 1): Classification of methods. *Science Periodical on Research and Technology in Sport: Physical Training/Strength* W-4 (August):1–12.

—. 1985b. Strength training (part 2): Structural analysis of motor strength qualities and its application to training. *Science Periodical on Research and Technology in Sport: Physical Training/Strength* W-4 (September):1–10.

—. 1987. Applying the theory of strength development. *Track and Field Quarterly Review* 87(3): 4–44.

—. 1992. Training for power events. In *Strength and power in sports*, ed. P.V. Komi. Oxford: Blackwell Scientific Publications.

Schneider, W. 1985. Training high-performance skills: Fallacies and guidelines. *Human Factors* 27(3):285–300.

Schot, P.K., and K.M. Knutzen. 1992. A biomechanical analysis of four sprint start positions. *Research Quarterly for Exercise and Sport* 63(2):137–147.

Schwartz, S.I., R.C. Lillehei, G.T. Shires, F.C. Spencer, and E.H. Storer, eds. 1974. *Principles of surgery*. 2nd ed. New York: McGraw-Hill.

Sherwood, L. 1993. *Human physiology: From cells to systems*. 2nd ed. St. Paul: West.

Siff, M.C., and Y.V. Verkhoshansky. 1999. *Supertraining: Strength training for sporting excellence*. 4th ed. Littleton, CO: Supertraining International.

Singer, R.N. 1980. *Motor learning and human performance*. 3rd ed. New York: Macmillan.

Starzynski, T., and H. Sozanski. 1999. *Explosive power and jumping ability for all sports*. Island Pond, VT: Stadion.

Stone, M.H. 1982. Considerations in gaining a strength-power training effect (machines vs. free weights). *National Strength and Conditioning Association Journal* 4(1):22–24, 54.

—. 1993. Literature review: Explosive exercises and training. *National Strength and Conditioning Association Journal* 15(3):7–15.

Stone, M.H., and R.A. Borden. 1997. Modes and methods of resistance training. *Strength and Conditioning* 19(4):18–24.

Stone, M.H., T.J. Chandler, M.S. Conley, J.B. Kramer, and M.E. Stone. 1996. Training to muscular failure: Is it necessary? *Strength and Conditioning* 18(3):44–48.

Stone, M.H., D. Collins, S.S. Plisk, G. Haff, and M.E. Stone. 2000. Training principles: Evaluation of modes and methods of resistance training. *Strength and Conditioning Journal* in press.

Stone, M.H., S.J. Fleck, W.J. Kraemer, and N.T. Triplett. 1991. Health and performance related adaptations to resistive training. *Sports Medicine* 11(4):210–231.

Stone M., and J. Garhammer. 1981. Some thoughts on strength and power. *National Strength and Conditioning Association Journal* 3(5):24–25, 47.

Stone, M.H., and H. O'Bryant. 1987. *Weight training: A scientific approach*. Minneapolis: Bellwether Press/Burgess International Group.

Stone M.H., H. O'Bryant, and J. Garhammer. 1981. A hypothetical model for strength training. *Journal of Sports Medicine* 21:342–351.

Stone, M.H., H.S. O'Bryant, K.C. Pierce, G.G. Haff, A.J. Kock, B.K. Schilling, and R.L. Johnson. 1999a. Periodization: Effects of manipulating volume and intensity: Part 1. *Strength and Conditioning Journal* 21(2):56–62.

—. 1999b. Periodization: Effects of manipulating volume and intensity: Part 2. *Strength and Conditioning Journal* 21(3):54–60.

Stone, M.H., S.S. Plisk, M.E. Stone, B.K. Schilling, H.S. O'Bryant, and K.C. Pierce. 1998. Athletic performance development: Volume load—One set vs. multiple sets, training velocity, and training variation. *Strength and Conditioning* 20(6):22–31.

Stowers, T., 1983. The short term effects of three different strength-power training methods. *National Strength and Conditioning Association Journal* 5(3):24–27.

Thomas, C.L., ed. 1993. *Taber's Cyclopedic Medical Dictionary*. 17th ed. Philadelphia: Davis.

Tidow, G. Aspects of strength training in athletics. 1990. *New Studies in Athletics* 5(1):93–110.

Tippett, S.R., and M.L. Voight. 1995. Functional progressions for sport rehabilitation. Champaign, IL: Human Kinetics.

Verhoshansky, Y. 1986a. Speed-strength preparation and development of strength endurance of athletes in various specializations (part 1). *Soviet Sports Review* 21(2):82–85.

—. 1986b. Speed-strength preparation and development of strength endurance of athletes in various specializations (part 2). *Soviet Sports Review* 21(3):120–124.

—. 1988. Development of local muscular endurance. *Soviet Sports Review* 23(4):206–208.

—. 1986. *Fundamentals of special strength training on sports*. Livonia, MI: Sportivny Press.

Vermeil, A. 1998. Personal communication.

Viru, A. 1995. *Adaptation in sports training*. Boca Raton, FL: CRC Press.

Viru, A., and M. Viru. 1993. The specific nature of training on muscle: A review. *Sports Medicine, Training and Rehabilitation* 4(2):79–98.

Vorobyev, A.N. 1978. *A textbook on weightlifting*. Budapest: International Weightlifting Federation.

Wainwright, S.A., W.D. Bigg, J.D. Currey, and J.M. Gosline. 1976. *Mechanical design in organisms*. Princeton: Princeton University Press.

Ward, B., and G.B. Dintiman. 1993. *Speed and explosion*. Kill Devil Hills, NC: National Association of Speed and Explosion. Video.

Wathen, D. 1993. Literature review: Explosive/plyometric exercises. *National Strength and Conditioning Association Journal* 15(3):17–19.

Waxman, S.G. 1996. *Correlative Neuroanatomy*. 2nd ed. Stanford, CT: Appleton & Lange.

Weiss, L.W. 1991. The obtuse nature of muscular strength: The contribution of rest to its development and expression. *Journal of Applied Sport Science Research* 5(4):219–227.

Willoughby, D. 1993. The effects of mesocycle-length weight training programs involving periodization and partially equated volumes on upper and lower body strength. *Journal of Strength and Conditioning Research* 7:2–8.

Wilson, G. 1992. *State of the art review no. 29: Strength training for sport*. Canberra: Australian Sports Commission/National Sports Research Center.

Winter, D.A. 1979. *Biomechanics of human movement*. New York: Wiley.

Woo, S.L.Y., and J.A. Buckwalter. 1991. *Injury and repair of the musculoskeletal soft tissue*. Rosemont, IL: American Academy of Orthopaedic Surgeons.

Young, W.B. 1992. Neural activation and performance in power events. *Modern Athlete and Coach* 30(1):29–31.

—. 1993. Training for speed/strength: Heavy vs. light loads. *National Strength and Conditioning Association Journal* 15(5):34–42.

—. 1995. Strength qualities: What they are and what they mean to the coach. *Strength and Conditioning Coach* 3(4):13–16.

Zatsiorsky, V.M. 1992. Intensity of strength training facts and theory: Russian and Eastern European approach. *National Strength and Conditioning Association Journal* 14(5):46–57.

—. 1995. *Science and practice of strength training*. Champaign, IL: Human Kinetics.

Index

Note: The italicized letters *f* and *t* refer to figures and tables, respectively.

About the Editor

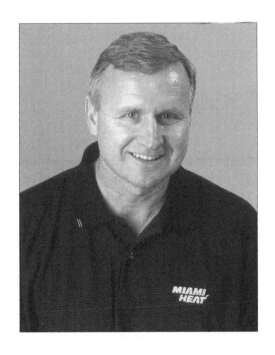

Bill Foran is in his thirteenth year as the strength and conditioning coach for the Miami Heat. Prior to his work with the Heat, he was the head strength and conditioning coach for the University of Miami and Washington State University. He has a master's degree in exercise physiology from Michigan State University and is a certified strength and conditioning specialist (CSCS). Foran resides in Pembroke Pines, Florida.

About the Contributors

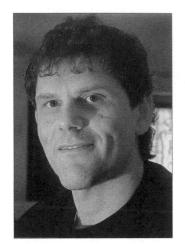

Nikos Apostolopoulos is the founder of Stretch Therapy® and micro-Stretching®. He is the director of the Serapis Stretch Therapy Clinic in Vancouver, British Columbia, Canada, the only clinic in the world pioneering the development of therapeutic stretching. The clinic uses Stretch Therapy and micro-Stretching—recovery regeneration techniques based on functional clinical anatomy—to treat many professional, elite, and amateur athletes and individuals suffering from various musculoskeletal disorders. Nikos graduated from the Faculty of Physical and Health Education at the University of Toronto with an emphasis in Sports Medicine. He has over 20 years experience in gross and functional anatomy and is a member of the American Association of Anatomists (AAA), American Association of Clinical Anatomists (AACA), American College of Sports Medicine (ACSM), and the International Association for the Study of Pain (IASP).

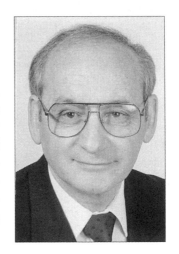

A professor emeritus at York University in Toronto, **Tudor O. Bompa, PhD,** has authored numerous articles on physical conditioning as well as eleven important books on the subject including four for Human Kinetics; *Serious Strength Training*; *Periodization: Theory and Methodology of Training*, *Periodization Training for Sports*, *and Total Training for Young Champions*. His work has been translated into 15 languages, and he has made presentations on training theories, planning, and periodization in more than 30 countries. Visit his website at **www.tudorbompa.com**. Bompa lives in Sharon, Ontario.

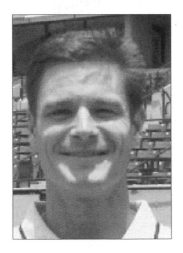

As the strength and conditioning coach for the USA Tennis Player Development Program, **Barrett Bugg**'s primary responsibility is the exercise testing, training, and tracking of the USA Tennis touring pro teams who are on the WTA and ATP tours. He also implements tennis-specific strength and conditioning programs for elite junior American tennis players. A certified strength and conditioning specialist (CSCS), Bugg earned a bachelor of science degree at Arizona State University in exercise science. Bugg has been with the USTA since September 1996 and frequently contributes strength and conditioning related articles for a variety of publications.

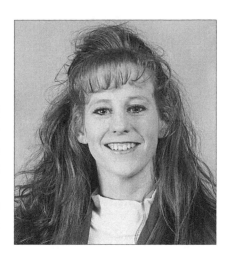

Courtney Carter is the first full-time female strength and conditioning coach ever at the University of Nebraska. Over the course of her career she has worked with 15 national championship/conference championship teams, covering five different sports. Carter has a masters in physical education and is a certified strength and conditioning coach (CSCS). A member of the NSCA, she lives in Lincoln, Nebraska.

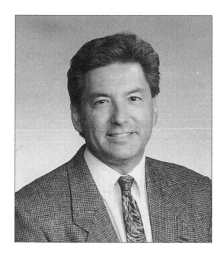

Donald Chu is a licensed physical therapist, a certified athletic trainer through the National Athletic Trainers' Association (NATA), and a CSCS through the NSCA. Dr. Chu, who earned a PhD in physical therapy and kinesiology from Stanford University, is the program director for the physical therapist assistant program at Ohlone College in Fremont, California. He is also a professor emeritus of kinesiology and physical education at California State University, Hayward. Chu, a former president of the NSCA, lives in Alameda, California.

Gray Cook is the director of orthopedic and sports physical therapy at Dunn, Cook and Associates. He is Reebok's first master coach, a position developed from his approach to conditioning based on motor learning. Cook has authored many book chapters on functional testing and exercise from a conditioning perspective. He received his master's in physical therapy (MSPT) from the University of Miami School of Medicine and holds a board cerfication as a specialist in orthopedic physical therapy (OCS). He is part of the faculty for the North American Sports Medicine Institute, where he co-teaches a course on Functional Exercise Training. Cook is also a Certified Strength and Conditioning Specialist (CSCS) who has published and presented nationally on the

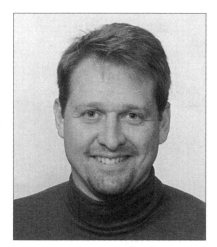

subjects of rehabilitation and high-level strength and conditioning practices and programs. He consults internationally with university research and athletic programs as well as professional sports organizations and elite individual athletes. Cook resides in Danville, Virginia.

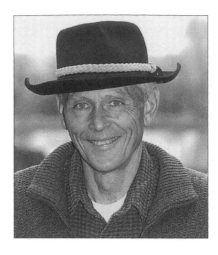

A running coach since the early 1960s, **Jack Daniels, PhD,** is currently a professor of physical education and is a distance running coach at State University of New York at Cortland. He received his doctoral degree in exercise physiology at the University of Wisconsin. Named "The World's Best Coach" by *Runner's World* magazine, he has led Cortland runners to seven NCAA Division III National Championships, 24 individual national titles, and more than 110 All-America awards. Daniels resides in Cortland, New York.

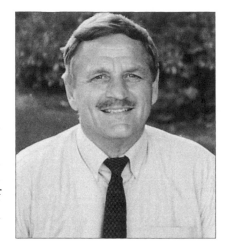

George Blough Dintiman, PhD, has more than 30 years of experience working on speed improvement with athletes at all levels—from beginners to the pros. The author of 30 books and three videos on speed improvement and health and wellness topics, Dintiman also is an NFL speed consultant and an internationally recognized authority on speed improvement for team sports. He is a board member of the International Sports Science Association and is president of the National Association of Speed and Explosion. Dintiman resides in Kill Devil Hills, North Carolina.

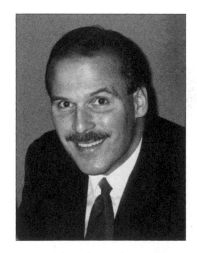

Pete Draovitch has been the personal physical therapist for PGA Tour star Greg Norman since 1993. He also serves as physical therapist and wellness consultant for Martin Memorial Medical Center; as president and CEO of The Bodyguards, Inc.; and as spring training physical therapy consultant for the St. Louis Cardinals baseball organization. Draovitch holds a master's degree in physical therapy and sports medicine/physical education. He is a member of the American Physical Therapy Association, the National Athletic Trainers' Association, and the NSCA.

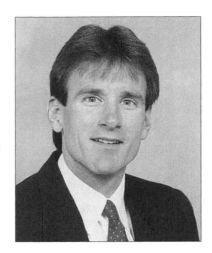

Todd Ellenbecker is a physical therapist and clinic director of Physiotherapy Associates Scottsdale Sports Clinic in Arizona. He is a certified sports clinical specialist, an orthopaedic clinical specialist, and a certified strength and conditioning specialist. Ellenbecker is also the manuscript reviewer for the *Journal of Orthopaedic and Sports Physical Therapy* and a member of the editorial board of the *Journal of Strength and Conditioning Research*. He has published many books with Human Kinetics, including *Complete Conditioning for Tennis* (1998). Ellenbecker resides in Scottsdale, Arizona.

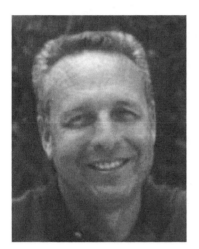

Vern Gambetta is the president of Gambetta Sports Training Systems. He served as the speed and conditioning coach for the Tampa Bay Mutiny major league soccer team (1996, 1997, and 1999) and the conditioning consultant to the U.S. men's World Cup soccer team (1998). Gambetta has been a conditioning consultant to the New England Revolution, The Chicago Fire, and University of North Carolina Women's Soccer. He was the director of conditioning for the Chicago White Sox from 1987 to 1996. Recognized internationally as an expert in training and conditioning for sport, he has lectured and conducted clinics in Canada, Japan, Australia, and Europe. Gambetta obtained his MA in education with an emphasis in physical education from Stanford University. He resides in Sarasota, Florida.

Ana Gómez, MS, is a doctoral fellow in the Department of Kinesiology in the Human Performance Lab of the University of Connecticut.

Kent Johnston is the strength and conditioning coach for the Seattle Seahawks. Johnston served under head Green Bay Packers coach Mike Holmgren as the strength and conditioning coach from 1992 through 1998. In 1997, Johnston was honored as Strength and Conditioning Coach of the Year by the Professional Football Strength and Conditioning Coaches' Society. Before joining the Packers, Johnston spent five years (1987-1991) in the weight room of the Tampa Bay Buccaneers and was a staff member at University of Alabama (1983-1986), where he helped develop NFL linebackers Cornelius Bennett and Derrick Thomas. Johnston earned his master's degree in physical education from the University of Alabama in 1984.

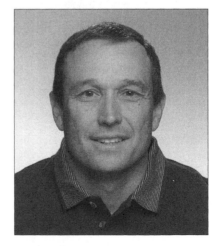

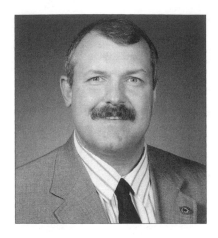

William Kraemer, PhD, is a professor and the director of research for the Neag School of Education and is the head of the Sports Medicine Research Division in the Human Performance Laboratory at the University of Connecticut. Dr. Kraemer is a former president and vice president of the NSCA; this association honored him with the Sport Scientist of the Year in 1992 and the Lifetime Achievement Award in 1994. He is also a fellow of the American College of Sports Medicine.

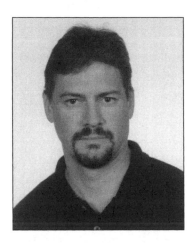

As the strength and conditioning director for the United States Olympic Committee, **Eric Lawson** oversees programs for resident athletes at the Colorado Springs, Lake Placid, and Chula Vista training facilities. Lawson is a member of the NSCA and has been published in *Skating Magazine, Olympic Coach, Conditioning Press,* and *USA Volleyball Magazine.* He is also slated to be the strength and conditioning physiologist at the 2000 Olympic Games in Sydney, Australia. Lawson resides in Monument, Colorado.

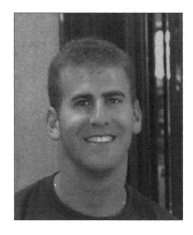

Brandon Marcello holds a masters degree in exercise physiology from Marshall University, where he taught anatomy and physiology and developed and implemented strength and conditioning programs for the varsity sports teams. Marcello's knowledge and training in the area of female athletic performance has been in constant demand by key college and professional athletes. He is also a recognized author whose work appears in a governing publication for the United States Olympic Committee and numerous periodicals. Marcello is certified by the National Strength and Conditioning Association and U.S. Weightlifting and is a coach at Athlete's Performance in Tempe, Arizona.

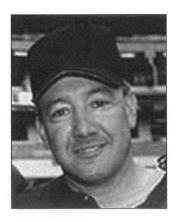

Fernando Montes is the long-time strength and conditioning coach for the Cleveland Indians, who were named Organization of the Year in 1992, his first year with the club. He previously served as strength and conditioning coach for the Stanford University department of athletics and was named head athletics trainer for the USA field hockey teams at the 1984 Olympic Games in Los Angeles. Montes is the founder and president of the Professional Baseball S&C Coach Society. He currently resides in North Ridgeville, Ohio.

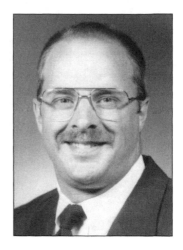

Steven Scott Plisk has been the director of sports conditioning at Yale University since 1997. He is a certified strength and conditioning specialist through the National Strength & Conditioning Association (NSCA) and a Level I Coach through USA Weightlifting. His current professional positions include member at large of the NSCA Board of Directors, associate editor of the Strength & Conditioning Journal Editorial Board, faculty member at the NSCA Coaches' College, and chapter author and symposium presenter at the NSCA Certification Commission.

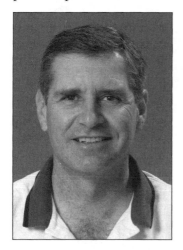

E. Paul Roetert is the former administrator of sport science for the United States Tennis Association (USTA) and is currently the executive director of the American Sport Education Program (ASEP) for Human Kinetics. Roetert received his PhD in biomechanics from the University of Connecticut and is a fellow in the American College of Sports Medicine. An accomplished writer, Roetert has coauthored *Complete Conditioning for Tennis* (Human Kinetics, 1998) and published articles in numerous scientific publications. Roetert lives in Miami, Florida.

Peter Twist has coached more than 500 professional athletes including Mark Messier, Pavel Bure, and Hakeem Olajuwan. He has authored dozens of articles and two books on the subjects of conditioning and quickness, including *Complete Conditioning for Ice Hockey* (1997 Human Kinetics). Having coached in the NHL for seven years, Twist is currently the president of the Hockey Conditioning Coaches Association and coeditor of the *Journal of Hockey Conditioning & Player Development*. Twist resides in North Vancouver, British Columbia, Canada.

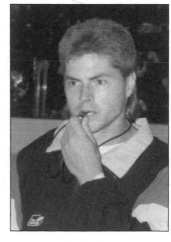

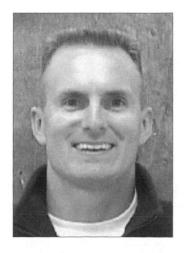

A leader in the field of performance training, **Mark Verstegen** has coached at Washington State University and served as Assistant Director of Player Development at Georgia Tech, where he implemented the most innovative and effective performance program in the school's history. Verstegen created, the International Performance Institute in Bradenton, Florida. He now directs Athletes' Performance, in Tempe, Arizona and is frequently a keynote speaker at international symposia, motivational seminars and coaching clinics. The effectiveness of Verstegen's work is best measured by his athletes' success: he has trained numerous first-round NFL draft picks, WTA Grand Slam Champions, top PGA/LPGA players, AL and NL Major League Rookies of the Year, MLB Batting Champions, NBA All-Stars, and other world-class athletes.

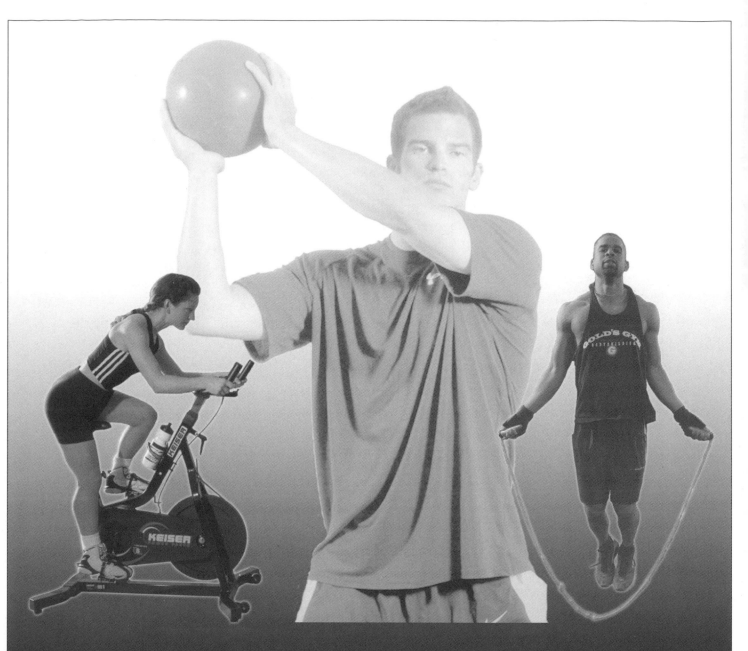
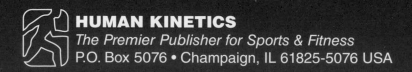